Thyroid Radiofrequency Ablation

Auh Whan Park • Giovanni Mauri • Ji-hoon Kim
Editors

# Thyroid Radiofrequency Ablation

## A Comprehensive Guide

Springer

*Editors*
Auh Whan Park
Department of Radiology, Division of Interventional Radiology
University of Texas Southwestern Medical Center
Dallas, TX, USA

Ji-hoon Kim
Department of Radiology
Seoul National University Hospital, Seoul National University College of Medicine
Seoul, South Korea

Giovanni Mauri
Unit of Diagnostic and Interventional Radiology
IRCCS Ospedale Galeazzi - Sant'Ambrogio
Milan, Italy

ISBN 978-3-031-65287-5 ISBN 978-3-031-65288-2 (eBook)
https://doi.org/10.1007/978-3-031-65288-2



This Springer imprint is published by the registered company Springer Nature Switzerland AG
The registered company address is: Gewerbestrasse 11, 6330 Cham, Switzerland

# Preface

A decade ago, I embarked on an exploration of thyroid radiofrequency ablation (RFA) with only a rudimentary understanding of the technique. Over the years, my appreciation for RFA as a viable alternative to traditional thyroid surgery has grown, especially for patients who might benefit from less invasive treatments. Historically, when medical therapies were insufficient, surgical removal of the thyroid was the primary solution. Now, thyroid ablation offers renewed hope to those who previously had limited options. The transition from predominantly surgical interventions to the inclusion of ablation techniques represents a pivotal shift in managing thyroid disorders. This shift challenges the physician to consider the possibility of preserving the thyroid gland whenever feasible.

Along this journey, I recognized a significant gap in educational resources that would support RFA as a treatment option. Driven by empathy for patients with treatable thyroid conditions and a firm belief in the benefits of RFA, I initially created a concise handbook to provide essential information and practical insights. However, the complexity of thyroid RFA soon necessitated a more detailed and comprehensive guide.

Compiling this textbook has been a challenging endeavor, largely because of the lack of any precedent. Therefore, it is the result of years of dedicated research and learning. While it may still be deficient in some areas, my hope is that it will be invaluable to those seeking to understand and implement thyroid RFA in clinical practice. The aim of this work is to share the accumulated knowledge of RFA's efficacy and adaptability, ultimately enhancing patient standard of care.

This textbook includes input from experts from around the world, who readily shared their knowledge and perspectives. I am profoundly grateful to all of them and to countless others who have contributed to this field. I am also grateful for the invaluable contributions of my co-editors, Dr. Giovanni Mauri and Dr. Ji-Hoon Kim, whose insights and expertise have greatly enriched this work. I am especially thankful to you, the reader, for embarking on this educational journey with me and allowing me the opportunity to contribute to our shared objective of improving the health and lives of those affected by thyroid conditions. I hope this textbook will not only serve as a fundamental educational resource but also encourage the broader application of thyroid RFA, leading to the best possible outcomes for our patients.

Dallas, TX, USA — Auh Whan Park
Milan, Italy — Giovanni Mauri
Seoul, South Korea — Ji-hoon Kim

# Contents

# Contributors

**Susana Calle** Department of Neuroradiology, Division of Diagnostic Imaging, University of MD Anderson Cancer Center, Houston, TX, USA

**Satyanarayana Chekuri** Department of Radiology, Division of Nuclear Medicine, University of Texas Southwestern Medical Center, Dallas, TX, USA

**Wen-Chieh Chen** Department of Internal Medicine, Division of Endocrinology and Metabolism, Kaohsiung Chang Gung Memorial Hospital, Kaohsiung, Taiwan

**Pi-Ling Chiang** Department of Diagnostic Radiology, Kaohsiung Chang Gung Memorial Hospital, Chang Gung University College of Medicine, Kaohsiung, Taiwan

Thyroid Head and Neck Ablation Center, Kaohsiung Chang Gung Memorial Hospital, Kaohsiung, Taiwan

**Michael Douek** Department of Interventional Radiology, UCLA, Los Angeles, CA, USA

**Steven P. Hodak** NYU Langone Health, New York, NY, USA

**Timothy C. Huber** Department of Vascular and Interventional Radiology, Jefferson Radiology, Hartford, CT, USA

**Iram Hussain** Department of Internal Medicine, Division of Endocrinology, Diabetes and Metabolism, University of Texas Southwestern Medical Center, Dallas, TX, USA

**Ana Kashfia Islam** Department of Surgery, Division of Endocrine Surgery, University of Texas Southwestern Medical Center, Dallas, TX, USA

**Diana Kaya** Department of Neuroradiology, Division of Diagnostic Imaging, University of Texas MD Anderson Cancer Center, Houston, TX, USA

**Dong Wook Kim** Department of Radiology, Busan Paik Hospital, Inje University College of Medicine, Busan, South Korea

**Ji-hoon Kim** Department of Radiology, Seoul National University Hospital, Seoul National University College of Medicine, Seoul, South Korea

**Seung Kwon Kim** Department of Radiology, Division of Interventional Radiology, University of Texas Southwestern Medical Center, Dallas, TX, USA

**Yoon-Jin Kim** Dotter Department of Interventional Radiology, Oregon Health and Sciences University, Portland, OR, USA

**Elizabeth M. Kurian** Department of Anatomic Pathology, University of Texas Southwestern Medical Center, Dallas, TX, USA

**Kim O. Learned** Department of Neuroradiology, Division of Diagnostic Imaging, University of Texas MD Anderson Cancer Center, Houston, TX, USA

**Ji Ye Lee** Department of Radiology, Seoul National University Hospital, Seoul National University College of Medicine, Seoul, South Korea

**Min Kyoung Lee** Department of Radiology, Yeouido St. Mary's Hospital, Catholic University of Korea School of Medicine, Seoul, South Korea

**Nincheng (Peter) Li, MD, MS** Department of Radiology, Division of Interventional Radiology, UMass Chan Medical School, Worcester, MA, USA

**Wan Ni Lin** Department of Otolaryngology Head and Neck Surgery, Chung Gung Memorial Hospital, Linkou Medical Center, Taoyuan, Taiwan

**Wei-Che Lin** Department of Diagnostic Radiology, Kaohsiung Chang Gung Memorial Hospital, Chang Gung University College of Medicine, Kaohsiung, Taiwan

Thyroid Head and Neck Ablation Center, Kaohsiung Chang Gung Memorial Hospital, Kaohsiung, Taiwan

College of Medicine, National Sun Yat-Sen University, Kaohsiung, Taiwan

**Giovanni Mauri** Unit of Diagnostic and Interventional Radiology, IRCCS Ospedale Galeazzi - Sant'Ambrogio, Milan, Italy

**Nghi C. Nguyen** Department of Radiology, Division of Nuclear Medicine, University of Texas Southwestern Medical Center, Dallas, TX, USA

**Orhan K. Öz** Department of Radiology, Division of Nuclear Medicine, University of Texas Southwestern Medical Center, Dallas, TX, USA

**Auh Whan Park** Department of Radiology, Division of Interventional Radiology, University of Texas Southwestern Medical Center, Dallas, TX, USA

**Brian J. Park, MD, MS** Dotter Department of Interventional Radiology, Oregon Health and Science University, Portland, OR, USA

**Kepal Patel** Department of Surgery, NYU Langone Health, New York, NY, USA

**Alan A. Sag** Department of Interventional Radiology, University of Miami Miller School of Medicine, Miami, FL, USA

**Jung Hee Shin** Samsung Medical Center, Seoul, South Korea

**Jung Suk Sim** Department of Radiology, Withsim Clinic, Seongnam-si, Gyeonggi-do, South Korea

**Ravi N. Srinivasa** Department of Radiology, Division of Interventional Radiology, University of California, Los Angeles, CA, USA

**Emily Steen** Kelsey-Seybold, Fort Bend Medical and Diagnostic Center, Sugar Land, TX, USA

**Jin Yong Sung** Department of Radiology, Thyroid Center, Daerim St. Mary's Hospital, Seoul, South Korea

**Gary Tse** Department of Interventional Radiology, UCLA, Los Angeles, CA, USA

**Ming-Hsun Wu** Department of Surgery, National Taiwan University Hospital, Taipei, Taiwan

# Part I
# Thyroid Nodules

# Chapter 1
# Current Diagnosis and Management of Thyroid Nodules

**Iram Hussain**

Thyroid nodules (TNs) can be detected in up to 68% of the general population when using high-resolution ultrasonography (US), although most are benign and asymptomatic [1]. A small percentage of TNs are clinically significant and will need intervention: they may be malignant (~5–10%), autonomously functioning (~5%), or cause compressive/cosmetic symptoms (~5–15%) [2–4]. The goal of thyroid nodule management is to identify this subset of patients, present all viable options to them, and decide on an individualized treatment plan that meets their needs [2, 5].

## Initial Evaluation

The initial evaluation focuses on determining the risk of malignancy and functional status of clinically evident or incidentally discovered TNs. This includes clinical history, physical examination, laboratory evaluation, and imaging [5]. Depending on the results, some nodules may require further diagnostic evaluation with needle biopsies and molecular marker testing [5].

I. Hussain (✉)
Department of Internal Medicine, Division of Endocrinology, Diabetes and Metabolism, University of Texas Southwestern Medical Center, Dallas, TX, USA
e-mail: iram.hussain@utsouthwestern.edu


A. W. Park et al. (eds.), *Thyroid Radiofrequency Ablation*,
https://doi.org/10.1007/978-3-031-65288-2_1

## *Clinical Evaluation*

The clinical history should include a detailed evaluation of symptoms as well as risk factors for thyroid cancer. Most TNs are asymptomatic; however, depending on the size and location of the nodule, patients' complaints may include globus sensation, dysphagia, hoarseness, and cosmetic issues [2, 6].

Risk factors for thyroid cancer include radiation exposure to the head and neck area and a family history of differentiated thyroid cancer (DTC), medullary thyroid cancer (MTC), or thyroid cancer syndromes including multiple endocrine neoplasia type 2 (MEN 2), Cowden syndrome, familial adenomatous polyposis, and Gardner syndrome [4, 6, 7]. Presentation at an age less than 14 years or over 70 years, persistent dysphonia, and male gender are also associated with an increased risk of malignancy [7]. Rapid enlargement of nodules could be due to bleeding into the nodule or an aggressive malignancy such as anaplastic thyroid cancer [2, 8].

Physical examination includes a visual assessment of the anterior neck, and palpation of the thyroid gland and cervical lymph nodes [2, 7]. Whether a thyroid nodule is visible and palpable depends on its size and location. Nodule size also correlates with symptoms [9]. The risk of malignancy is increased if the nodule is immobile or if there is evidence of vocal cord paralysis/paresis or cervical lymphadenopathy [6, 10].

## *Laboratory Evaluation*

Thyroid function tests should be performed in all patients with TNs and are interpreted as indicated in Table 1.1. If thyroid-stimulating hormone (TSH) is normal, it is not necessary to measure thyroxine (T4) and triiodothyronine (T3) levels. A suppressed TSH level is an indication for further testing to determine whether the patient has subclinical or overt hyperthyroidism [2, 4]. A higher TSH level is associated with a higher risk of malignancy [6]. Thyroid peroxidase antibody (TPO Ab) levels should also be measured in case of elevated TSH to evaluate for autoimmune

**Table 1.1** Interpretation of thyroid function tests

| TSH[a] | T4[b] | T3[c] | State |
|---|---|---|---|
| Normal | Normal | Normal | Euthyroid |
| Decreased | Normal | Normal | Subclinical hyperthyroidism |
| Increased | Normal | Normal | Subclinical hypothyroidism |
| Decreased | Increased | Increased | Primary hyperthyroidism |
| Increased | Decreased | Decreased | Primary hypothyroidism |
| Decreased | Normal | Increased | Primary hyperthyroidism (T3 thyrotoxicosis) |

[a] Thyroid-stimulating hormone or thyrotropin
[b] Thyroxine, either free or total (usually free thyroxine is measured)
[c] Triiodothyronine, either free or total (usually total triiodothyronine is measured when thyrotropin is suppressed; triiodothyronine does not need to be measured when thyrotropin is elevated)

chronic lymphocytic thyroiditis [2]. Calcitonin level is not routinely tested except in cases of suspected or confirmed MTC [2, 6].

## *Ultrasonography and Other Imaging*

### Neck Ultrasonography

Neck US is the imaging modality of choice to evaluate TNs; it should include an evaluation for cervical lymphadenopathy in both the central and lateral neck [4]. Point-of-care US acts as an extension of the physical examination and provides more information than still images [6]. Characteristics of the thyroid gland itself, thyroid nodules, and lymph nodes should be noted in the report as indicated in Table 1.2 [6].

Multiple risk-stratification systems have been developed based on the sonographic features of TNs. The goal is to identify those nodules that are at greatest risk of malignancy and to avoid unnecessary biopsy of nodules that are likely benign [6]. Most guidelines, including the American Thyroid Association (ATA) (Fig. 1.1), define risk by association of two or more nodule features, whereas the American College of Radiology Thyroid Imaging Reporting and Data System (ACR TI-RADS) individually assesses five nodule features expressed in a numerical score that is then assigned to a risk class based on the sum of the five scores (Fig. 1.2). A summary of commonly used systems is given in Table 1.3.

**Table 1.2** Information reported on thyroid ultrasonography

| Thyroid gland | Thyroid nodule | Lymph node |
|---|---|---|
| Size of each lobe | Size | Size |
| Isthmus thickness | Location (within thyroid) | Location (level of neck) |
| Echogenicity[a] | Echogenicity[a] | Echogenicity[a] |
| Texture[b] | Composition[c] | Shape |
| Vascularity | Margins[d] | Calcifications/cystic change |
| Tracheal deviation (±) | Echogenic foci[e] | Vascular pattern |
| | Vascular pattern | |

[a] Echogenicity can be anechoic, hypoechoic, isoechoic, or hyperechoic
[b] Texture can be heterogenous or homogenous
[c] Composition can be solid, mixed solid-cystic, or cystic
[d] Margins can be ill-defined, smooth, irregular, or with solid or continuous peripheral calcifications
[e] Nodule can have no echogenic foci, or echogenic foci representing colloid, or micro- or macro-calcifications

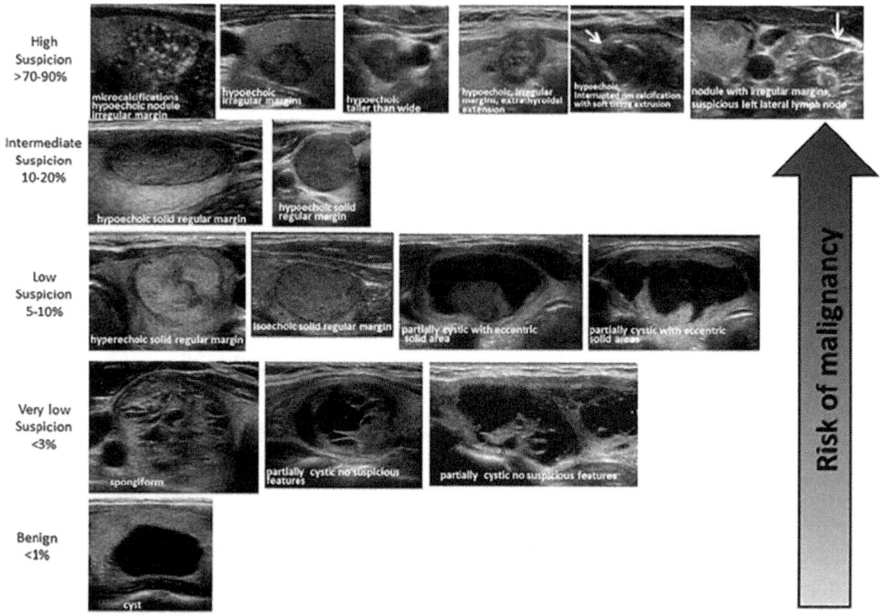


**Fig. 1.1** ATA nodule sonographic patterns and risk of malignancy. Image reproduced from the 2015 American Thyroid Association (ATA) management guidelines for adult patients with thyroid nodules and differentiated thyroid cancer [4] and shows the risk of malignancy with various sonographic patterns. An updated version of the ATA thyroid nodule guidelines is due for publication in 2024

## Cross-Sectional Imaging

Cross-sectional imaging [including computed tomography (CT), magnetic resonance imaging (MRI), and positron emission tomography (PET)] is not typically used to evaluate thyroid nodule characteristics; however, it may be useful for surgical staging in cases of known malignancy [14]. TNs are often identified incidentally on cross-sectional imaging done for other reasons, in which case US evaluation is usually recommended.

CT, and less commonly MRI, can be used preoperatively in both benign and malignant thyroid disease to evaluate substernal goiters and nodules, compression or displacement of surrounding structures, invasion of adjacent structures, cervical lymphadenopathy, and distant metastases [14].

## Thyroid Scintigraphy

Radionuclide scintigraphy using I-123 (iodine isotopes) or technetium-99 m pertechnetate provides information about the functional status of a thyroid nodule [6]. Thyroid scintigraphy needs to be performed in patients with subclinical or overt

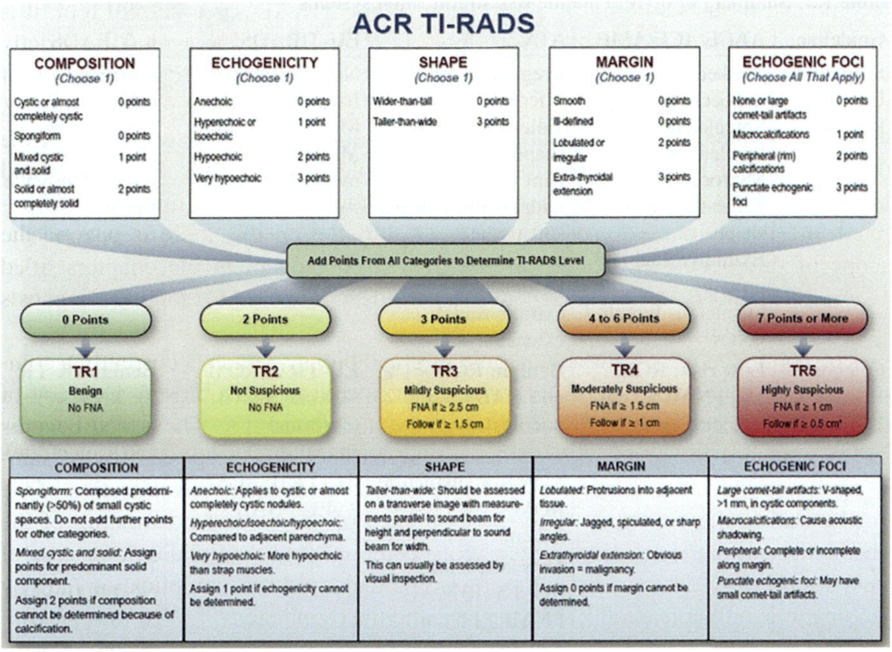


**Fig. 1.2** ACR TI-RADS system for risk assessment. Image reproduced from the American College of Radiology Thyroid Imaging, Reporting and Data System (TI-RADS): White Paper of the ACR TI-RADS Committee [11] and shows how risk is calculated, along with the size cut-offs when fine-needle aspiration (FNA) biopsy is considered for thyroid nodule with different risk scores

hyperthyroidism (suppressed TSH) to identify autonomously functioning thyroid nodules (AFTNs), as this may affect management.

## *Cytology and Molecular Marker Testing*

### Cytology

Based on clinical features and imaging, a determination is made as to whether a thyroid nodule needs to be biopsied. If the nodule meets the criteria for biopsy, then this is usually performed via ultrasound-guided fine-needle aspiration (FNA) [4]. Core needle biopsies may also be performed in select cases; however, they are much less common.

The most commonly used reporting system for thyroid biopsy results is The Bethesda System for Reporting Thyroid Cytopathology (TBSRTC), summarized in Table 1.4 [15]. In cases of indeterminate results (Bethesda III and IV, and sometimes V), molecular marker testing may need to be performed to determine the next course of action.

**Table 1.3** Summary of thyroid nodule risk stratification systems

| Guideline | AACE/ACE/AME | ATA | EU-TIRADS | K-TIRADS |
|---|---|---|---|---|
| Suspicious US features | Marked hypoechogenicity<br>Spiculated/ lobulated margins<br>Microcalcification<br>Taller-than-wide shape<br>Extrathyroidal growth<br>Suspicious lymph nodes | Irregular margins<br>Microcalcification<br>Taller-than-wide shape<br>Rim calcifications with small extrusive soft-tissue component<br>Evidence of extrathyroidal extension | Non-oval shape<br>Irregular margins<br>Microcalcification<br>Marked hypoechogenicity | Punctate echogenic foci<br>Nonparallel orientation (taller-than-wide shape)<br>Irregular margin |
| Category | **Low risk:** ROM 1%, FNAB >2 cm (selected cases) | **Benign:** ROM <1%, no FNAB (cystic nodules) | **EU-TR 2:** ROM ~0%, no FNAB (cysts and spongiform) | **Benign (K-TR 2):** ROM <3%, no FNAB (cysts and spongiform) |
| | | **Very low suspicion:** ROM <3%, FNAB ≥2 cm | **EU-TR 3:** ROM 2–4%, FNAB >2 cm | |
| | | **Low suspicion:** ROM 5–10%, FNAB ≥1.5 cm | | **Low suspicion (K-TR 3):** ROM 3–10%, FNAB >2 cm |
| | **Intermediate risk:** ROM 5–15%, FNAB >2 cm | **Intermediate suspicion:** ROM 10–20%, FNAB ≥1 cm | **EU-TR 4:** ROM 6–17%, FNAB >1.5 cm | **Intermediate suspicion (K-TR 4):** ROM 10–40%, FNAB >1–1.5 cm |
| | **High risk:** ROM 50–90%, FNAB ≥1 cm | **High suspicion:** ROM >70–90%, FNAB ≥1 cm | **EU-TR 5:** ROM 26–87%, FNAB >1 cm | **High suspicion (K-TR 5):** ROM >60%, FNAB >1 cm |

This table provides a summary of the risk of malignancy and the indications for fine-needle aspiration biopsy for different organizations [4, 11–13]. The American College of Radiology Thyroid Imaging, Reporting, and Data System is also widely used but is described separately in Fig. 1.2
Abbreviations: *AACE* American Association of Clinical Endocrinology, *ACE* American College of Endocrinology, *AME* Associazione Medici Endocrinologi, *ATA* American Thyroid Association, *EU-TIRADS* European Thyroid Imaging, Reporting, and Data System, *K-TIRADS* Korean Thyroid Imaging, Reporting and Data System, *US* ultrasonography, *ROM* risk of malignancy, *FNAB* fine-needle aspiration biopsy

**Table 1.4** The Bethesda system for reporting thyroid cytopathology

| Diagnostic category | ROM[a] if NIFTP is t CA mean (%) (range, %) | ROM if NIFTP is excluded mean (%) | Usual management[b] |
|---|---|---|---|
| **Bethesda I:** Nondiagnostic | 13 (5–20) | 12 | Repeat US-guided FNAB |
| **Bethesda II:** Benign | 4 (2–7) | 2 | Clinical and US follow-up |
| **Bethesda III:** Atypia of undetermined significance | 22 (13–30) | 18 | Repeat FNAB, molecular testing, diagnostic lobectomy, or surveillance |
| **Bethesda IV:** Follicular neoplasm | 30 (23–34) | 23 | Molecular testing or diagnostic lobectomy |
| **Bethesda V:** Suspicious for malignancy | 74 (67–83) | 65 | Molecular testing, lobectomy, or near-total thyroidectomy |
| **Bethesda VI:** Malignant | 97 (97–100) | 94 | Lobectomy or near-total thyroidectomy |

This table provides a summary of the categories in the 2023 Bethesda System for Reporting Thyroid Cytopathology, along with the implied risk of malignancy with expected ranges based on follow-up of surgically resected nodules with the recommended clinical management, and the estimated final risk of malignancy, if excluding nodules diagnosed by surgical pathologic examination as noninvasive follicular thyroid neoplasm with papillary-like nuclear features [15]

Abbreviations: *ROM* risk of malignancy, *%* percentage, *NIFTP* noninvasive follicular thyroid neoplasm with papillary-like nuclear features, *CA* cancer, *FNAB* fine-needle aspiration biopsy, *US* ultrasound

[a] Risk of malignancy varies with the type and structure of the nodule

[b] The usual management is only a suggested course of action; the actual management will depend on the overall clinical picture. In addition, molecular testing may dictate the extent of surgery and further guide management. The classification applies to primary thyroid malignancies, so if metastatic malignancies are noted then management may be different with surgery not necessarily indicated

## Molecular Marker Testing

Molecular markers are gene mutations seen in cancer and can be used to identify the risk of malignancy in indeterminate thyroid nodules. If molecular marker testing indicates that the thyroid nodule is likely benign then it can be treated as a Bethesda II (benign) nodule and surgery can be avoided. The outcomes of various companies offering measurement of molecular markers in thyroid biopsy specimens are summarized in Table 1.5 [16–22].

**Table 1.5** A comparison of molecular marker testing companies

| Company | Type | Sensitivity and specificity (%) | NPV and PPV (%) | False negative rate (%) |
|---|---|---|---|---|
| Thyroseq v3™ | Gene sequencing test, evaluating five classes of genetic alterations in 112 genes | 94 and 82 | 97 and 66 | 3 |
| Mir-THYpe™ | mRNA-based classifier test | 94.6 and 81 | 95.9 and 76.1 | ~ 2.1 |
| Afirma GSC™ | Gene sequencing of RNA and machine learning algorithms | 91 and 68 | 96 and 47 | ~ 2.1 |
| miR*Inform*/ ThyraMIR/ ThyGenX™ | miRNA-based classifier test | 88.6 and 85.1 | 94 and 73.8 | ~ 3.6 |
| RosettaGX reveal™ | miRNA-based assay | 85.2 and 71.9 | 91.1 and 59.1 | ~ 4.7 |
| ThyroidPrint™ | A 10-gene thyroid genetic classifier | 96–87 | 97.5 and 77.8 | NR |

This table provides a summary of available molecular marker testing companies, along with results of studies assessing their performance [16, 18–22]
Abbreviations: *NPV* negative predictive value, *PPV* positive predictive value, *mRNA* messenger ribonucleic acid, *miRNA* microribonucleic acid; *NR* not reported

## Management of Thyroid Nodules

Further management of thyroid nodules depends on their malignant potential, functional status, and symptomatology. Clinically insignificant nodules do not need any intervention. Multiple options for treatment are available and sometimes more than one treatment modality may be used in the same patient to achieve the desired therapeutic effect.

### *Management of Benign Nodules*

Asymptomatic nodules that are confirmed to be benign do not need to be followed sonographically [2]. Nodules that have the potential to grow or cause symptoms in the future may be monitored for stability with periodic neck US (usually every 12 months) [23]. TNs with a suspicious appearance on imaging may need to be monitored more frequently; or may need a repeat FNA biopsy to confirm that they are benign [4, 23, 24].

Symptomatic and clinically significant nodules require intervention; however, treatment may differ depending on whether the nodule is autonomously functioning (AF) [2]. AFTNs can cause biochemical subclinical or overt hyperthyroidism, in addition to symptoms [2, 3, 25]. Treatment of subclinical hyperthyroidism is only indicated if the patient is over 65 years old, has cardiovascular risk factors or disease, has osteoporosis, or is a postmenopausal woman not on estrogen or bisphosphonates [26]. Overt hyperthyroidism will always need to be treated. Options for the management of benign thyroid nodules are as follows:

- Medical management.
- Radioactive iodine ablation.
- Surgery.
- Chemical ablation.
- Thermal ablation.

## Medical Management

There are no recommended medical options for shrinking thyroid nodules; however thionamides, namely methimazole (MMI), carbimazole, and propylthiouracil (PTU), can be used to treat hyperthyroidism secondary to AFTN, though only MMI and PTU are available in the United States. MMI is preferred over PTU unless the patient is in the first trimester of pregnancy, primarily due to the risk of significant hepatotoxicity with PTU, resulting in safety-related warnings issued by the Food and Drug Administration (FDA), the European Medicines Agency, and the United Kingdom Medicines and Healthcare Regulatory Agency in 2009 [26].

Patients with overt hyperthyroidism need to have their thyroid function normalized as soon as possible to prevent cardiovascular morbidity and mortality [27]. Symptomatic patients with a heart rate over 90 beats per minute or with coexisting cardiovascular disease should also be treated with a beta blocker [26].

AFTNs do not go into remission; therefore, MMI would need to be administered long term. This is appropriate in some cases, such as in elderly patients on a low dose, but definitive therapy is usually recommended [26].

## Radioactive Iodine Ablation

Radioactive iodine (RAI) ablation can be used to treat subclinical or overt hyperthyroidism caused by AFTNs. The hyperthyroidism resolves over time after treatment.

In patients with toxic multinodular goiter (TMNG), the response rate is 80% by 6 months, and up to 20% of patients may need re-treatment, with an overall success rate of 81% [28–31]. Those with a single AFTN have a response rate of 89% by 1 year, and 6–18% have persistent hyperthyroidism after treatment requiring a second dose, with an overall success rate of 93.7% [31, 32]. Patients can develop hypothyroidism after treatment with risk increasing over time—60–64% of patients may be hypothyroid 20–24 years later [32, 33].

RAI is usually not the best choice to treat patients with compressive symptoms, as significant shrinkage is not achieved and nodules may need continued surveillance [4, 34, 35]. Patients of advanced age or those who are poor surgical candidates may favor RAI therapy [26].

## Surgery

The most common approach used to treat symptomatic, benign thyroid nodules is partial thyroidectomy [4, 36]. In cases of bilateral symptomatic thyroid nodules, or TMNG, total thyroidectomy may need to be performed. High-volume surgeons typically have lower complication rates, and partial thyroidectomies are less likely to result in complications compared to total thyroidectomies [37, 38].

Thyroidectomies are usually performed under general anesthesia, with associated complications; however, they can also be performed under local anesthesia with monitored anesthesia care [39]. Approximately 11–50% of patients may develop hypothyroidism after partial thyroidectomy; those with a higher preoperative TSH and positive TPO Ab are at increased risk [40, 41]. In cases of AFTNs, the goal of partial thyroidectomy is to normalize thyroid function, and only 2–3% develop hypothyroidism [26]. Surgery is the fastest way to correct the thyrotoxic state [26].

Both conventional thyroidectomy and minimally invasive video-assisted thyroidectomy (MIVAT) result in a permanent scar on the neck [42]. For scarless surgery, patients may undergo a transoral endoscopic thyroidectomy vestibular approach (TOETVA) [43]. Another option is an endoscopic thyroidectomy via an axillary approach that would result in less visible scarring [44, 45]. Although there is limited data showing the long-term safety and feasibility of these approaches, early data is promising.

## Chemical Ablation

Chemical ablation is most effective for cystic or predominantly cystic nodules, although it has been used to treat solid nodules [46]. Ethanol is the most common agent used; however, there are some studies with other agents including tetracycline hydrochloride, polidocanol, and OK-432 [47–49].

Thyroid cysts can become symptomatic if they are large enough. The first step in management is usually percutaneous drainage to relieve symptoms; however, 10–80% of cysts will recur [50]. Recurrent cysts can be managed with surgery or chemical ablation [4]. Ethanol ablation (EA) has been shown to be superior to simple aspiration, and several studies have shown safety and efficacy [46, 50–52].

Treatment of solid nodules with EA does result in volume decrease and, in the case of AFTNs, improvement of hyperthyroidism; although it is harder to achieve a therapeutic effect if the nodule is larger [53, 54]. When treating cystic nodules, the ethanol is confined to the cystic space; however, using EA for treating solid nodules can cause possible leakage, leading to complications and uneven distribution of ethanol necessitating more treatment sessions [54, 55].

For these reasons, chemical ablation is recommended for the initial treatment of cystic or predominantly cystic nodules, and thermal ablation is preferred for solid or predominantly solid nodules [56]. Mixed solid-cystic nodules can sometimes be treated with a combination of chemical and thermal ablation.

#### Thermal Ablation

Ultrasound-guided thermal ablation techniques, as listed below, have been shown to be effective for treating benign, symptomatic nodules:

- Radiofrequency ablation (RFA).
- Laser ablation (LA).
- Microwave ablation (MWA).
- High-intensity focused ultrasound (HIFU).

  Thermal ablation was initially used as an option in patients who did not want surgery or who were poor surgical candidates; however, it has been gaining popularity in recent years [57, 58]. RFA and LA are the two most widely used and studied techniques, with MWA and HIFU being less common.

  Although all thermal ablation techniques are relatively safe and effective, RFA has shown the greatest volume reduction with sustained long-term benefit over 3–5 years in the literature, with LA also showing sustained benefit over 10 years [56, 59–65]. The goal of therapy is to achieve resolution of symptoms, and in the case of AFTNs, normalization of thyroid function tests, so clinical efficacy may be achieved with all techniques. Therapy should be selected based on clinical context, availability, expertise, cost, and patient preference, rather than volume reduction alone.

  The functional status of the nodule does not influence volume reduction; however, smaller nodules do show a better response [65–67]. The response rate of AFTNs treated with RFA is 60–90%, which is comparable to that of RAI ablation [65, 68–70].

  The advantages of thermal ablation are as follows: no surgical scar, possible to perform under local anesthesia, and no to low risk of hypothyroidism when compared to RAI ablation or surgery.

### *Management of Indeterminate Nodules*

Indeterminate nodules (Bethesda III and IV) are a therapeutic challenge since their malignant potential cannot be ignored, yet an aggressive treatment strategy may be unnecessary if they do turn out to be benign. Typical management strategies are already outlined in Table 1.4 [15].

Molecular marker testing can aid in risk stratification. Nodules that are likely benign after testing are treated with a partial thyroidectomy. If molecular marker testing is suspicious for malignancy, then the patient may opt for a partial or total thyroidectomy, depending on personal preference and factors such as the presence of contralateral nodules and the likelihood of thyroid hormone supplementation postoperatively.

If molecular marker testing is not available, a repeat FNA biopsy or core biopsy is performed, and if the cytopathology is indeterminate again, then a partial thyroidectomy is performed [4]. The final surgical pathology will determine whether patients require a completion thyroidectomy. There is limited data on the use of thermal ablation for indeterminate nodules (with or without molecular testing), with no long-term follow-up studies, so this is not currently recommended [71].

## *Management of Malignant Nodules*

Nodules confirmed to be malignant or likely malignant typically undergo surgery although alternative approaches are sometimes considered. Possible treatment strategies include:

- Surgery.
- Active surveillance.
- Thermal ablation.
- Chemical ablation.

### Surgery

Surgical resection is the standard of care for malignant thyroid nodules [4]. The extent of surgery, i.e., total thyroidectomy versus partial thyroidectomy, depends on whether there are high-risk features present such as large nodule, aggressive cytopathology, extra-thyroidal extension, or cervical lymphadenopathy.

A total or near-total thyroidectomy is recommended if the nodule is greater than 4 cm, there is gross extra-thyroidal extension, clinically evident nodal involvement, or distant metastasis [4]. A partial thyroidectomy can be considered in lower-risk tumors less than 4 cm in size, depending on patient preference and the plan for future monitoring [4, 72, 73]. Thyroglobulin is unreliable as a tumor marker in case of partial thyroidectomy, so monitoring for recurrence is done using neck US alone [74, 75]. The need for postoperative radioactive iodine is an indication for a total thyroidectomy [4].

### Active Surveillance

Active surveillance with neck ultrasonography may be considered in known or suspected malignancy in patients with very low-risk tumors, poor surgical candidates, or those with a relatively short life span as intervention may not improve morbidity or mortality [4, 24]. A small percentage of patients with papillary thyroid microcarcinoma (PTMC) may develop clinically significant regional or distant metastasis; unfortunately, there are no clinical features that indicate which of these very low-risk patients will go on to develop clinically significant disease [4].

### Ablation

There is limited data describing chemical and thermal ablation being used to treat primary thyroid carcinoma; however, it has been suggested in patients with low-risk tumors who cannot get or do not want surgery or active surveillance [76].

There is limited data on the use of EA to treat primary thyroid carcinoma, with published data showing the complete disappearance of the tumor in less than 50% of cases [77–79]. Therefore, EA for primary thyroid cancer is not recommended [54].

Ultrasound-guided thermal ablation techniques, including RFA, LA, and MWA, show more promise, although current society guidelines worldwide do not yet recommend thermal ablation for primary thyroid cancers, except in selected cases [80–84]. A systemic review and meta-analysis show that although all thermal ablation techniques were safe and effective, RFA achieved the highest mean volume reduction [85]. It is also noted thermal ablation may have limited efficacy in multifocal cancers and in controlling regional microscopic metastasis [76, 86, 87].

## References

1. Kant R, Davis A, Verma V. Thyroid nodules: advances in evaluation and management. Am Fam Physician. 2020;102(5):298–304.
2. Durante C, Grani G, Lamartina L, Filetti S, Mandel SJ, Cooper DS. The diagnosis and management of thyroid nodules: a review. JAMA. 2018;319(9):914–24.
3. Durante C, Costante G, Lucisano G, Bruno R, Meringolo D, Paciaroni A, et al. The natural history of benign thyroid nodules. JAMA. 2015;313(9):926–35.
4. Haugen BR, Alexander EK, Bible KC, Doherty GM, Mandel SJ, Nikiforov YE, et al. 2015 American thyroid association management guidelines for adult patients with thyroid nodules and differentiated thyroid cancer: the American thyroid association guidelines task force on thyroid nodules and differentiated thyroid cancer. Thyroid. 2016;26(1):1–133.
5. Grani G, Sponziello M, Pecce V, Ramundo V, Durante C. Contemporary thyroid nodule evaluation and management. J Clin Endocrinol Metab. 2020;105(9):2869–83.
6. Maxwell C, Sipos JA. Clinical diagnostic evaluation of thyroid nodules. Endocrinol Metab Clin N Am. 2019;48(1):61–84.
7. Nambron R, Rosenthal R, Bahl D. Diagnosis and evaluation of thyroid nodules-the clinician's perspective. Radiol Clin North Am. 2020;58(6):1009–18.
8. Salehian B, Liem SY, Mojazi Amiri H, Maghami E. Clinical trials in management of anaplastic thyroid carcinoma; progressions and set backs: a systematic review. Int J Endocrinol Metab. 2019;17(1):e67759.
9. Eng OS, Potdevin L, Davidov T, Lu SE, Chen C, Trooskin SZ. Does nodule size predict compressive symptoms in patients with thyroid nodules? Gland Surg. 2014;3(4):232–6.
10. Hamming JF, Goslings BM, van Steenis GJ, van Ravenswaay CH, Hermans J, van de Velde CJ. The value of fine-needle aspiration biopsy in patients with nodular thyroid disease divided into groups of suspicion of malignant neoplasms on clinical grounds. Arch Intern Med. 1990;150(1):113–6.
11. Gharib H, Papini E, Garber JR, Duick DS, Harrell RM, Hegedus L, et al. American association of clinical endocrinologists, American college of endocrinology, and associazione medici endocrinologi medical guidelines for clinical practice for the diagnosis and management of thyroid nodules—2016 update. Endocr Pract. 2016;22(5):622–39.

12. Russ G, Bonnema SJ, Erdogan MF, Durante C, Ngu R, Leenhardt L. European thyroid association guidelines for ultrasound malignancy risk stratification of thyroid nodules in adults: the EU-TIRADS. Eur Thyroid J. 2017;6(5):225–37.
13. Ha EJ, Chung SR, Na DG, Ahn HS, Chung J, Lee JY, et al. 2021 Korean thyroid imaging reporting and data system and imaging-based management of thyroid nodules: Korean society of thyroid radiology consensus statement and recommendations. Korean J Radiol. 2021;22(12):2094–123.
14. Traylor KS. Computed tomography and MR imaging of thyroid disease. Radiol Clin North Am. 2020;58(6):1059–70.
15. Ali SZ, Baloch ZW, Cochand-Priollet B, Schmitt FC, Vielh P, VanderLaan PA. The 2023 Bethesda system for reporting thyroid cytopathology. Thyroid®. 2023;33(9):1039–44.
16. Steward DL, Carty SE, Sippel RS, Yang SP, Sosa JA, Sipos JA, et al. Performance of a multigene genomic classifier in thyroid nodules with indeterminate cytology: a prospective blinded multicenter study. JAMA Oncol. 2019;5(2):204–12.
17. Harrell RM, Eyerly-Webb SA, Golding AC, Edwards CM, Bimston DN. Statistical comparison of Afirma Gsc and Afirma Gec outcomes in a community endocrine surgical practice: early findings. Endocr Pract. 2019;25(2):161–4.
18. Santos MTD, Buzolin AL, Gama RR, Silva E, Dufloth RM, Figueiredo DLA, et al. Molecular classification of thyroid nodules with indeterminate cytology: development and validation of a highly sensitive and specific new miRNA-based classifier test using fine-needle aspiration smear slides. Thyroid. 2018;28(12):1618–26.
19. Patel KN, Angell TE, Babiarz J, Barth NM, Blevins T, Duh QY, et al. Performance of a genomic sequencing classifier for the preoperative diagnosis of cytologically indeterminate thyroid nodules. JAMA Surg. 2018;153(9):817–24.
20. Labourier E, Shifrin A, Busseniers AE, Lupo MA, Manganelli ML, Andruss B, et al. Molecular testing for miRNA, mRNA, and DNA on fine-needle aspiration improves the preoperative diagnosis of thyroid nodules with indeterminate cytology. J Clin Endocrinol Metab. 2015;100(7):2743–50.
21. Lithwick-Yanai G, Dromi N, Shtabsky A, Morgenstern S, Strenov Y, Feinmesser M, et al. Multicentre validation of a microRNA-based assay for diagnosing indeterminate thyroid nodules utilising fine needle aspirate smears. J Clin Pathol. 2017;70(6):500–7.
22. Gonzalez HE, Martinez JR, Vargas-Salas S, Solar A, Veliz L, Cruz F, et al. A 10-gene classifier for indeterminate thyroid nodules: development and multicenter accuracy study. Thyroid. 2017;27(8):1058–67.
23. Tessler FN, Middleton WD, Grant EG, Hoang JK, Berland LL, Teefey SA, et al. ACR thyroid imaging, reporting and data system (TI-RADS): white paper of the ACR TI-RADS committee. J Am Coll Radiol. 2017;14(5):587–95.
24. Yi KH. The revised 2016 Korean thyroid association guidelines for thyroid nodules and cancers: differences from the 2015 American thyroid association guidelines. Endocrinol Metab (Seoul). 2016;31(3):373–8.
25. Chami R, Moreno-Reyes R, Corvilain B. TSH measurement is not an appropriate screening test for autonomous functioning thyroid nodules: a retrospective study of 368 patients. Eur J Endocrinol. 2014;170(4):593–9.
26. Ross DS, Burch HB, Cooper DS, Greenlee MC, Laurberg P, Maia AL, et al. 2016 American thyroid association guidelines for diagnosis and management of hyperthyroidism and other causes of thyrotoxicosis. Thyroid. 2016;26(10):1343–421.
27. Ryodi E, Metso S, Huhtala H, Valimaki M, Auvinen A, Jaatinen P. Cardiovascular morbidity and mortality after treatment of hyperthyroidism with either radioactive iodine or thyroidectomy. Thyroid. 2018;28(9):1111–20.
28. Erkan ME, Demirin H, Asik M, Celbek G, Yildirim M, Aydin Y, et al. Efficiency of radioactive I-131 therapy in geriatric patients with toxic nodular goiter. Aging Clin Exp Res. 2012;24(6):714–7.
29. Nygaard B, Hegedus L, Ulriksen P, Nielsen KG, Hansen JM. Radioiodine therapy for multinodular toxic goiter. Arch Intern Med. 1999;159(12):1364–8.

30. Erickson D, Gharib H, Li H, van Heerden JA. Treatment of patients with toxic multinodular goiter. Thyroid. 1998;8(4):277–82.
31. Tarantini B, Ciuoli C, Di Cairano G, Guarino E, Mazzucato P, Montanaro A, et al. Effectiveness of radioiodine (131-I) as definitive therapy in patients with autoimmune and non-autoimmune hyperthyroidism. J Endocrinol Investig. 2006;29(7):594–8.
32. Ceccarelli C, Bencivelli W, Vitti P, Grasso L, Pinchera A. Outcome of radioiodine-131 therapy in hyperfunctioning thyroid nodules: a 20 years' retrospective study. Clin Endocrinol. 2005;62(3):331–5.
33. Holm LE, Lundell G, Israelsson A, Dahlqvist I. Incidence of hypothyroidism occurring long after iodine-131 therapy for hyperthyroidism. J Nucl Med. 1982;23(2):103–7.
34. Porterfield JR Jr, Thompson GB, Farley DR, Grant CS, Richards ML. Evidence-based management of toxic multinodular goiter (Plummer's disease). World J Surg. 2008;32(7):1278–84.
35. Nygaard B, Hegedus L, Nielsen KG, Ulriksen P, Hansen JM. Long-term effect of radioactive iodine on thyroid function and size in patients with solitary autonomously functioning toxic thyroid nodules. Clin Endocrinol. 1999;50(2):197–202.
36. Patel KN, Yip L, Lubitz CC, Grubbs EG, Miller BS, Shen W, et al. The American association of endocrine surgeons guidelines for the definitive surgical management of thyroid disease in adults. Ann Surg. 2020;271(3):e21–93.
37. Meltzer C, Hull M, Sundang A, Adams JL. Association between annual surgeon total thyroidectomy volume and transient and permanent complications. JAMA Otolaryngol Head Neck Surg. 2019;145:830–7.
38. Hauch A, Al-Qurayshi Z, Randolph G, Kandil E. Total thyroidectomy is associated with increased risk of complications for low- and high-volume surgeons. Ann Surg Oncol. 2014;21(12):3844–52.
39. Snyder SK, Roberson CR, Cummings CC, Rajab MH. Local anesthesia with monitored anesthesia care vs general anesthesia in thyroidectomy: a randomized study. Arch Surg. 2006;141(2):167–73.
40. Kandil E, Krishnan B, Noureldine SI, Yao L, Tufano RP. Hemithyroidectomy: a meta-analysis of postoperative need for hormone replacement and complications. ORL J Otorhinolaryngol Relat Spec. 2013;75(1):6–17.
41. Verloop H, Louwerens M, Schoones JW, Kievit J, Smit JW, Dekkers OM. Risk of hypothyroidism following hemithyroidectomy: systematic review and meta-analysis of prognostic studies. J Clin Endocrinol Metab. 2012;97(7):2243–55.
42. Sahm M, Otto R, Pross M, Mantke R. Minimally invasive video-assisted thyroidectomy: a critical analysis of long-term cosmetic results using a validated tool. Ann R Coll Surg Engl. 2019;101(3):180–5.
43. Jongekkasit I, Jitpratoom P, Sasanakietkul T, Anuwong A. Transoral endoscopic thyroidectomy for thyroid cancer. Endocrinol Metab Clin N Am. 2019;48(1):165–80.
44. Phan HH, Nguyen TH, Vo HL, Le NT, Tran NL. Single-port access endoscopic thyroidectomy via axillary approach for the benign thyroid tumor: new aspects from Vietnam. Int J Gen Med. 2021;14:1853–64.
45. Yulian ED, Kurnia A, Kartini D, Melati PA. Endoscopic thyroidectomy via axillary-breast-shoulder approach: early experience of 42 cases. Surg Oncol. 2020;34:318–23.
46. de Alcantara-Jones DM, Borges LMB, Nunes TFA, Pita GB, Rocha VB, Lavinas JM, et al. Percutaneous injection of ethanol for thyroid nodule treatment: a comparative study. Arch Endocrinol Metab. 2021;65(3):322–7.
47. Giammarile F, Bielli E, Fattapposta A, Ventura T, Baschieri I. Sclerotherapy of thyroid cysts with tetracycline hydrochloride. Minerva Endocrinol. 1994;19(3):143–7.
48. Chang HS, Yoon JH, Chung WY, Park CS. Sclerotherapy with OK-432 for recurrent cystic thyroid nodule. Yonsei Med J. 1998;39(4):367–71.
49. Lin Y, Li P, Shi YP, Tang XY, Ding M, He Y, et al. Sequential treatment by polidocanol and radiofrequency ablation of large benign partially cystic thyroid nodules with solid components: efficacy and safety. Diagn Interv Imaging. 2020;101(6):365–72.

50. Bennedbaek FN, Hegedus L. Treatment of recurrent thyroid cysts with ethanol: a randomized double-blind controlled trial. J Clin Endocrinol Metab. 2003;88(12):5773–7.
51. Yasuda K, Ozaki O, Sugino K, Yamashita T, Toshima K, Ito K, et al. Treatment of cystic lesions of the thyroid by ethanol instillation. World J Surg. 1992;16(5):958–61.
52. Cesareo R, Tabacco G, Naciu AM, Crescenzi A, Bernardi S, Romanelli F, et al. Long-term efficacy and safety of percutaneous ethanol injection (PEI) in cystic thyroid nodules: a systematic review and meta-analysis. Clin Endocrinol. 2021;96:97–106.
53. Di Lelio A, Rivolta M, Casati M, Capra M. Treatment of autonomous thyroid nodules: value of percutaneous ethanol injection. AJR Am J Roentgenol. 1995;164(1):207–13.
54. Hahn SY, Shin JH, Na DG, Ha EJ, Ahn HS, Lim HK, et al. Ethanol ablation of the thyroid nodules: 2018 consensus statement by the Korean Society of Thyroid Radiology. Korean J Radiol. 2019;20(4):609–20.
55. Gharib H, Hegedus L, Pacella CM, Baek JH, Papini E. Clinical review: nonsurgical, image-guided, minimally invasive therapy for thyroid nodules. J Clin Endocrinol Metab. 2013;98(10):3949–57.
56. Papini E, Monpeyssen H, Frasoldati A, Hegedus L. 2020 European thyroid association clinical practice guideline for the use of image-guided ablation in benign thyroid nodules. Eur Thyroid J. 2020;9(4):172–85.
57. Negro R, Trimboli P. Thermal ablation for benign, non-functioning thyroid nodules: a clinical review focused on outcomes, technical remarks, and comparisons with surgery. Electromagn Biol Med. 2020;39(4):347–55.
58. Mainini AP, Monaco C, Pescatori LC, De Angelis C, Sardanelli F, Sconfienza LM, et al. Image-guided thermal ablation of benign thyroid nodules. J Ultrasound. 2017;20(1):11–22.
59. Cesareo R, Pacella CM, Pasqualini V, Campagna G, Iozzino M, Gallo A, et al. Laser ablation versus radiofrequency ablation for benign non-functioning thyroid nodules: six-month results of a randomized, parallel, open-label, trial (LARA trial). Thyroid. 2020;30(6):847–56.
60. Cheng Z, Che Y, Yu S, Wang S, Teng D, Xu H, et al. US-guided percutaneous radiofrequency versus microwave ablation for benign thyroid nodules: a prospective multicenter study. Sci Rep. 2017;7(1):9554.
61. Korkusuz Y, Groner D, Raczynski N, Relin O, Kingeter Y, Grunwald F, et al. Thermal ablation of thyroid nodules: are radiofrequency ablation, microwave ablation and high intensity focused ultrasound equally safe and effective methods? Eur Radiol. 2018;28(3):929–35.
62. Deandrea M, Trimboli P, Garino F, Mormile A, Magliona G, Ramunni MJ, et al. Long-term efficacy of a single session of RFA for benign thyroid nodules: a longitudinal 5-year observational study. J Clin Endocrinol Metab. 2019;104(9):3751–6.
63. Volpi E. Thermal treatment options for benign thyroid nodules—the role of radio-frequency ablation and laser therapy. Clin Thyroidol. 2021;33(1):17–20.
64. Gambelunghe G, Stefanetti E, Avenia N, De Feo P. Percutaneous ultrasound-guided laser ablation of benign thyroid nodules: results of 10-year follow-up in 171 patients. J Endocr Soc. 2021;5(7):bvab081.
65. Hussain I, Zulfiqar F, Li X, Ahmad S, Aljammal J. Safety and efficacy of radiofrequency ablation of thyroid nodules-expanding treatment options in the United States. J Endocr Soc. 2021;5(8):bvab110.
66. Cesareo R, Palermo A, Pasqualini V, Cianni R, Gaspa G, Manfrini S, et al. Radiofrequency ablation for the management of thyroid nodules: a critical appraisal of the literature. Clin Endocrinol. 2017;87(6):639–48.
67. Cesareo R, Pasqualini V, Simeoni C, Sacchi M, Saralli E, Campagna G, et al. Prospective study of effectiveness of ultrasound-guided radiofrequency ablation versus control group in patients affected by benign thyroid nodules. J Clin Endocrinol Metab. 2015;100(2):460–6.
68. Cesareo R, Palermo A, Benvenuto D, Cella E, Pasqualini V, Bernardi S, et al. Efficacy of radiofrequency ablation in autonomous functioning thyroid nodules. A systematic review and meta-analysis. Rev Endocr Metab Disord. 2019;20(1):37–44.
69. de Boer H, Bom W, Veendrick P, Bom E, van Borren M, Joosten F. Hyperactive thyroid nodules treated by radiofrequency ablation: a Dutch single-centre experience. Neth J Med. 2020;78(2):64–70.

70. Cervelli R, Mazzeo S, Boni G, Boccuzzi A, Bianchi F, Brozzi F, et al. Comparison between radioiodine therapy and single-session radiofrequency ablation of autonomously functioning thyroid nodules: a retrospective study. Clin Endocrinol. 2019;90(4):608–16.
71. Li X, Lan Y, Li N, Yan L, Xiao J, Zhang M, et al. Ultrasound-guided thermal ablation of Bethesda IV thyroid nodules: a pilot study. Front Endocrinol (Lausanne). 2021;12:674970.
72. Mendelsohn AH, Elashoff DA, Abemayor E, St John MA. Surgery for papillary thyroid carcinoma: is lobectomy enough? Arch Otolaryngol Head Neck Surg. 2010;136(11):1055–61.
73. Nixon IJ, Ganly I, Patel SG, Palmer FL, Whitcher MM, Tuttle RM, et al. Thyroid lobectomy for treatment of well differentiated intrathyroid malignancy. Surgery. 2012;151(4):571–9.
74. Ritter A, Mizrachi A, Bachar G, Vainer I, Shimon I, Hirsch D, et al. Detecting recurrence following lobectomy for thyroid cancer: role of thyroglobulin and thyroglobulin antibodies. J Clin Endocrinol Metab. 2020;105(6):dgaa152.
75. Park S, Jeon MJ, Oh HS, Lee YM, Sung TY, Han M, et al. Changes in serum thyroglobulin levels after lobectomy in patients with low-risk papillary thyroid cancer. Thyroid. 2018;28(8):997–1003.
76. Jeong SY, Baek JH, Choi YJ, Lee JH. Ethanol and thermal ablation for malignant thyroid tumours. Int J Hyperth. 2017;33(8):938–45.
77. Goletti O, Lenziardi M, De Negri F, Fiorini I, Lippolis PV, Cristofani E, et al. Inoperable thyroid carcinoma: palliation with percutaneous injection of ethanol. Eur J Surg. 1993;159(11–12):639–41.
78. Isozaki T, Kiba T, Numata K, Saito S, Shimamura T, Kitamura T, et al. Medullary thyroid carcinoma with multiple hepatic metastases: treatment with transcatheter arterial embolization and percutaneous ethanol injection. Intern Med. 1999;38(1):17–21.
79. Akasu H, Shimizu K, Kitagawa W, Naito Z, Kawanami O, Tanaka S. Histological study of papillary thyroid carcinoma treated with percutaneous ethanol injection therapy. Pathol Int. 2002;52(5–6):406–9.
80. Zhang M, Luo Y, Zhang Y, Tang J. Efficacy and safety of ultrasound-guided radiofrequency ablation for treating low-risk papillary thyroid microcarcinoma: a prospective study. Thyroid. 2016;26(11):1581–7.
81. Zhou W, Jiang S, Zhan W, Zhou J, Xu S, Zhang L. Ultrasound-guided percutaneous laser ablation of unifocal T1N0M0 papillary thyroid microcarcinoma: preliminary results. Eur Radiol. 2017;27(7):2934–40.
82. Yue W, Wang S, Yu S, Wang B. Ultrasound-guided percutaneous microwave ablation of solitary T1N0M0 papillary thyroid microcarcinoma: initial experience. Int J Hyperth. 2014;30(2):150–7.
83. Kim JH, Baek JH, Sung JY, Min HS, Kim KW, Hah JH, et al. Radiofrequency ablation of low-risk small papillary thyroid carcinoma: preliminary results for patients ineligible for surgery. Int J Hyperth. 2017;33(2):212–9.
84. Hussain I, Andrade A, Ahmad S, Aljammal J, Nakhle S. North American society of interventional endocrinologists (NASOIE) consensus statement on thermal and chemical ablation of thyroid nodules and neck lesions. 2022.
85. Choi Y, Jung SL. Efficacy and safety of thermal ablation techniques for the treatment of primary papillary thyroid microcarcinoma: a systematic review and meta-analysis. Thyroid. 2020;30(5):720–31.
86. Valcavi R, Piana S, Bortolan GS, Lai R, Barbieri V, Negro R. Ultrasound-guided percutaneous laser ablation of papillary thyroid microcarcinoma: a feasibility study on three cases with pathological and immunohistochemical evaluation. Thyroid. 2013;23(12):1578–82.
87. Ahmad S, Aljammal J, Orozco I, Raashid S, Zulfiqar F, Nikravan SP, Hussain I. Radiofrequency ablation of cervical thyroid cancer metastases-experience of endocrinology practices in the United States. J Endocr Soc. 2023;7(7):bvad066. https://doi.org/10.1210/jendso/bvad066. PMID: 37287647; PMCID: PMC10243860.

# Chapter 2
# Imaging Diagnosis of Thyroid Nodules

**Ji Ye Lee**

## Introduction

Thyroid nodules are commonly encountered in clinical practice, with a prevalence of approximately 5–15% being malignant [1]. The incidence of thyroid cancer is on the rise due to various factors. To aid in the differential diagnosis of thyroid nodules, several imaging techniques and procedures have been developed, including ultrasonography (US), computed tomography (CT), and magnetic resonance imaging (MRI). Imaging plays multiple roles based on the histology and specific clinical situations of thyroid nodules. Differentiated thyroid carcinoma (DTC) originating from thyroid follicular epithelial cells constitutes the majority of thyroid cancers. In patients with DTC, imaging plays a crucial role in preoperative staging, operative planning, surveillance after treatment, and cases of suspected recurrence [2].

## Initial Evaluation of Patients Suspected with or Known Thyroid Nodules

### *Ultrasonography*

For patients with clinically suspected thyroid nodules, US of the thyroid and neck is recommended to determine the origin of the mass and assess associated changes in the thyroid gland and neck. US is a highly sensitive method for detecting thyroid nodules, enabling size and morphological feature assessment, as well as evaluation

J. Y. Lee (✉)
Department of Radiology, Seoul National University Hospital, Seoul National University College of Medicine, Seoul, South Korea



A. W. Park et al. (eds.), *Thyroid Radiofrequency Ablation*,
https://doi.org/10.1007/978-3-031-65288-2_2

of nodal involvement [3–8]. With the increasing incidence of thyroid nodules and thyroid cancer, the utilization of thyroid fine-needle aspiration (FNA) has significantly risen [9, 10]. Although FNA is a simple and safe diagnostic tool for thyroid nodules, it can cause patient discomfort, and additional costs are associated with repeat biopsies or ancillary tests [11, 12]. Therefore, identifying optimal candidates for FNA based on US features is crucial. Morphological features and nodule size assessed by US are used to guide decisions and perform biopsies, which are widely implemented in various US-based risk stratification systems (RSSs) for thyroid nodules. Several US-based RSSs have been developed to guide physicians in determining indications for US-guided biopsy and further evaluations [13–18].

US features associated with malignancy include solid composition, hypoechogenicity, irregular margins, and the presence of punctate echogenic foci (microcalcifications) (Fig. 2.1) [13–19]. The American Thyroid Association (ATA) guidelines also consider a nodule surrounded by interrupted rim calcifications with evidence of soft tissue extrusion as likely to be an infiltrative cancer [13]. Conversely, colloid or pure cysts and nodules with a spongiform appearance (defined as more than 50% of volume consisting of microcystic lesions) are unlikely to be malignant (malignancy risk <2%). Solid nodules that are either isoechoic or hyperechoic (similar or brighter echo compared to normal thyroid) without suspicious US features have a low cancer risk (<5–10%).

Multiple professional societies dedicated to thyroid research have developed risk stratification systems (RSSs) that, while similar, are not exactly alike. These systems classify nodules based on ultrasound (US) features that indicate a risk of malignancy and propose size thresholds for biopsy (Table 2.1) [14–16, 18]. Various guidelines have also been created to identify nodule patterns [13–16, 18]. These guidelines offer estimated cancer risks for each category based on patterns.

The American College of Radiology (ACR) suggested a scoring system to assess thyroid nodule imaging, known as ACR-TIRADS (Thyroid Imaging Reporting and Data System) [17]. In this system, points are allocated based on five US features, and the sum total determines the TIRADS classification of the nodule, its estimated cancer risk, and the recommendation for biopsy or monitoring. Across all classification systems, malignancy risk assessments based on US appearance are fairly

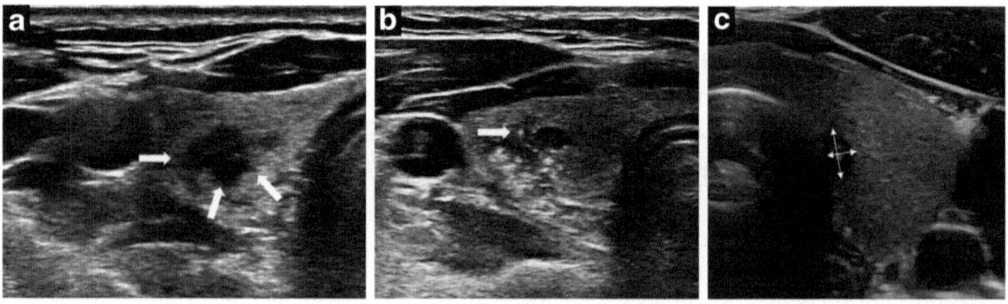


**Fig. 2.1** US features associated with malignancy. (**a**) Solid nodule with hypoechogenicity and irregular margin. (**b**) Solid hypoechoic nodule with multiple punctate echogenic foci (microcalcifications). (**c**) Solid hypoechoic nodule with nonparallel (taller-than-wide) orientation

**Table 2.1** Risk stratification systems from various society guidelines for risk based biopsy in thyroid nodules

| AACE, ACE and AME | ATA | EU-TIRADS | ACR TIRADS | K-TIRADS |
|---|---|---|---|---|
| Low risk<br>ROM <1%<br>FNA >20 mm (selective)<br>Cystic (fluid >80%)<br>Mostly cystic with reverberation artifact and no suspicious US signs<br>Isoechoic spongiform | Benign<br>ROM <1%<br>FNA not indicated<br>Purely cysts (no solid component) | Benign<br>ROM, 0%<br>FNA not indicated<br>Pure, anechoic cysts<br>Entirely spongiform | Benign<br>ROM, 2%<br>FNA not indicated<br>Spongiform<br>Pure cyst | Benign<br>ROM <3%<br>FNA not indicated<br>Iso-hyperechoic spongiform<br>Partially cystic with intracystic EF and CTA, pure cyst |
| | Very low-suspicion<br>ROM <3%<br>FNA >20 mm or observation<br>Spongiform/partially cystic with eccentric solid area without microcalcifications, irregular margin, ETE, taller than wide shape | Low risk<br>ROM 2–4%<br>Oval, smooth margin, iso- or hyperechoic, without high risk feature | Not suspicious<br>ROM, 2%<br>FNA not indicated<br>Mixed cystic/solid noncalcified nodules with smooth margins and oval shape | Low suspicion<br>ROM 3–10%<br>FNA >2.0 cm<br>Partially cystic or iso–/hyperechoic nodule without any of the three suspicious US features |
| Intermediate risk<br>ROM 5–15%<br>FNA >20 mm<br>Slightly hypoechoic or<br>Isoechoic with ovoid-round shape, smooth or ill-defined margins | Low suspicion<br>ROM 5–10%<br>FNA ≥15 mm<br>Isoechoic/hyperechoic solid | | Mildly suspicious<br>ROM, 5%<br>FNA ≥25 mm<br>Isoechoic solid/hypoechoic cystic<br>Noncalcified nodules with smooth margins and oval shape | |
| | Intermediate suspicion<br>ROM 10–20%<br>FNA ≥10 mm<br>Hypoechoic solid, smooth margin, without microcalcification, ETE or taller than wide shape | Intermediate risk<br>ROM 6–17%<br>FNA >15 mm<br>Oval shape, smooth margins, mildly hypoechoic, without any feature of high risk | Moderately suspicious<br>ROM 5–20%<br>FNA >15 mm<br>Hypoechoic solid, noncalcified with oval shape and either smooth or irregular/microlobulated margins<br>Isoechoic solid/mixed noncalcified with either nonparallel orientation, lobulated/irregular margins, or PEF | Intermediate suspicion<br>ROM 10–40%<br>FNA >1.0–1.5 cm<br>Solid hypoechoic nodules without any of three suspicious US features<br>Partially cystic or iso–/hyperechoic with any of the three suspicious US features<br>Entirely calcified nodule |

(continued)

**Table 2.1** (continued)

| AACE, ACE and AME | ATA | EU-TIRADS | ACR TIRADS | K-TIRADS |
|---|---|---|---|---|
| High risk<br>ROM 50–90%<br>FNA ≥10 mm<br>Nodules with ≥1 of:<br>Marked hypoechogenicity<br>Spiculated/lobulated margin<br>Microcalcifications<br>Taller-than-wide shape<br>Extrathyroidal growth<br>Pathologic adenopathy | High suspicion<br>ROM >70–90%<br>FNA ≥10 mm<br>Solid hypoechoic or solid hypoechoic component of partially cystic nodule with ≥1 of the following:<br>Irregular margin (infiltrative, microlobulated)<br>Microcalcifications<br>Taller than wide shape<br>Rim calcifications with small extrusive soft tissue<br>ETE | High risk<br>ROM 26–87%<br>FNA ≥10 mm<br>Nodule with ≥ of the following:<br>Nonoval shape<br>Irregular margin<br>Microcalcifications<br>Marked hypoechogenicity | Suspicious<br>ROM >20%<br>FNA >10 mm<br>Hypoechoic solid nodule with any of the following<br>Nonparallel orientation (taller than wide)<br>ETE<br>PEF<br>Isoechoic solid with irregular or microlobulated margins and either peripheral rim calcifications or PEF | High suspicion<br>ROM >60%<br>FNA >1.0 cm<br>Solid hypoechoic nodule with any of suspicious US features (punctate echogenic foci, nonparallel, orientation, irregular margins) |

Abbreviations: *ROM* risk of malignancy, *FNA* fine needle aspiration biopsy, *AACE/ACE/AME* American Association of Clinical Endocrinologists, American college of Endocrinology, and Associazione Medici Endocrinologi, *ACR* American College of Radiologists, *ATA* American Thyroid Association, *EU-TIRADS* European Thyroid Imaging Reporting and Data System, *FNAB* fine-needle aspiration biopsy, *ACR-TR* American College of Radiologists Thyroid Imaging Reporting and Data System, *ETE* extrathyroidal extension, *PEF* punctate echogenic foci, *US* ultrasonography, *EF* echogenic foci, *CTA* comet tail artifact consistent. However, the detailed lexicons and suggested size cutoffs for biopsy vary (Table 2.1) [20]. Currently, there is no universally accepted RSS, and the International Thyroid Imaging Reporting and Data System (I-TIRADS) is in the process of being drafted, building upon the consensus of numerous professional organizations.

### *Neck CT and Neck MRI*

The ability of CT and MRI to differentiate thyroid cancers from benign nodules is insufficient unless there is evidence of local tumor invasion or metastasis [21, 22]. However, cross-sectional imaging modalities can help determine the extent of large goiters with intrathoracic or retropharyngeal extension. They may be used as additional modalities when there is suspicion of advanced thyroid cancer associated with aerodigestive tract or recurrent laryngeal nerve invasion and lymph node (LN) metastasis [14, 23]. CT is more effective than US in defining the degree of tracheal compression. While MRI can serve as an alternative to CT, CT is preferred due to its lower risk of respiratory motion artifacts, shorter scan time, and higher resolution [2, 24].

## Preoperative Evaluation of Thyroid Cancer

The primary goals of initial therapy for DTC are the removal of the primary tumor, treatment of disease extending beyond the thyroid capsule, and management of clinically significant LN metastases [13]. The completeness of surgical resection significantly influences outcomes, as residual metastatic LNs are the most common site of persistent disease or recurrence. Therefore, accurate preoperative staging is crucial for surgical planning.

### *Ultrasonography*

Preoperative US is recommended for patients with thyroid cancer to assess the site and size of the primary tumor, contralateral lobe, gross extrathyroidal extension (ETE), and LN metastasis in the neck [2, 25–31]. US is accurate in predicting ETE and detecting cancer in the contralateral lobe [32–38]. In the eighth edition of the American Joint Committee on Cancer staging system, minor ETE to perithyroidal soft tissue no longer constitutes a T category. Gross ETE to the strap muscle is classified as category T3b, while ETE to major neck structures is categorized as T4. The latest guidelines from the Korean Society of Thyroid Radiology (KSThR) have outlined ultrasound (US) features indicative of extrathyroidal extension (ETE) (Table 2.2 and Fig. 2.2) [16, 38].

**Table 2.2** Recommended US criteria for diagnosing gross ETE of thyroid cancer

| Category | US feature | Description |
|---|---|---|
| **Gross ETE** | | |
| Strap muscle | Replacement of strap muscle | Cancer protruding into the strap muscle, with indistinct strap muscle margins |
| RLN | Protrusion into TEG | Protrusion of thyroid cancer into the TEG, beyond the expected margin of the normal thyroid gland |
| Trachea | Obtuse angle | Obtuse angle formed by the surfaces of thyroid cancer and tracheal cartilage |

*ETE* extrathyroidal extension, *RLN* recurrent laryngeal nerve, *TEG* tracheoesophageal groove, *US* ultrasonography

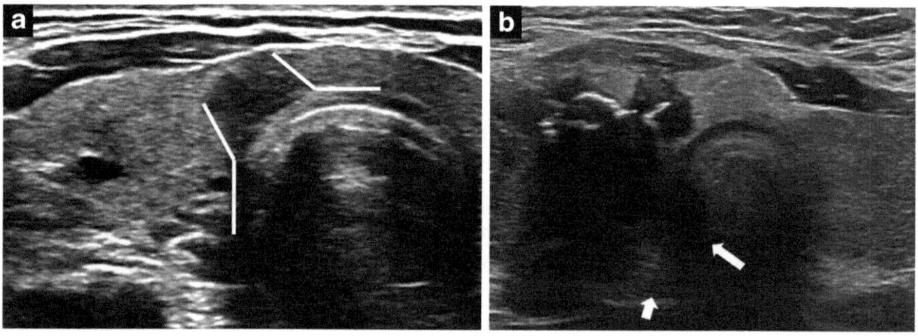


**Fig. 2.2** US feature of extrathyroidal extension of thyroid cancer to the (**a**) trachea and (**b**) recurrent laryngeal nerve. (**a**) An obtuse angle (white line) was formed between the surface of the trachea and thyroid cancer. (**b**) Protrusion of thyroid cancer into the tracheoesophageal groove

For strap muscle invasion, the replacement of strap muscle (protrusion of thyroid cancer into the strap muscle with indistinct margins) is the most predictive of gross ETE. In cases where the thyroid cancer abuts the tracheal wall, tracheal invasion can be assessed based on the angle formed by the surface of the cancer and the trachea on US. An obtuse angle between the cancer and trachea demonstrates the highest sensitivity for tracheal invasion. The risk of recurrent laryngeal nerve (RLN) invasion can be evaluated based on the presence of normal thyroid tissue between the tracheoesophageal groove (TEG) and the cancer, as well as the protrusion of the cancer into the TEG. Protrusion of the cancer into the TEG exhibits the highest accuracy for predicting RLN invasion compared to other US features [16, 38].

US demonstrates excellent resolution and diagnostic accuracy in detecting cervical LN metastasis [39–46], particularly in the lateral neck [47]. Regarding the risk of LN metastasis, cervical LNs can be classified as suspicious, indeterminate, or probably benign based on their US features (Table 2.3, Fig. 2.3). In the KSThR guideline, LNs with features such as cystic changes, echogenic foci (calcifications), cortical hyperechogenicity (focal/diffuse), or abnormal vascularity (peripheral or diffuse) are considered suspicious, as these features are highly specific for LN metastases from thyroid cancer. Indeterminate LNs are those without imaging

**Table 2.3** US- based criteria for the diagnosis of lymph node metastasis in patients with thyroid cancer

| ETA | | K-TIRADS | | |
|---|---|---|---|---|
| Category | US | Category | US | CT |
| **Suspicious for malignancy** | At least one of the following:<br>1. Microcalcifications<br>2. Partially cystic appearance<br>3. Peripheral/diffusely increased vascularization<br>4. Hyperechoic tissue looking like thyroid | **Suspicious** | Any of the four suspicious features<br>Cystic change<br>Calcifications<br>Hyperechogenicity<br>Abnormal vascularity | Any of the three suspicious features<br>Cystic change<br>Calcifications<br>Strong/heterogeneous enhancement |
| **Indeterminate** | Absence of hilum and at least one of the following:<br>1. Round shape<br>2. Increased SD ≥8 mm in level II and ≥5 mm in levels III and IV<br>3. Increased central vascularization | **Indeterminate** | Loss of echogenic hilum and hilar vascularity | Loss of hilar fat and vessel enhancement, with no suspicious CT features |
| **Normal** | 1. Normal hilum<br>2. Ovoid shape and normal size<br>3. Absent or hilar vascularization<br>4. No suspicious feature | **Probably benign** | Echogenic hilum<br>Hilar vascularity | Presence of hilar fat or vessel enhancement and no suspicious CT features |

*SD* short axis diameter, *ETA* European Thyroid Association, *K-TIRADS* Korean Thyroid Imaging Reporting and Data System

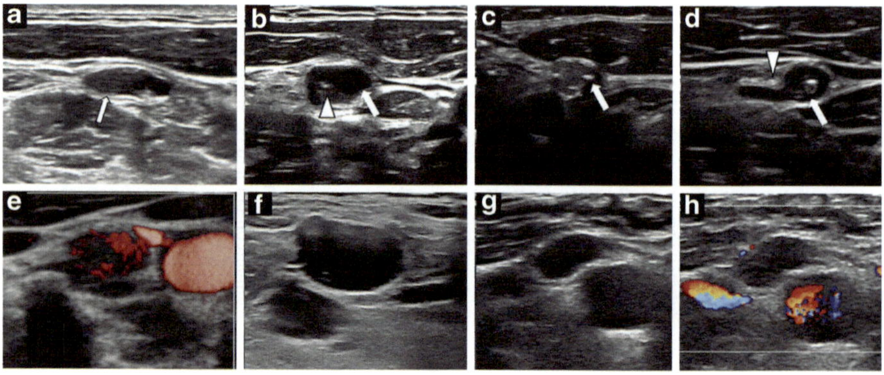


**Fig. 2.3** Ultrasound features of cervical lymph nodes. (**a**) Suspicious LN with hyperechogenicity (arrow), (**b**) suspicious LN with cystic change (arrow), hyperechogenicity and echogenic foci (arrowhead), (**c**) suspicious LN with hyperechogenicity and calcification (arrow, large echogenic foci), (**d**) suspicious LN with focal hyperechogenicity (arrow), echogenic foci (calcification), and preserved hilum (arrowhead), (**e**) suspicious LN with abnormal diffuse vascularity, (**f**) suspicious LN with cystic change, (**g**, **h**) indeterminate LN with loss of hilum, (**g**) and loss of hilar vascularity (**h**)

features of suspicious or probably benign LNs. They may exhibit a loss of echogenic hilum and hilar vascularity on US and can have various shapes (ovoid or round). However, these imaging features for indeterminate LNs are not specific to metastatic nodes. Recent node-by-node studies in preoperative thyroid cancer patients have shown that the malignancy risk of indeterminate LNs is significantly higher than that of probably benign LNs but lower than that of suspicious LNs [48–50].

The European Thyroid Association (ETA) has proposed a similar three-tiered system for cervical LNs in patients with thyroid cancer, classifying them as 'normal,' 'indeterminate,' and 'suspicious for malignancy' [39]. Table 2.3 summarizes the imaging-based classification systems for neck lesions in thyroid cancer patients.

According to the KSThR guideline, US-guided biopsy is recommended for suspicious cervical LNs (≥3–5 mm) and indeterminate LNs (>5 mm in short diameter) detected by US, particularly in cases where biopsy results may impact surgical management [9]. The addition of fine needle aspiration-thyroglobulin washout to the evaluation of cervical LNs increases the sensitivity for diagnosing cervical LN metastasis.

## *Neck CT and Neck MRI*

Recent studies have demonstrated that the combination of CT with US has a higher diagnostic performance for detecting cervical LN metastasis compared to US alone [40–46, 48, 51]. In accordance with the KSThR guideline, cervical LNs can be classified into three categories based on their malignancy risk determined by CT

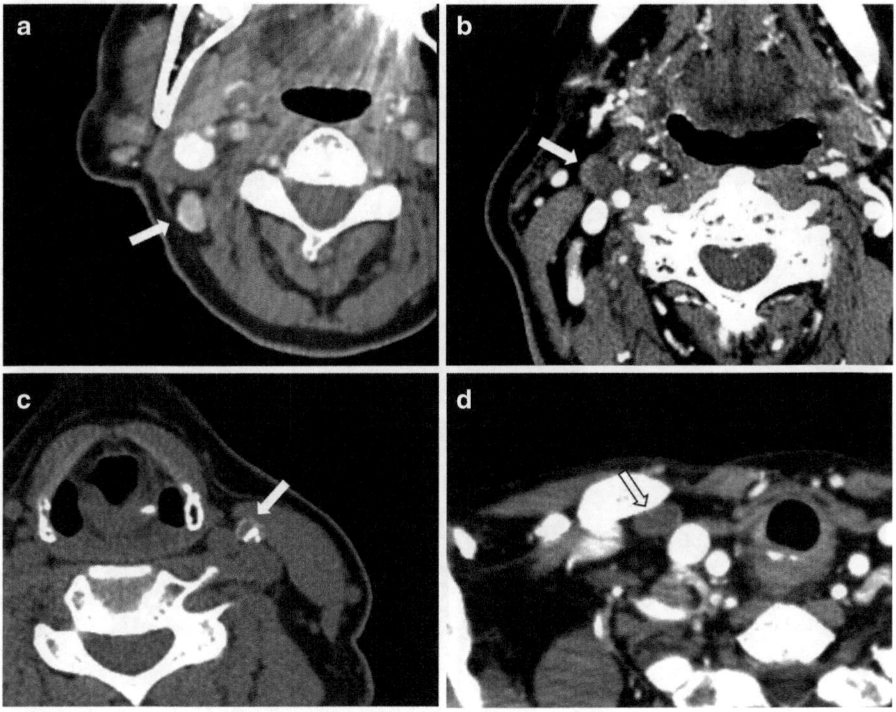


**Fig. 2.4** CT features of suspicious LNs. (**a**) Metastastic LN with diffuse strong contrast enhancement, (**b**) metastatic LN with heterogeneous enhancement, (**c**) metastatic LN with calcifications, and (**d**) metastatic LN with cystic change

features: suspicious, indeterminate, and probably benign [16]. Suspicious LNs are characterized by features such as cystic changes, calcifications, and strong (focal/diffuse) or heterogeneous enhancement (Fig. 2.4). Indeterminate LNs do not exhibit imaging features indicative of either suspicious or benign LNs.

CT is useful for evaluating suspicious metastatic neck LNs detected by US. It can detect LN metastasis in the retropharyngeal or superior mediastinal compartments that may be missed by US [23, 40, 48]. Imaging studies with intravenous (IV) contrast injection are necessary to assess LN metastases with strong or heterogeneous contrast enhancement, as well as cystic changes [2]. A recent meta-analysis indicated that the CT protocol used is an important factor affecting diagnostic accuracy and suggested that arterial phase scans and thin reconstruction slices might improve sensitivity [52]. In cases where biopsy may impact surgical management, the KSThR guideline recommends US-guided biopsy for suspicious cervical LNs (≥3–5 mm) and indeterminate LNs (>5 mm in short diameter) detected by CT [16] (Fig. 2.5).

Neck MRI can be comparable to CT in evaluating sites that are not visible on US and in detecting hyperenhancing lesions after IV contrast injection. MRI offers superior soft-tissue resolution, and the use of gadolinium-based contrast medium

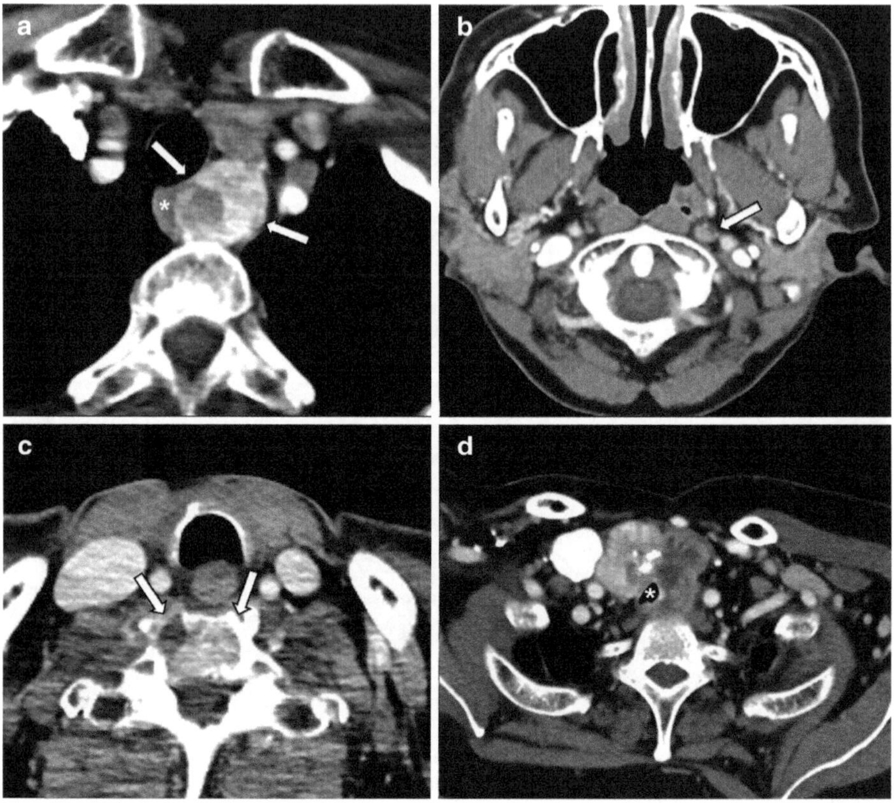


**Fig. 2.5** Detection of thyroid cancers on CT, which were not evaluable with US. (**a**) Axial contrast-enhanced CT image depicts recurrent tumor (arrow) in the upper mediastinum, compressing the esophagus (asterisk), (**b**) CT shows metastatic LNs in the left retropharyngeal area (arrow), (**c**) CT shows enhancing osteolytic bone metastasis (arrow) in the cervical vertebral body from thyroid cancer, and (**d**) CT shows invasive advanced thyroid cancer encircling and invading the trachea, causing luminal narrowing (asterisk)

does not interfere with future radioiodine administration. However, conventional MRI techniques may have lower sensitivity than CT for detecting small macroscopic metastatic lesions (<2 mm) and LN metastases with diameters less than 10 mm [53]. Additionally, MRI may be less sensitive than CT in detecting calcified metastatic LNs. Therefore, neck CT is often considered the primary cross-sectional imaging modality for detecting LN metastasis in differentiated thyroid carcinoma (DTC) [2].

Invasive DTC occurs in 10–15% of patients [13]. For these patients, contrast-enhanced cross-sectional imaging, such as MRI or CT, is instrumental in accurately assessing the extent of aerodigestive tract invasion and vascular involvement [2, 13, 16]. Both MRI and CT exhibit similar degrees of accuracy in predicting local invasion of the esophagus, trachea, and recurrent laryngeal nerve [54–57].

## Postoperative Evaluation of Thyroid Cancer

### *Neck US*

After definitive treatment for thyroid cancer, imaging modalities, particularly US, play a crucial role in detecting, classifying, and localizing potentially abnormal lesions in the neck. For any structural lesion detected in the neck through imaging, decisions regarding further management (active surveillance, revision surgery, local ablation therapy, or radioactive iodine treatment) should be made based on the lesion's location and individual clinical factors [13, 16, 47]. Imaging is essential for delineating the extent and location of the disease before additional treatment.

US is capable of detecting and characterizing recurrent tumors in the neck [28, 58–60], and US scans should include evaluation of both the thyroidectomy bed and cervical lymph nodes [39]. Several US features suggestive of recurrent tumor in the thyroid bed have been identified in previous studies (Fig. 2.6), and the ETA has defined a US-based classification for thyroid bed lesions based on these features

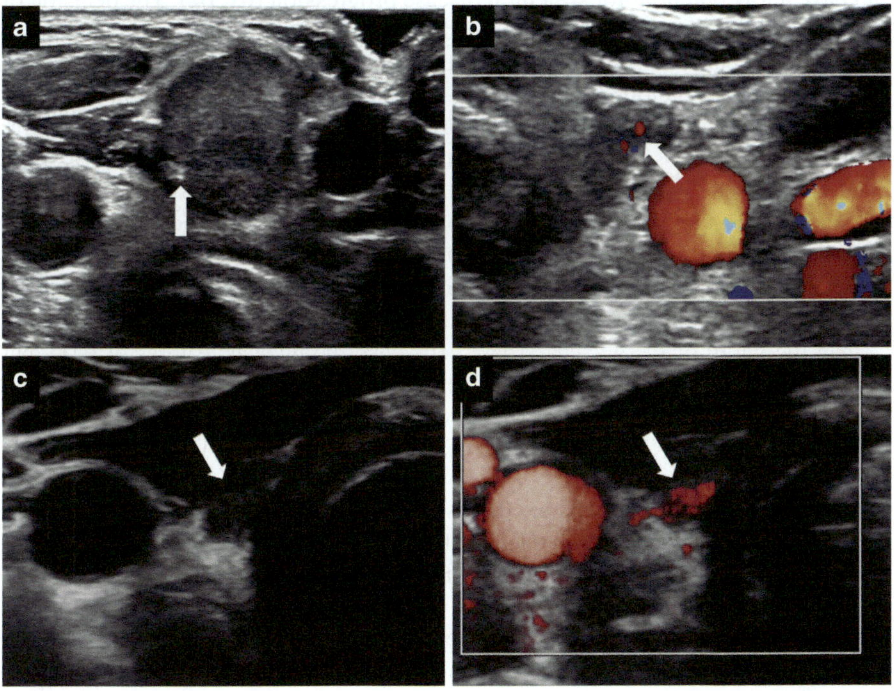


**Fig. 2.6** Ultrasound features of recurrent tumors in the thyroid bed. (**a**) Recurrent tumor in the left lower thyroid bed with hyperechogenicity, echogenic foci (arrow) and nonparallel orientation, (**b**) recurrent tumor with hyperechogenicity and abnormal vascularity (arrow), (**c**) recurrent tumor (arrow) with hypoechogenicity (**c**), but with abnormal diffuse vascularity (**d**)

**Table 2.4** US criteria for diagnosis of tumor recurrence in the thyroid bed after thyroidectomy for thyroid cancer

| ETA | Description |
|---|---|
| Suspicious | Taller-than-wide orientation<br>Irregular margins<br>Microcalcifications<br>Cystic changes<br>Increased vascularization |
| Indeterminate | Lesions displaying hypoechogenicity alone |
| Normal | Triangular or flattened area, uniformly hyperechoic or isoechoic vs surrounding muscle/tissue |

*ETE* extrathyroidal extension

(Table 2.4) [39]. Regarding cervical lymph nodes, the imaging features are the same as those used in the preoperative classification system, with LNs classified as suspicious (suspicious for malignancy), indeterminate, or probably benign (normal) (Table 2.3) [16, 39]. Recent studies have shown that suspicious metastatic lesions in the thyroid bed or lateral neck detected after surgery usually exhibit stable behavior and have a low potential for structural disease progression [61, 62]. The decision of whether and when to perform US-guided FNA for suspicious recurrent lesions in postoperative patients with thyroid cancer should be based on the location of the lymph node or suspicious lesion and the management plan (reoperation, nonsurgical ablation therapy, or active surveillance). Considering the high risk of postoperative complications associated with repeat surgery, FNA may be deferred for small indeterminate or suspicious lymph nodes measuring <8–10 mm (short diameter on US and CT images) in postoperative patients if US surveillance is considered instead of reoperation or ablation therapy for suspicious recurrent lesions [16, 63]. The addition of FNA-thyroglobulin washout to cytology increases the sensitivity of evaluating recurrent cancers in the neck.

## *Neck CT or MRI*

In cases where suspected recurrent disease is not clearly delineated on US or when the suspected recurrent disease involves the aerodigestive tract, CT can be a valuable imaging modality. CT may also be employed when US is unable to adequately visualize disease recurrence, particularly in patients with high levels of serum thyroglobulin (Tg) or Tg antibodies and negative US findings [2, 13, 23]. A recent study demonstrated the additional benefit of CT in conjunction with US for detecting recurrent thyroid cancer [64]. Before revision surgery or image-guided interventions, it is essential to accurately identify the target lesion using both US and CT [2, 16]. Cross-sectional imaging of other body regions, such as the lungs and mediastinum, may complement neck US and CT when they are unable to localize any recurrent tumor [13, 16].

## References


1. Hegedüs L. Clinical practice. The thyroid nodule. N Engl J Med. 2004;351(17):1764–71.
2. Lee JY, Baek JH, Ha EJ, Sung JY, Shin JH, Kim JH, et al. 2020 imaging guidelines for thyroid nodules and differentiated thyroid cancer: Korean society of thyroid radiology. Korean J Radiol. 2021;22(5):840–60.
3. Brito JP, Gionfriddo MR, Al Nofal A, Boehmer KR, Leppin AL, Reading C, et al. The accuracy of thyroid nodule ultrasound to predict thyroid cancer: systematic review and meta-analysis. J Clin Endocrinol Metab. 2014;99(4):1253–63.
4. Smith-Bindman R, Lebda P, Feldstein VA, Sellami D, Goldstein RB, Brasic N, et al. Risk of thyroid cancer based on thyroid ultrasound imaging characteristics: results of a population-based study. JAMA Intern Med. 2013;173(19):1788–96.
5. Solbiati L, Osti V, Cova L, Tonolini M. Ultrasound of thyroid, parathyroid glands and neck lymph nodes. Eur Radiol. 2001;11(12):2411–24.
6. Chiofalo MG, Signoriello S, Fulciniti F, Avenia N, Ristagno S, Lombardi CP, et al. Predictivity of clinical, laboratory and imaging findings in diagnostic definition of palpable thyroid nodules. A multicenter prospective study. Endocrine. 2018;61(1):43–50.
7. Lee YH, Kim DW, In HS, Park JS, Kim SH, Eom JW, et al. Differentiation between benign and malignant solid thyroid nodules using an US classification system. Korean J Radiol. 2011;12(5):559–67.
8. Mandel SJ. Diagnostic use of ultrasonography in patients with nodular thyroid disease. Endocr Pract. 2004;10(3):246–52.
9. Sosa JA, Hanna JW, Robinson KA, Lanman RB. Increases in thyroid nodule fine-needle aspirations, operations, and diagnoses of thyroid cancer in the United States. Surgery. 2013;154(6):1420–6; discussion 6–7
10. Zevallos JP, Hartman CM, Kramer JR, Sturgis EM, Chiao EY. Increased thyroid cancer incidence corresponds to increased use of thyroid ultrasound and fine-needle aspiration: a study of the veterans affairs health care system. Cancer. 2015;121(5):741–6.
11. Bongiovanni M, Spitale A, Faquin WC, Mazzucchelli L, Baloch ZW. The Bethesda system for reporting thyroid cytopathology: a meta-analysis. Acta Cytol. 2012;56(4):333–9.
12. Na DG, Kim JH, Sung JY, Baek JH, Jung KC, Lee H, et al. Core-needle biopsy is more useful than repeat fine-needle aspiration in thyroid nodules read as nondiagnostic or atypia of undetermined significance by the Bethesda system for reporting thyroid cytopathology. Thyroid. 2012;22(5):468–75.
13. Haugen BR, Alexander EK, Bible KC, Doherty GM, Mandel SJ, Nikiforov YE, et al. 2015 American thyroid association management guidelines for adult patients with thyroid nodules and differentiated thyroid cancer: the American thyroid association guidelines task force on thyroid nodules and differentiated thyroid cancer. Thyroid. 2016;26(1):1–133.
14. Gharib H, Papini E, Garber JR, Duick DS, Harrell RM, Hegedüs L, et al. American association of clinical endocrinologists, American college of endocrinology, and associazione medici endocrinologi medical guidelines for clinical practice for the diagnosis and management of thyroid nodules—2016 update. Endocr Pract. 2016;22(5):622–39.
15. Shin JH, Baek JH, Chung J, Ha EJ, Kim JH, Lee YH, et al. Ultrasonography diagnosis and imaging-based management of thyroid nodules: revised Korean society of thyroid radiology consensus statement and recommendations. Korean J Radiol. 2016;17(3):370–95.
16. Ha EJ, Chung SR, Na DG, Ahn HS, Chung J, Lee JY, et al. 2021 Korean thyroid imaging reporting and data system and imaging-based management of thyroid nodules: Korean society of thyroid radiology consensus statement and recommendations. Korean J Radiol. 2021;22(12):2094–123.
17. Tessler FN, Middleton WD, Grant EG, Hoang JK, Berland LL, Teefey SA, et al. ACR thyroid imaging, reporting and data system (TI-RADS): white paper of the ACR TI-RADS committee. J Am Coll Radiol. 2017;14(5):587–95.

18. Russ G, Bonnema SJ, Erdogan MF, Durante C, Ngu R, Leenhardt L. European thyroid association guidelines for ultrasound malignancy risk stratification of thyroid nodules in adults: the EU-TIRADS. Eur Thyroid J. 2017;6(5):225–37.
19. Moon WJ, Baek JH, Jung SL, Kim DW, Kim EK, Kim JY, et al. Ultrasonography and the ultrasound-based management of thyroid nodules: consensus statement and recommendations. Korean J Radiol. 2011;12(1):1–14.
20. Yoon SJ, Na DG, Gwon HY, Paik W, Kim WJ, Song JS, et al. Similarities and differences between thyroid imaging reporting and data systems. AJR Am J Roentgenol. 2019;213(2):W76–w84.
21. Hoang JK, Langer JE, Middleton WD, Wu CC, Hammers LW, Cronan JJ, et al. Managing incidental thyroid nodules detected on imaging: white paper of the ACR incidental thyroid findings committee. J Am Coll Radiol. 2015;12(2):143–50.
22. Shetty SK, Maher MM, Hahn PF, Halpern EF, Aquino SL. Significance of incidental thyroid lesions detected on CT: correlation among CT, sonography, and pathology. AJR Am J Roentgenol. 2006;187(5):1349–56.
23. Hoang JK, Oldan JD, Mandel SJ, Policeni B, Agarwal V, Burns J, et al. ACR appropriateness criteria(®) thyroid disease. J Am Coll Radiol. 2019;16(5s):S300–s14.
24. Hoang JK, Branstetter BF, Gafton AR, Lee WK, Glastonbury CM. Imaging of thyroid carcinoma with CT and MRI: approaches to common scenarios. Cancer Imaging. 2013;13(1):128–39.
25. Pacini F, Basolo F, Bellantone R, Boni G, Cannizzaro MA, De Palma M, et al. Italian consensus on diagnosis and treatment of differentiated thyroid cancer: joint statements of six Italian societies. J Endocrinol Investig. 2018;41(7):849–76.
26. Eun NL, Son EJ, Kim JA, Gweon HM, Kang JH, Youk JH. Comparison of the diagnostic performances of ultrasonography, CT and fine needle aspiration cytology for the prediction of lymph node metastasis in patients with lymph node dissection of papillary thyroid carcinoma: a retrospective cohort study. Int J Surg. 2018;51:145–50.
27. Jiang HJ, Wu CW, Chiang FY, Chiou HC, Chen IJ, Hsiao PJ. Reliable sonographic features for nodal thyroglobulin to diagnose recurrent lymph node metastasis from papillary thyroid carcinoma. Clin Otolaryngol. 2018;43(4):1065–72.
28. Leboulleux S, Girard E, Rose M, Travagli JP, Sabbah N, Caillou B, et al. Ultrasound criteria of malignancy for cervical lymph nodes in patients followed up for differentiated thyroid cancer. J Clin Endocrinol Metab. 2007;92(9):3590–4.
29. O'Connell K, Yen TW, Quiroz F, Evans DB, Wang TS. The utility of routine preoperative cervical ultrasonography in patients undergoing thyroidectomy for differentiated thyroid cancer. Surgery. 2013;154(4):697–701; discussion 701-3
30. Rosário PW, de Faria S, Bicalho L, Alves MF, Borges MA, Purisch S, et al. Ultrasonographic differentiation between metastatic and benign lymph nodes in patients with papillary thyroid carcinoma. J Ultrasound Med. 2005;24(10):1385–9.
31. Stulak JM, Grant CS, Farley DR, Thompson GB, van Heerden JA, Hay ID, et al. Value of preoperative ultrasonography in the surgical management of initial and reoperative papillary thyroid cancer. Arch Surg. 2006;141(5):489–94; discussion 94–6
32. Lee CY, Kim SJ, Ko KR, Chung KW, Lee JH. Predictive factors for extrathyroidal extension of papillary thyroid carcinoma based on preoperative sonography. J Ultrasound Med. 2014;33(2):231–8.
33. Kwak JY, Kim EK, Youk JH, Kim MJ, Son EJ, Choi SH, et al. Extrathyroid extension of well-differentiated papillary thyroid microcarcinoma on US. Thyroid. 2008;18(6):609–14.
34. Choi JS, Chung WY, Kwak JY, Moon HJ, Kim MJ, Kim EK. Staging of papillary thyroid carcinoma with ultrasonography: performance in a large series. Ann Surg Oncol. 2011;18(13):3572–8.
35. Park JS, Son KR, Na DG, Kim E, Kim S. Performance of preoperative sonographic staging of papillary thyroid carcinoma based on the sixth edition of the AJCC/UICC TNM classification system. AJR Am J Roentgenol. 2009;192(1):66–72.
36. Moon SJ, Kim DW, Kim SJ, Ha TK, Park HK, Jung SJ. Ultrasound assessment of degrees of extrathyroidal extension in papillary thyroid microcarcinoma. Endocr Pract. 2014;20(10):1037–43.

37. Kuo EJ, Thi WJ, Zheng F, Zanocco KA, Livhits MJ, Yeh MW. Individualizing surgery in papillary thyroid carcinoma based on a detailed sonographic assessment of extrathyroidal extension. Thyroid. 2017;27(12):1544–9.
38. Chung SR, Baek JH, Choi YJ, Sung TY, Song DE, Kim TY, et al. Sonographic assessment of the extent of extrathyroidal extension in thyroid cancer. Korean J Radiol. 2020;21(10):1187–95.
39. Leenhardt L, Erdogan MF, Hegedus L, Mandel SJ, Paschke R, Rago T, et al. 2013 European thyroid association guidelines for cervical ultrasound scan and ultrasound-guided techniques in the postoperative management of patients with thyroid cancer. Eur Thyroid J. 2013;2(3):147–59.
40. Lee Y, Kim JH, Baek JH, Jung SL, Park SW, Kim J, et al. Value of CT added to ultrasonography for the diagnosis of lymph node metastasis in patients with thyroid cancer. Head Neck. 2018;40(10):2137–48.
41. Ahn JE, Lee JH, Yi JS, Shong YK, Hong SJ, Lee DH, et al. Diagnostic accuracy of CT and ultrasonography for evaluating metastatic cervical lymph nodes in patients with thyroid cancer. World J Surg. 2008;32(7):1552–8.
42. Kim E, Park JS, Son KR, Kim JH, Jeon SJ, Na DG. Preoperative diagnosis of cervical metastatic lymph nodes in papillary thyroid carcinoma: comparison of ultrasound, computed tomography, and combined ultrasound with computed tomography. Thyroid. 2008;18(4):411–8.
43. Suh CH, Baek JH, Choi YJ, Lee JH. Performance of CT in the preoperative diagnosis of cervical lymph node metastasis in patients with papillary thyroid cancer: a systematic review and meta-analysis. AJNR Am J Neuroradiol. 2017;38(1):154–61.
44. Yang SY, Shin JH, Hahn SY, Lim Y, Hwang SY, Kim TH, et al. Comparison of ultrasonography and CT for preoperative nodal assessment of patients with papillary thyroid cancer: diagnostic performance according to primary tumor size. Acta Radiol. 2020;61(1):21–7.
45. Lesnik D, Cunnane ME, Zurakowski D, Acar GO, Ecevit C, Mace A, et al. Papillary thyroid carcinoma nodal surgery directed by a preoperative radiographic map utilizing CT scan and ultrasound in all primary and reoperative patients. Head Neck. 2014;36(2):191–202.
46. Bongers PJ, Verzijl R, Dzingala M, Vriens MR, Yu E, Pasternak JD, et al. Preoperative computed tomography changes surgical management for clinically low-risk well-differentiated thyroid cancer. Ann Surg Oncol. 2019;26(13):4439–44.
47. Yi KH, Lee EK, Kang H-C, Kim SW, Kim IJ, Park SY, et al. Revised Korean thyroid association management guidelines for patients with thyroid nodules and thyroid cancer. IJT. 2016;9(2):59–126.
48. Yoo RE, Kim JH, Hwang I, Kang KM, Yun TJ, Choi SH, et al. Added value of computed tomography to ultrasonography for assessing LN metastasis in preoperative patients with thyroid cancer: node-by-node correlation. Cancers (Basel). 2020;12(5):1190.
49. Chung SR, Baek JH, Rho YH, Choi YJ, Sung T-Y, Song DE, et al. Sonographic diagnosis of cervical lymph node metastasis in patients with thyroid cancer and comparison of European and Korean guidelines for stratifying the risk of malignant lymph node. Korean J Radiol. 2022;23(11):1102–11.
50. Lee JY, Yoo RE, Rhim JH, Lee KH, Choi KS, Hwang I, et al. Validation of ultrasound risk stratification systems for cervical lymph node metastasis in patients with thyroid cancer. Cancers (Basel). 2022;14(9):2106.
51. Lee DH, Kim YK, Yu HW, Choi JY, Park SY, Moon JH. Computed tomography for detecting cervical lymph node metastasis in patients who have papillary thyroid microcarcinoma with tumor characteristics appropriate for active surveillance. Thyroid. 2019;29(11):1653–9.
52. Cho SJ, Suh CH, Baek JH, Chung SR, Choi YJ, Lee JH. Diagnostic performance of MRI to detect metastatic cervical lymph nodes in patients with thyroid cancer: a systematic review and meta-analysis. Clin Radiol. 2020;75(7):562.e1–562.e1.e10.
53. Choi JY, Choi YS, Park YH, Kim JH. Experience and analysis of level VII cervical lymph node metastases in patients with papillary thyroid carcinoma. J Korean Surg Soc. 2011;80(5):307–12.
54. Seo YL, Yoon DY, Lim KJ, Cha JH, Yun EJ, Choi CS, et al. Locally advanced thyroid cancer: can CT help in prediction of extrathyroidal invasion to adjacent structures? AJR Am J Roentgenol. 2010;195(3):W240–4.

55. Takashima S, Takayama F, Wang J, Kobayashi S, Kadoya M. Using MR imaging to predict invasion of the recurrent laryngeal nerve by thyroid carcinoma. AJR Am J Roentgenol. 2003;180(3):837–42.
56. Wang J, Takashima S, Matsushita T, Takayama F, Kobayashi T, Kadoya M. Esophageal invasion by thyroid carcinomas: prediction using magnetic resonance imaging. J Comput Assist Tomogr. 2003;27(1):18–25.
57. Wang JC, Takashima S, Takayama F, Kawakami S, Saito A, Matsushita T, et al. Tracheal invasion by thyroid carcinoma: prediction using MR imaging. AJR Am J Roentgenol. 2001;177(4):929–36.
58. Pacini F, Molinaro E, Castagna MG, Agate L, Elisei R, Ceccarelli C, et al. Recombinant human thyrotropin-stimulated serum thyroglobulin combined with neck ultrasonography has the highest sensitivity in monitoring differentiated thyroid carcinoma. J Clin Endocrinol Metab. 2003;88(8):3668–73.
59. Torlontano M, Crocetti U, Augello G, D'Aloiso L, Bonfitto N, Varraso A, et al. Comparative evaluation of recombinant human thyrotropin-stimulated thyroglobulin levels, 131I whole-body scintigraphy, and neck ultrasonography in the follow-up of patients with papillary thyroid microcarcinoma who have not undergone radioiodine therapy. J Clin Endocrinol Metab. 2006;91(1):60–3.
60. Lepoutre-Lussey C, Maddah D, Golmard JL, Russ G, Tissier F, Trésallet C, et al. Post-operative neck ultrasound and risk stratification in differentiated thyroid cancer patients with initial lymph node involvement. Eur J Endocrinol. 2014;170(6):837–46.
61. Robenshtok E, Fish S, Bach A, Domínguez JM, Shaha A, Tuttle RM. Suspicious cervical lymph nodes detected after thyroidectomy for papillary thyroid cancer usually remain stable over years in properly selected patients. J Clin Endocrinol Metab. 2012;97(8):2706–13.
62. Rondeau G, Fish S, Hann LE, Fagin JA, Tuttle RM. Ultrasonographically detected small thyroid bed nodules identified after total thyroidectomy for differentiated thyroid cancer seldom show clinically significant structural progression. Thyroid. 2011;21(8):845–53.
63. Kim JH, Baek JH, Lim HK, Ahn HS, Baek SM, Choi YJ, et al. 2017 thyroid radiofrequency ablation guideline: Korean society of thyroid radiology. Korean J Radiol. 2018;19(4):632–55.
64. Hong EK, Kim JH, Lee J, Yoo RE, Kim SC, Kim MJ, et al. Diagnostic value of computed tomography combined with ultrasonography in detecting cervical recurrence in patients with thyroid cancer. Head Neck. 2019;41(5):1206–12.

# Chapter 3
# Fine-Needle Aspiration and Core Needle Biopsy of Thyroid Nodules

**Susana Calle, Diana Kaya, and Kim O. Learned**

## Introduction

Thyroid nodules are common among older adults with approximately 60% harboring one or more nodules, although only 5% are malignant [1]. Thyroid nodules are usually asymptomatic and are most often discovered incidentally during other diagnostic imaging tests or can occasionally present as a palpable abnormality. Ultrasound is considered the imaging modality of choice for the evaluation of the thyroid gland and can help to identify clinically significant thyroid nodules that meet the criteria for tissue sampling.

The precise patient selection and methodology with which thyroid nodule biopsies are performed varies greatly among institutions and depends on several factors including, but not limited to, resources, patient population, referring services, radiologist preference, and experience. Patient selection, particularly in the community setting, often relies on American College of Radiology (ACR) Thyroid Imaging Reporting and Data Systems (TIRADS) or other similar systems developed by the Korean Thyroid Association (KTA), American Thyroid Association (ATA), and British Thyroid Association (BTA). Many of these systems demonstrate similar sensitivity, specificity, and negative predicative values in prediction of malignancy in histologically proven thyroid nodules [2].

The TIRADS algorithm aims to stratify thyroid nodules by ultrasound features into different categories depending on the degree of suspicion. This system facilitates the radiologist's judgment process and it presents a framework with which to

S. Calle (✉)
Department of Neuroradiology, Division of Diagnostic Imaging,
University of MD Anderson Cancer Center, Houston, TX, USA
e-mail: SCalle@mdanderson.org

D. Kaya · K. O. Learned
Department of Neuroradiology, Division of Diagnostic Imaging,
University of Texas MD Anderson Cancer Center, Houston, TX, USA


A. W. Park et al. (eds.), *Thyroid Radiofrequency Ablation*,
https://doi.org/10.1007/978-3-031-65288-2_3

recommend tissue sampling or observation. While TIRADS is a helpful tool, it is important to note that it should not represent a rigid model that must be strictly adhered to. Patient history is paramount and should include the determination of risk factors for the development of thyroid malignancy, including family history, exposure to ionizing radiation, and hereditary syndromes. Such factors influence the decision-making process as they lower the threshold for both active surveillance and biopsy [1]. Also, the context of each case and patient preference must be incorporated into the ultimate disposition. A full discussion on this topic is beyond the scope of this document and is discussed in further detail in the chapters titled "Current Diagnosis and Management of Thyroid Nodules" and "Imaging Diagnosis of Thyroid Nodules" of this series.

The combined use of ultrasound guidance and biopsy, which is currently a common practice, is associated with a significant increase in diagnostic accuracy of thyroid biopsies compared to palpation-guided techniques [3]. The added benefits of US guidance over palpation-guided technique includes the possibility of sampling of non-palpable, small, or posteriorly located nodules, the visualization of the needle during the procedure, and the assurance of the correct positioning of the needle tip within the solid, most suspicious component of the nodule in the case of mixed solid/cystic lesions. Furthermore, US guidance reduces complication rates by helping to avoid large vessels, the trachea, and the esophagus.

The effectiveness of the US-guided procedures depends on the skills of the operator, the experience of the cytopathologist interpreting the smears, the vascularity of the nodule, and the presence of cystic or calcified components within the nodule. A comprehensive diagnostic ultrasound scan which includes evaluation of the thyroid and cervical nodes should be performed prior to the biopsy. The detection of abnormal lymph nodes necessitates the biopsy of suspicious thyroid nodules and of cervical adenopathy for appropriate staging and surgical planning purposes.

## Clinical Evaluation of Patients

### *Pre-Procedural Evaluation*

Ultrasound-guided biopsy of the thyroid is a minimally invasive procedure without any absolute contraindications. The major relative contraindications include significant coagulopathy, severely compromised cardiopulmonary function or hemodynamic instability, and inability of the patient to cooperate or tolerate the procedure. Other relative contraindications may include skin infection at the site of needle entry and the presence of a low riding thyroid gland with retrosternal thyroid nodules that may hinder ultrasound visualization of the needle tract.

The failure of the patient to maintain a supine position, vigorous respiration and anxiety may preclude safe ultrasound-guided thyroid biopsy. Giving detailed information regarding procedural steps, including low level of expected discomfort, possible referred pain to the ipsilateral ear and jaw, employment of very thin needles, and short procedural time can help alleviate the patient's anxiety.

There are no established thresholds for when the procedure can be performed safely in patients with hypertension. The operator must evaluate the patient on an individual basis, assessing severity, chronicity, and symptomatology of hypertension, while considering the risk and benefits of the procedure.

Any history of cardiac or pulmonary disease, usage of anticoagulants, and history of allergic reaction to local anesthetics should be reviewed and addressed. A thorough evaluation of the patient's history and a focused physical examination should be performed with relative contraindications addressed before the procedure.

## *Patients on Anticoagulation Therapy*

A sizable portion of patients referred for US-guided fine-needle aspiration (FNA) of the thyroid take 1 or 2 antithrombotic agents, such as aspirin and clopidogrel, or anticoagulant medications, such as warfarin and heparin. Several studies have shown that FNA of the thyroid can be safely performed in patients taking antithrombotic and anticoagulants without the risk of hematoma formation [4, 5]. The overall incidence of hematoma development associated with thyroid FNA taking antithrombotic/anticoagulant agents was at about 1% in these studies. The Society of Interventional Radiology Guidelines designates FNA of the thyroid as a low bleeding risk procedure. Pre-procedural PT/INR, hemoglobin, and platelet count check is not routinely recommended for FNA or core needle biopsy (CNB) [6]. The guideline does not recommend discontinuation of the antithrombotic or anticoagulant agents in low-risk procedures. However, if lab results are available, platelet transfusions are recommended for platelet counts less than 20,000 and correction of INR to <3 is considered appropriate [1].

Furthermore, it is not necessary to interrupt novel anticoagulants such as dabigatran, rivaroxaban, and apixaban used in stroke prevention for nonvalvular atrial fibrillation and venous thrombosis prophylaxis prior to or following US-guided FNA [7].

Additionally, the risk of bloody specimens resulting in nondiagnostic cytology results is not significantly higher in patients on anticoagulation therapy [8]. However, in one retrospective study, a threefold increase of nondiagnostic specimens was seen in patients receiving aspirin. While routine cessation of aspirin in all patients undergoing a first thyroid FNA is likely not necessary, some authors suggest a possible benefit to withholding aspirin in patients with low cardiovascular risk in order to increase the likelihood of yielding a diagnostic sample [9].

Our current institutional guideline recommends withdrawal of aspirin for 7 days, clopidogrel for 5 days, warfarin for 5 days, and heparin for 1 day.

## Fine-Needle Aspiration

FNA of the thyroid is a widely available, low-cost, and safe procedure which, in capable hands, provides diagnostic-quality cellular sampling without significant blood contamination and with minimal patient discomfort. FNA of the thyroid was first described in 1930 by Martin and Ellis who originally used an 18-gauge-needle [10]. However, due to initial concerns regarding tumor seeding, the technique did not gain wide acceptance until the 1970s–1980s with the use of smaller 21- to 27-gauge needles [11]. Implementation of thyroid FNA ultimately led to the reduction in the number of thyroid surgeries as well as in an increase in the number of cancers detected during surgery [12].

The success of thyroid nodule FNA is determined by a low false-negative rate (FNR) and a high true positive rate [13]. While a low FNR relies on the quality of the sample obtained and the skillset of the proceduralist, a high true positive rate depends on the quality of the interpretation of the biopsy [13]. Consequently, implementation of evidence-guided appropriate device selection and technique directly influences diagnostic accuracy.

### *Devices/Materials*

A wide range of needle lengths and gauges are currently available for use in thyroid nodule FNA. Needle size should allow for the passage of follicular cells while minimizing the risk of hemorrhagic complications and bloody samples. Follicular cell nuclei are similar in size to that of red blood cells and lymphocytes, which is approximately 8–10 μm [13]. Commonly used 25- and 27-gauge needles have internal diameters of 191–241 μm, which represent roughly 20–50 times the diameter of follicular cell nuclei and allow for sampling of small stromal-epithelial fragments and intact follicles with an average three-dimensional diameter of approximately 200 μm [13]. Larger needles, particularly those larger than 23 gauge and used in combination with the aspiration method, increase the incidence of bloody samples without contributing substantially to the number of cells obtained [14]. FNA can be attempted with the smaller gauge needle with progression to larger needles if needed and depending on the incidence of dry samples as evidenced on direct inspection of the unstained slides.

Regular long bevel needles with an angle of 14° or less are preferred over short bevel needles as they allow for high cellular yield and effective tissue cutting at both the leading and trailing edges. Furthermore, unlike short bevel needles, longer bevel needles are not as easily occluded by muscle and other soft tissues present along the biopsy tract.

The need to apply suction or aspiration during FNA thyroid nodule sampling is a topic of considerable debate. While the broader term FNA has been more widely utilized, two distinct methodologies have been described. The term aspiration biopsy refers to the application of negative pressure by creating suction using a syringe or other special syringe holder while moving through a target lesion [15]. A second technique, more accurately termed fine needle nonaspiration cytology, introduces cellular material into the bore of the needle by the scraping effect of the needle bevel combined with the repeated back-and-forth excursions within the nodule [15]. Additionally, capillary effect, which is greater at smaller needle diameters, further contributes to cellular yield and the resultant surface tension often obviates the need for suction [13]. When comparing blood, number of cells, and preserved architecture, a series of 200 patients with thyroid nodules showed no statistically significant difference between the aspiration and nonaspiration techniques [16]. Other studies, including a meta-analysis and a series of 150 patients with thyroid gland enlargement, favored the nonaspiration technique with varying degrees of statistical significance [17, 18]. The disadvantages to each technique include the increased incidence of bloody samples, which impair interpretation in the case of aspiration biopsies, and the suboptimal yield of cellular material in the case of the nonaspiration technique. A meta-analysis that reviewed 2221 samples collected with both modalities concluded that both techniques may be useful and that a combination approach may be applied [19]. Suction may be indicated in fibrotic nodules or when cyst evacuation is required [15].

At our institution, thyroid biopsies are generally performed with high-frequency, linear transducers. These probes provide excellent image resolution of the thyroid gland which is a relatively superficial anatomic structure. Depending on the exact position of the nodule in question, the proceduralist may elect to apply the trapezoidal imaging function which extends the lateral field of view of the image in order to include specific structures along the projected course of the biopsy tract.

Occasionally, a micro-convex transducer may be selected for instances where a smaller footprint is preferred. The micro-convex probe may prove useful for lesions located near the suprasternal compartment, adjacent to bony prominences, or in deep locations that require a steeper angle of entry.

## *Procedure Technique*

Prior to beginning the biopsy, an informed consent must be obtained, and a time-out should be performed. Real-time sonographic evaluation of the thyroid lesion by the primary proceduralist is recommended and should be directed at establishing the route of entry, transducer selection, and optimal patient position.

Patient positioning is paramount to a successful procedure and must ensure the comfort of both the patient and the proceduralist throughout the duration of the biopsy. A mild hyperextension of the neck can be achieved by placing a pillow beneath the lower neck/upper back of the patient; this position allows the thyroid gland to be displaced anteriorly [15]. Mild hyperextension also better exposes and flattens the entry site and stretches the soft tissues of the neck for ease of access. A history of prior cervical spine pain or manipulation, as well as poor tolerance of the patient to remain in a decubitus position, should be taken into consideration when selecting the patient's position.

When first evaluating the nodule with ultrasound, the proceduralist must consider the depth of the lesion, the angle of entry, and the structures present along the projected course of the needle to determine the approach. The ideal trajectory for the biopsy is that which allows the safest and shortest access to the lesion [15]. In general, the nodule may be accessed from lateral-to-medial (sternocleidomastoid muscle side to trachea) or from medial-to-lateral depending on these factors and on the proceduralist's preference.

A biopsy tray is set up to include the necessary items required during the procedure (Fig. 3.1). Materials are placed on a sterile surface at an easily accessible height and distance from the proceduralist. Items included at our institution are as follows: sterile gauze pads, sterile drapes for dressing, small bowl with 70% isopropyl alcohol, medication labels and marker, sharps disposal pad, disposable 10-mL syringes, disposable 20-mL syringes, 3.8 cm (1.5 in.) long 25-gauge needles, Lidocaine 10 mg/mL (1%) injection 5 mL, glass slides for preparation of cytology smears, and sterile transducer cover.

The moments taken before the biopsy begins should not be underestimated as they set the stage for a smooth process and a successful outcome.

The ultrasound transducer is selected, and a sterile cover is placed. The patient's skin needs only to be cleansed with a simple alcohol preparation since the needle size used is similar to that of intramuscular injections and blood draws [13]. Although elaborate sterile draping of the patient is not necessary [13], it provides a clean surface on which to rest the transducer and contributes to the asepsis of the procedure.

In general, large, superficial, palpable nodules may be comfortably sampled without the use of local anesthetics. On the other hand, local anesthesia is recommended for deep nodules that may foreseeably require more involved probing to reach or when a greater number of passes will be required if no immediate cytologic

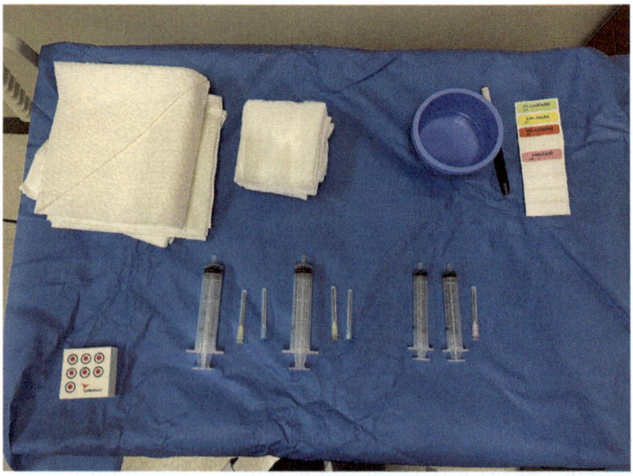

**Fig. 3.1** Example FNA biopsy tray

assessment is available. Ultimately, the use of local anesthesia is within the discretion of the operator with the agreement of the patient. At our institution, we elect to administer local anesthesia in nearly all patients in order to comfortably obtain repeat biopsies, if required, and minimize patient discomfort. The agent of choice for local anesthesia is 1–2% lidocaine with or without epinephrine [13]. A volume of approximately 0.5–1.5 mL is to be slowly administered into the subcutaneous fat and down to the thyroid capsule. While some proceduralists opt to create a wheal at the dermis, others rely on back infiltration of the subcutaneous anesthesia to the dermis, obviating the need for a painful dermal wheal [13, 15]. Allergic reactions to lidocaine have been rarely reported at this small dose and the effect of the anesthetic lasts 0.5–1.5 h [13].

Two commonly used techniques for ultrasound-guided FNA include the parallel and perpendicular techniques. In the parallel technique, preferred at our institution, the needle is inserted into the skin, adjacent to the probe footprint and oriented parallel to the long axis of the transducer. With this technique, the entire length of the needle is visualized from the surface of the skin, through the soft tissues along the biopsy trajectory, and ultimately to the target (Figs. 3.2 and 3.3) [15, 20]. The perpendicular or short axis approach, more commonly used for vascular access by interventional radiology, is performed by inserting the needle along the middle of the transducer at its short axis. In this technique, only the tip of the needle is visualized. Doppler ultrasound can be implemented to identify small vessels to be avoided overlying the thyroid gland.

Once the tip of the needle is confirmed within the target nodule, slow, deliberate excursions within the lesion are performed. A dwell time of 2–5 s within the nodule is recommended with approximately three back and forward motions to maximize

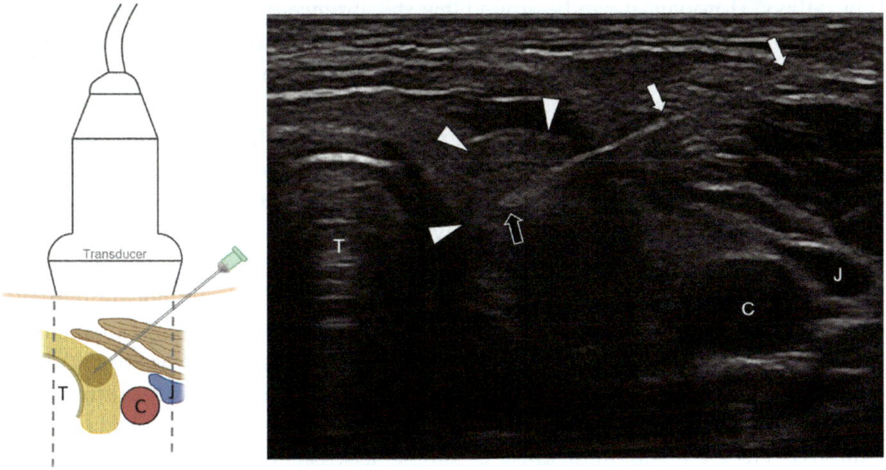


**Fig. 3.2** Schematic illustration and still ultrasound image demonstrating a lateral-to-medial, parallel approach ultrasound-guided fine needle biopsy of a left thyroid lobe nodule with the entire length of the needle in view (white arrows) and the needle tip (black arrow) within the nodule (white arrowheads). *T* trachea, *C* carotid artery, *J* jugular vein

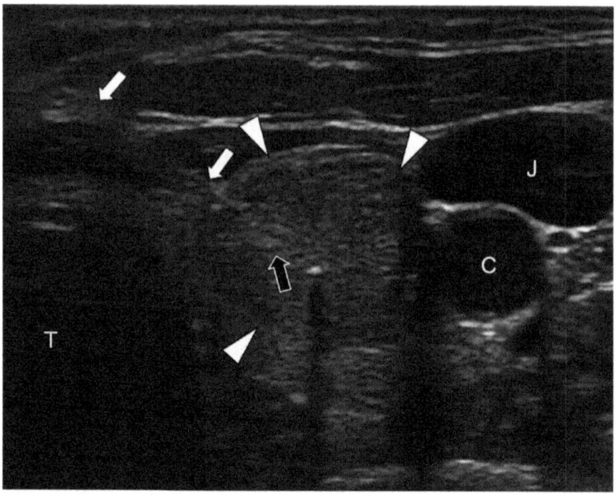


**Fig. 3.3** Still ultrasound image demonstrating a medial-to-lateral, parallel approach ultrasound-guided fine needle biopsy of a left thyroid lobe nodule with the entire length of the needle in view (white arrows) and the needle tip (black arrow) within the nodule (white arrowheads). *T* trachea, *C* carotid artery, *J* jugular vein

the diagnostic yield [13]. This technique effectively produces 1–2 slides per pass [13]. Rotation of the needle within the lesion may aid in loosening the sample with the sharp beveled edge, allowing for the introduction of cellular material to the bore of the needle [15]. Careful attention to the hub of the needle is suggested and once a drop of blood is evident, no further excursions should be undertaken so as to minimize blood contamination of the specimen [15]. The obtained material is then smeared on slides for fixation, staining, and interpretation. Additionally, the needle is flushed in CytoLyt solution for cell block analysis.

Real-time cytologic evaluation of samples for specimen adequacy positively influence the diagnostic yield of the procedure, occasionally at the expense of workflow delays. However, it can be argued that the absence of sample verification may ultimately result in greater costs to the system due to the increased need for repeat procedures and surgery [15]. Furthermore, over time, immediate feedback provided by the cytopathologist or cytopathology technologist may alter the procedural technique and reduce the number of nondiagnostic samples. However, immediate cytopathology assessment is not always feasible due to resource availability. For this reason, an increased number of passes can be obtained when immediate cytology evaluation is not possible. In a study analyzing the rate of nondiagnostic samples as a function of the number of passes, results concluded that an optimal number of six passes yielded a nondiagnostic rate of 1.4% and that this rate did not substantially decline in those with greater than six passes [21]. Conversely, in a comparison of studies where the number of passes was evaluated, the small increase of diagnostic accuracy above five passes was deemed negligible and did not outweigh the increased morbidity [13]. For this reason, the consensus was to perform no more than five passes when immediate cytologic assessment was not available and approximately two passes from different sites within the nodule when rapid interpretation was possible [13].

## Complications

Complications related to FNA are generally rare [20] and increase with increasing needle gauge [13]. A 30-min postprocedural observation period is recommended to evaluate for early warning signs. The most commonly encountered complications are local pain and bruising at the biopsy site. Following ultrasound-guided FNA, local compression and icing can minimize bleeding and inflammation, and acetaminophen may be given for pain relief [13, 20]. Small hematomas are usually asymptomatic and tend to resolve spontaneously. Rare instances of life-threatening hematomas have been reported necessitating surgical evacuation. Vasovagal reactions, while alarming, are usually self-limited and resolve with reclining the patient, cold compresses, and offering juice or crackers [13]. Postprocedural infection is uncommon, even in the immunocompromised patient [13, 20]. Other rare complications reported in the literature include transient recurrent laryngeal nerve paralysis and tumor seeding, with tumor seeding occurring more commonly with a larger needle gauge [13].

## Core Needle Biopsy

The rationale for employing core needle biopsy (CNB) for the diagnosis of thyroid nodule lies in overcoming certain limitations of the fine needle technique, namely the rates of inconclusive or nondiagnostic results [22]. Indeterminate cytologic results have been reported to range from 14% to 52% and nondiagnostic samples are calculated at 10–33.6% [23].

CNB provides a larger sample of tissue which provides further information on architectural structures within the nodule and allows for immunochemical staining [22]. FNA and CNB share high specificity (74–91%, respectively) and high sensitivity (100–99%, respectively) rates [24]. However, in a meta-analysis pooling 4580 patients with 4746 thyroid nodules, CNB was shown to have a markedly lower proportion of nondiagnostic and inconclusive results, 5.5% vs. 22.6% and 8% vs. 40.2%, respectively [24]. Most guidelines suggest CNB to be considered as a complementary method to FNA, which is still the standard diagnostic tool due to its cost-effectiveness, low complication rate, and high patient tolerance [13, 25]. In general, CNB may be performed in cases where FNA has produced an indeterminate result [22, 24].

Although one proposed benefit to the implementation of CNB is the potential for elucidation of indeterminate follicular lesions, several authors have concluded that CNB is similar to FNA in distinguishing between follicular adenoma and follicular carcinoma [13]. CNB is reportedly helpful when there is suspicion of rarer thyroid malignancies such as lymphoma, anaplastic carcinoma, and medullary carcinomas [15, 22, 24]. In a single-center study analyzing 104 patients with thyroid lymphoma and anaplastic thyroid carcinoma, CNB was found to increase the diagnostic sensitivity and positive predictive values over FNA [22]. Also, a review of 191 patients with medullary carcinoma similarly found higher positive predictive value (PPV) and sensitivity using CNB relative to FNA [26].

## *Devices/Materials*

Core biopsy devices used for thyroid nodule biopsy consist of spring-activated, single- or double-action needles with excursion lengths of 1.1–2.0 cm, 6–10 cm needle lengths, and variable internal diameters. Needle diameters proposed in the literature range from 14 to 22 gauge with 18–21- gauge needles used more commonly [22]. To our knowledge, there is currently no solid evidence supporting a particular choice of needle gauge for thyroid nodule CNB [22]. However, ultimately, the sample size will depend on both the inner diameter of the needle and the length of the specimen notch [22].

The mechanism of core needles is that of an inner stylet and an outer cutting cannula. The stylet has a 2-mm angled tip with a specimen notch for holding the tissue sample [22]. The outer cannula serves to transect the nodule, cut the tissue, and place it on the specimen notch [22] (Fig. 3.4). In double-action or automated needles, both the stylet and the cannula are spring-activated, which allow for penetration of tougher tissue at the expense of less control on the advance of the device and a greater propensity to neighboring tissue damage [22]. On the other hand, single-action or semi-automated needles rely on the manual introduction of the inner stylet followed by the spring-activated advancement of the cutting cannula [22]. A coaxial or guiding needle may be introduced through which the core needle device may be inserted. This may be of particular use when multiple samples are required as it minimizes the insertion of the needle through the soft tissues overlying the lesion, improving both accuracy and efficiency [22].

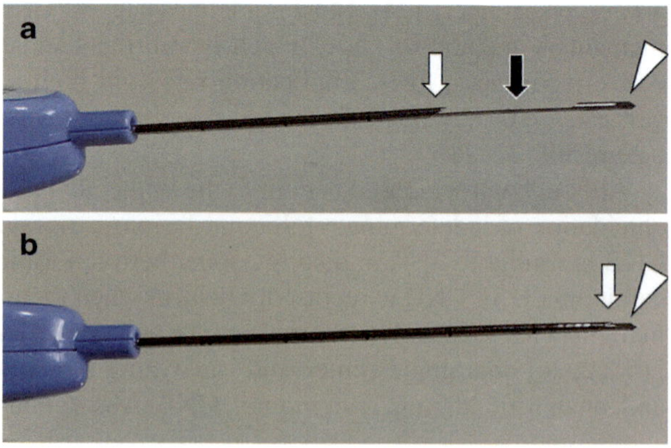


**Fig. 3.4** Semi-automated core needle biopsy device with a 2 mm angled tip (arrowhead), inner stylet with a specimen notch (black arrow), and outer cutting cannula prior to (**a**) and following (**b**) the spring-activated trigger

## *Procedure Technique*

The CNB technique shares several similarities with the FNA method, namely the ultrasound transducers used, the biopsy tray set up, and the completion of appropriate informed consent and time-out procedures. The reader may refer to the prior section on FNA for further detail. Also, as previously discussed, the experienced operator is encouraged to evaluate the target prior to the commencement of the procedure to assess for appropriate needle size and planned route of entry, which in turn influences both the safety and diagnostic accuracy of the biopsy [22]. Vessel mapping with Doppler ultrasound performed prior to the procedure also aids in avoiding vessel injury. The proceduralist should aim to elect a needle with a specimen notch length similar to the diameter of the nodule [22].

The patient is placed in the supine position with mild extension of the neck. Unlike FNA where a simple alcohol preparation is sufficient for skin cleansing, with the introduction of larger needle sizes (18 gauge or larger), the use of an iodine solution may be a reasonable addition [13]. Local anesthesia with lidocaine is administered with a finer needle along the biopsy route down to the thyroid capsule. Skin puncture may be performed to allow for greater maneuverability of the device. This may be achieved via a small superficial skin nick using a sharp scalpel or with the use of the core needle itself by employing a precise snapping movement of the wrist [22]. As with FNA, CNB may be performed from lateral-to-medial or medial-to-lateral, with the parallel/longitudinal method favored over the vertical approach to ensure complete visualization of the needle along the biopsy tract. Also, a trans-isthmic approach has been described as a suitable and recommended approach for CNB of thyroid nodules [22].

If the double-action or automated needle is used, the operator must ensure the entire length of the needle is within the field of view. Additionally, the tip of the needle may be placed in a safe location, often at the level of the thyroid capsule. The calculated trajectory of the triggered device should be anticipated and must be clear of vital structures with the depth of sample precisely predicted. Once these details have been established, the needle may be fired and the sampling site confirmed by imaging. Ideally, the sample is to include the normal thyroid parenchyma, the nodule-thyroid interface, and the nodule tissue itself when feasible [22].

With semi-automated devices, the stylet is advanced under ultrasound guidance within the nodule and the cutting cannula is fired while constantly maintaining the entire needle length within view (Fig. 3.5).

Once the sample has been obtained, a visual assessment of the biopsy specimen should be performed, which in turn allows for immediate feedback and predicts the need for additional samples. Macroscopically, the thyroid parenchyma will appear as a reddish soft tissue while most neoplasms will have a whiter appearance. Subsequently, the tissue sample is to immediately be fixed in a formalin preparation. For standard diagnostic purposes, one to two adequate samples are considered sufficient [22]. However, additional tissue may be required for molecular testing or for research purposes.

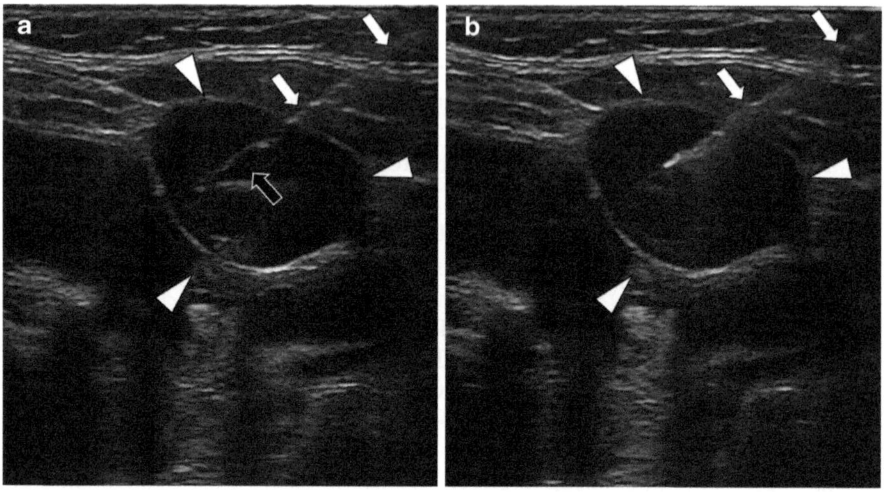


**Fig. 3.5** Still ultrasound images demonstrating a lateral-to-medial, parallel approach ultrasound-guided semi-automated CNB of a left thyroid lobe nodule with the entire length of the needle in view (white arrows). The specimen notch of the core needle device is seen within the nodule (black arrow in **a**). Visualization of the needle is maintained, and the cutting cannula is triggered while confirming its trajectory in image **b**

If the thyroid mass or nodule is markedly heterogeneous by ultrasound, it is recommended that samples be taken from different sites within the lesion. When coaxial devices are utilized, the guiding needle is inserted through the skin to the surface of the lesion and the biopsy needle is then placed within its bore. For subsequent samples, the angle of the guiding needle may be slightly adjusted to allow for different sample sites. When confronted with a hard nodule that does not easily allow for the puncture by the core needle, several methods may be attempted. These include the use of an automated device, the probing of the nodule surface to evaluate for sites of weakness, and the modification of the direction of the stylet direction [22].

Following completion of the procedure, direct compression of the biopsy site is recommended for approximately 20–30 min.

## *Complications*

The overall complication rate of US-guided CNB is low when performed by skilled proceduralists. In a meta-analysis analyzing the pooled proportion of complications following CNB for thyroid nodules, the incidence was calculated at 1.1%, with major complications estimated at only 0.06%, namely hematomas requiring hospitalization, permanent voice changes, and pseudoaneurysm formation [27].

Hemorrhagic complications account for the most common complications following thyroid CNB, with hematoma representing the most common type and vascular injury occurring in up to 3.9%, an incidence similar to FNA [22, 27, 28]. The majority of hematomas are effectively managed with direct compression of the neck for 30–120 min and generally are reabsorbed in 1–2 weeks [22]. Other examples were less frequently encountered, including pseudoaneurysm and arteriovenous fistula formation [22]. The risk of bleeding may be minimized by weighing risk-benefit ratios in patients with increased risk of hemorrhage, such as those on anticoagulants and those with clotting deficiencies. Also, the careful pre-procedural analysis of vascular structures and an appropriate technique further decrease the risk of bleeding [22].

Pain both during and following the procedure was one of the most frequently encountered complications. A study analyzing pain and satisfaction scores among 167 patients who had undergone thyroid FNA or CNB shows no significant difference between the groups both during and after the procedure [25].

Voice changes, both temporary and permanent, secondary to injury to the recurrent laryngeal nerve, have been reported in up to 1.9% of cases [29]. The use of the trans-isthmic approach has been reported to decrease the risk of direct injury to the recurrent laryngeal nerve [22].

The rich blood supply and lymphatic draining of the thyroid gland are protective factors against infection. However, rare cases of thyroid infection and abscess have been reported. Measures that may be taken to decrease the likelihood of infection include proper cleansing of the skin and careful evaluation of the ultrasound anatomy to prevent accidental puncture of the esophagus [22].

## Molecular Testing

### *FNA Results and Molecular Testing*

The Bethesda System for Reporting Thyroid Cytopathology (TBSRTC) was first published in 2010 for standardized reporting of thyroid cytology. Currently on its third edition published in 2023, the revised system assigns a single name for each of six diagnostic categories. These categories are (i) nondiagnostic, (ii) benign, (iii) atypia of indeterminate significance (AUS), (iv) follicular neoplasm, (v) suspicious for malignancy, and (vi) malignant. Nomenclature has been updated to align with the 2022 World Health Organization Classification of Thyroid Neoplasms. With further data gathered with the second edition published in 2017, the 2023 edition also includes the updated average risk of malignancy (ROM) and recommended clinical management addressing the significant and expanded use of molecular and ancillary testing in thyroid cytopathology, as included in Table 3.1.

The sample adequacy criteria by TBSRTC 2023 continues to be a minimum of 6 groups of well-preserved follicular cells and each group in turn must consist of at

**Table 3.1** The Bethesda system for reporting thyroid cytopathology 2023

| Category | ROM mean (%) | Recommended management |
|---|---|---|
| I. Nondiagnostic | 13 | Repeat FNA with US guidance |
| II. Benign | 4 | Clinical and US follow-up |
| III. Atypia of undetermined significance | 22 | Repeat FNA, molecular testing, lobectomy, or surveillance |
| IV. Follicular neoplasm | 30 | Molecular testing, lobectomy |
| V. Suspicious for malignancy | 74 | Molecular testing, lobectomy, or near-total thyroidectomy |
| VI. Malignant | 97 | Near-total thyroidectomy or lobectomy |

least 10 cells. The major drawbacks of FNA of the thyroid are indeterminate and nondiagnostic results, which do not render definitive cytologic diagnosis. The Bethesda Indeterminate cytologic results, consisting of Bethesda categories III and IV lesions, should theoretically occur in 7% of cases or less as proposed by TBSRTC. However, in practice, this result may vary more widely among individual pathologists and different institutions. Nondiagnostic samples or Bethesda class I account for average 10–20% with associated malignancy risk of 1–4% [30].

Further steps to overcome these predicaments in thyroid nodule characterization include repeat biopsy FNA, core biopsy, molecular testing, and diagnostic lobectomy. After an initial nondiagnostic cytology result, repeating the biopsy with US FNA yields a satisfactory specimen in 50–62% of cases [31]. In a study evaluating repeat FNA of nodules previously classified as Bethesda category I and III, 60% of nodules remained a category I or III following repeat FNA, and 40% changed category. Specifically, of the 40% prior category I nodules that changes category on repeat FNA, 95% became benign category II, 1% became suspicious follicular neoplasm category IV and suspicious for malignancy category V, and 4% became malignant category VI. Of the changed category III nodules on repeat FNA, 75% became benign, and 25% became malignant [32].

The 2015 ATA guidelines recommend molecular testing as an alternative for AUS/FLUS cytology (category III), follicular neoplasm or suspicious for a follicular neoplasm (category IV), and suspicious for malignancy cytology (category V) if such result would be expected to alter surgical decision-making [33]. Broadly, there are three methods for molecular testing: testing for somatic mutations, gene expression evaluation, and microRNA-based classifiers. Several commercially available methods are available on the market worldwide (Afirma GSC, Thyroseq V3, ThyGeNEX-ThyraMir, MirThy-pe) with the goal to improve the accuracy of preoperative diagnosis of cytologically indeterminate thyroid nodules.

The Afirma gene expression classifier (GEC, Veracyte, South San Francisco, CA) was introduced in January 2011 and was based on microarray analysis of mRNA expression profiles. The result of Afirma (GEC) classifies the specimen as "Afirma benign" (Afirma-B) or "Afirma suspicious" (Afirma-S). The Afirma (GEC) test demonstrated high sensitivity and a negative predictive value (NPV) of 94–95% among Bethesda III and IV thyroid nodules [34], but a relatively low specificity of approximately 50% and positive predictive value (PPV) of approximately 38% and poor performance with Hurtle cell lesions [35]. To overcome previous diagnostic limitations, the newer edition of Afirma was developed. The updated version, Afirma Genomic Sequencing Classifier (GSC), commercially available since 2017, now includes 12 classifiers and 7 additional components to identify parathyroid lesions, Hürthle cell lesions, BRAFV600E mutations, RET/PTC1–3 fusions, and medullary carcinoma utilizing next-generation RNA sequencing and machine learning algorithms. Validation studies demonstrated that Afirma GSC reclassify more indeterminate modules as benign and improved the specificity (68.3%) and PPV of the test (47.1%) [36].

ThyroSeq V3 (Thyroid Sequencing version 3) is a DNA- and RNA-based next-generation sequencing analysis that tests 112 cancer-related genes for more than 12,000 mutation hotspots. The test analyzes five different types of molecular alterations, including genetic alterations such as insertions and deletions, gene fusions, gene expression alterations, copy number alterations, and mutations (single nucleotide variants) [37]. ThyroSeq was validated in a prospective, blinded, multicenter cohort study on 286 cytologically indeterminate nodules with surgical pathology reports. It demonstrated high sensitivity (94%) and specificity (82%), with a negative predictive value of 97%, a positive predictive value of 66%, and a residual cancer risk of 3% in test-negative nodules. The study results showed that the ThyroSeq V3 molecular test can preclude diagnostic surgeries in up to 61% of patients with indeterminate Bethesda III to IV cytology nodules and 82% of all benign nodules with indeterminate cytology diagnosis [38]. In regard to Bethesda category V cytology results, which include suspicious for papillary carcinoma, medullary carcinoma, poorly differentiated carcinomas, anaplastic carcinomas, and metastatic carcinoma thyroid nodules, ThyroSeq V3 further improves cancer prediction and detects RAS-like, BRAF-like, and potentially targetable alterations which can alter patient management. It demonstrates a high sensitivity of 90% and specificity of 77% with high positive predictive values of 95% in suspicious for malignancy cytology. In addition, it provides information which can help in the planning of surgery extent. For example, the presence of TERT and TP 53 mutations may require more extensive surgery. Finding NTRK and RET fusions as well as BRAF V600E mutations can be targeted with new FDA-approved therapeutic agents [39].

The molecular tests successfully rule out malignancy of indeterminate cytology Bethesda III–IV (5–30% estimated risk of malignancy) with a high negative predictive value, similar to the benign Bethesda II cytology diagnosis (3% estimated risk of malignancy), hence preventing unnecessary diagnostic surgeries in about 60% of patients [38].

## Conclusion

US-guided FNA remains the gold standard technique for first-line cytologic diagnosis of thyroid nodules. The incorporation of high-resolution ultrasound evaluation, skillful procedural technique, and experienced pathology interpretation results in both a low false-negative rate and a high true positive rate with low risk of associated complications. Careful patient selection with guidance from ACR-TIRADS or similar models, along with evidence-based technique reduces the proportion of nondiagnostic samples. Complementary CNB and/or molecular testing may serve as an adjunct to elucidate indeterminate cytology results. Familiarity with Bethesda categories and clinical implications also aids in establishing a practice framework and determining the next appropriate step in management.

## References

1. Smith T, Kaufman CS. Ultrasound guided thyroid biopsy. Tech Vasc Interv Radiol. 2021;24(3):100768. https://doi.org/10.1016/j.tvir.2021.100768.
2. Chng CL, Tan HC, Too CW, et al. Diagnostic performance of ATA, BTA and TIRADS sonographic patterns in the prediction of malignancy in histologically proven thyroid nodules. Singapore Med J. 2018;59(11):578–83. https://doi.org/10.11622/smedj.2018062.
3. Tarigan TJE, Anwar BS, Sinto R, Wisnu W. Diagnostic accuracy of palpation versus ultrasound-guided fine needle aspiration biopsy for diagnosis of malignancy in thyroid nodules: a systematic review and meta-analysis. BMC Endocr Disord. 2022;22(1):181. https://doi.org/10.1186/s12902-022-01085-5.
4. Khadra H, Kholmatov R, Monlezun D, Kandil E. Do anticoagulation medications increase the risk of haematoma in ultrasound-guided fine needle aspiration of thyroid lesions? Cytopathology. 2018;29(6):565–8. https://doi.org/10.1111/cyt.12608.
5. Abu-Yousef MM, Larson JH, Kuehn DM, Wu AS, Laroia AT. Safety of ultrasound-guided fine needle aspiration biopsy of neck lesions in patients taking antithrombotic/anticoagulant medications. Ultrasound Q. 2011;27(3):157–9. https://doi.org/10.1097/RUQ.0b013e31822b5681.
6. Patel IJ, Rahim S, Davidson JC, et al. Society of interventional radiology consensus guidelines for the periprocedural management of thrombotic and bleeding risk in patients undergoing percutaneous image-guided interventions-part II: recommendations: endorsed by the Canadian association for interventional radiology and the cardiovascular and interventional radiological society of Europe. J Vasc Interv Radiol. 2019;30(8):1168–1184.e1. https://doi.org/10.1016/j.jvir.2019.04.017.
7. Lyle MA, Dean DS. Ultrasound-guided fine-needle aspiration biopsy of thyroid nodules in patients taking novel oral anticoagulants. Thyroid. 2015;25(4):373–6. https://doi.org/10.1089/thy.2014.0307.
8. Denham SLW, Ismail A, Bolus DN, Lockhart ME. Effect of anticoagulation medication on the thyroid fine-needle aspiration pathologic diagnostic sufficiency rate. J Ultrasound Med. 2016;35(1):43–8. https://doi.org/10.7863/ultra.15.03044.
9. Khan TS, Sharma E, Singh B, et al. Aspirin increases the risk of nondiagnostic yield of fine-needle aspiration and biopsy of thyroid nodules. Eur Thyroid J. 2018;7(3):129–32. https://doi.org/10.1159/000488451.
10. Martin HE, Ellis EB. Biopsy by needle puncture and aspiration. Ann Surg. 1930;92(2):169–81. https://doi.org/10.1097/00000658-193008000-00002.
11. Caplan RH, Kisken WA, Strutt PJ, Wester SM. Fine-needle aspiration biopsy of thyroid nodules. Postgrad Med. 1991;90(1):183–90. https://doi.org/10.1080/00325481.1991.11700990.
12. Hamberger B, Gharib H, Melton LJ, Goellner JR, Zinsmeister AR. Fine-needle aspiration biopsy of thyroid nodules. Impact on thyroid practice and cost of care. Am J Med. 1982;73(3):381–4.
13. Pitman MB, Abele J, Ali SZ, et al. Techniques for thyroid FNA: a synopsis of the National cancer institute thyroid fine-needle aspiration state of the science conference. Diagn Cytopathol. 2008;36(6):407–24. https://doi.org/10.1002/dc.20829.

14. Degirmenci B, Haktanir A, Albayrak R, et al. Sonographically guided fine-needle biopsy of thyroid nodules: the effects of nodule characteristics, sampling technique, and needle size on the adequacy of cytological material. Clin Radiol. 2007;62(8):798–803. https://doi.org/10.1016/j.crad.2007.01.024.
15. Dahiya N, Patel MD, Young SW. Neck procedures: thyroid and parathyroid. Radiol Clin North Am. 2020;58(6):1085–98. https://doi.org/10.1016/j.rcl.2020.07.005.
16. Haddadi-Nezhad S, Larijani B, Tavangar SM, Nouraei SM. Comparison of fine-needle-nonaspiration with fine-needle-aspiration technique in the cytologic studies of thyroid nodules. Endocr Pathol. 2003;14(4):369–73. https://doi.org/10.1385/ep:14:4:369.
17. Rizvi SAA, Husain M, Khan S, Mohsin M. A comparative study of fine needle aspiration cytology versus non-aspiration technique in thyroid lesions. Surg J R Coll Surg Edinb Irel. 2005;3(4):273–6. https://doi.org/10.1016/s1479-666x(05)80091-5.
18. Pothier DD, Narula A. Should we apply suction during fine needle cytology of thyroid lesions? A systematic review and meta-analysis. Ann R Coll Surg Engl. 2006;88(7):643–5. https://doi.org/10.1308/003588406X149147.
19. Song H, Wei C, Li D, et al. Comparison of fine needle aspiration and fine needle nonaspiration cytology of thyroid nodules: a meta-analysis. Biomed Res Int. 2015;2015:796120. https://doi.org/10.1155/2015/796120.
20. Langer JE, Baloch ZW, McGrath C, Loevner LA, Mandel SJ. Thyroid nodule fine-needle aspiration. Semin Ultrasound CT MRI. 2012;33(2):158–65. https://doi.org/10.1053/j.sult.2011.12.002.
21. Zhu W, Michael CW. How important is on-site adequacy assessment for thyroid FNA? An evaluation of 883 cases. Diagn Cytopathol. 2007;35(3):183–6. https://doi.org/10.1002/dc.20552.
22. Na DG, Baek JH, Jung SL, et al. Core needle biopsy of the thyroid: 2016 consensus statement and recommendations from Korean society of thyroid radiology. Korean J Radiol. 2017;18(1):217–37. https://doi.org/10.3348/kjr.2017.18.1.217.
23. Yoon JH, Kim EK, Kwak JY, Moon HJ. Effectiveness and limitations of core needle biopsy in the diagnosis of thyroid nodules: review of current literature. J Pathol Transl Med. 2015;49(3):230–5. https://doi.org/10.4132/jptm.2015.03.21.
24. Suh CH, Baek JH, Lee JH, et al. The role of core-needle biopsy in the diagnosis of thyroid malignancy in 4580 patients with 4746 thyroid nodules: a systematic review and meta-analysis. Endocrine. 2016;54(2):315–28. https://doi.org/10.1007/s12020-016-0991-9.
25. Jin Kim H, Koon Kim Y, Hoon Moon J, Young Choi J, Il CS. Thyroid core needle biopsy: patients' pain and satisfaction compared to fine needle aspiration. Endocrine. 2019;65(2):365–70. https://doi.org/10.1007/s12020-019-01973-2.
26. Ha EJ, Baek JH, Na DG, et al. The role of core needle biopsy and its impact on surgical management in patients with medullary thyroid cancer: clinical experience at 3 medical institutions. AJNR Am J Neuroradiol. 2015;36(8):1512–7. https://doi.org/10.3174/ajnr.A4317.
27. Ha EJ, Suh CH, Baek JH. Complications following ultrasound-guided core needle biopsy of thyroid nodules: a systematic review and meta-analysis. Eur Radiol. 2018;28(9):3848–60. https://doi.org/10.1007/s00330-018-5367-5.
28. Karstrup S, Balslev E, Juul N, Eskildsen PC, Baumbach L. US-guided fine needle aspiration versus coarse needle biopsy of thyroid nodules. Eur J Ultrasound. 2001;13(1):1–5. https://doi.org/10.1016/s0929-8266(01)00116-1.
29. Park KT, Ahn SH, Mo JH, et al. Role of core needle biopsy and ultrasonographic finding in management of indeterminate thyroid nodules. Head Neck. 2011;33(2):160–5. https://doi.org/10.1002/hed.21414.
30. Cibas ES, Ali SZ, NCI Thyroid FNA State of the Science Conference. The Bethesda system for reporting thyroid cytopathology. Am J Clin Pathol. 2009;132(5):658–65. https://doi.org/10.1309/AJCPPHLWMI3JV4LA.
31. Chow LS, Gharib H, Goellner JR, van Heerden JA. Nondiagnostic thyroid fine-needle aspiration cytology: management dilemmas. Thyroid. 2001;11(12):1147–51. https://doi.org/10.1089/10507250152740993.

32. Allen L, Al Afif A, Rigby MH, et al. The role of repeat fine needle aspiration in managing indeterminate thyroid nodules. J Otolaryngol Head Neck Surg. 2019;48(1):16. https://doi.org/10.1186/s40463-019-0338-7.
33. Haugen BR, Alexander EK, Bible KC, et al. 2015 American thyroid association management guidelines for adult patients with thyroid nodules and differentiated thyroid cancer: the American thyroid association guidelines task force on thyroid nodules and differentiated thyroid cancer. Thyroid. 2015;26(1):1–133. https://doi.org/10.1089/thy.2015.0020.
34. Patel KN, Angell TE, Babiarz J, et al. Performance of a genomic sequencing classifier for the preoperative diagnosis of cytologically indeterminate thyroid nodules. JAMA Surg. 2018;153(9):817–24. https://doi.org/10.1001/jamasurg.2018.1153.
35. Alexander EK, Kennedy GC, Baloch ZW, et al. Preoperative diagnosis of benign thyroid nodules with indeterminate cytology. N Engl J Med. 2012;367(8):705–15. https://doi.org/10.1056/NEJMoa1203208.
36. San Martin VT, Lawrence L, Bena J, et al. Real-world comparison of Afirma GEC and GSC for the assessment of cytologically indeterminate thyroid nodules. J Clin Endocrinol Metab. 2020;105(3):dgz099. https://doi.org/10.1210/clinem/dgz099.
37. Nikiforov YE, Baloch ZW. Clinical validation of the ThyroSeq v3 genomic classifier in thyroid nodules with indeterminate FNA cytology. Cancer Cytopathol. 2019;127(4):225–30. https://doi.org/10.1002/cncy.22112.
38. Steward DL, Carty SE, Sippel RS, et al. Performance of a multigene genomic classifier in thyroid nodules with indeterminate cytology: a prospective blinded multicenter study. JAMA Oncol. 2019;5(2):204–12. https://doi.org/10.1001/jamaoncol.2018.4616.
39. Skaugen JM, Taneja C, Liu JB, et al. Performance of a multigene genomic classifier in thyroid nodules with suspicious for malignancy cytology. Thyroid. 2022;32(12):1500–8. https://doi.org/10.1089/thy.2022.0282.

# Chapter 4
# Thyroid Pathology

**Elizabeth M. Kurian**

This chapter introduces surgical pathology of the thyroid with a focus on major malignant subtypes, clinical course, and key histologic features. The objective of this chapter is to provide a broad overview and foundation of basic thyroid tumor pathology.

## Normal Thyroid

The thyroid is an endocrine organ composed of two ovoid lobes connected by a narrow bridge of thyroid tissue called the isthmus, see Fig. 4.1a. A normal thyroid is surrounded by a thin fibrous capsule and can be oriented by gross examination. The upper poles are usually pointed, the inferior poles are rounded, the anterior surface appears nodular, and the posterior surface (which abuts the anterior trachea) is usually smooth. In 40–75% of cases, an accessory pyramidal lobe may be present as a narrow conical projection from the isthmus, often from the left side [1, 2].

Histologically, the thyroid is composed of follicular cells that form small and large circles, called follicles, with intraluminal colloid. A microfollicle is approximately 6–12 follicular cells arranged in a circular formation, whereas a macrofollicle contains a greater number of cells (see Fig. 4.1b). The thyroid is a highly vascularized organ, and on histology, there are small vessels within the stroma surrounding the follicles.

Normal follicular cells are flat to cuboidal in shape with round nuclei, scant cytoplasm, and inconspicuous nucleoli. Oncocytes (or Hurthle cells) are rare in a

E. M. Kurian (✉)
Department of Anatomic Pathology, University of Texas Southwestern Medical Center, Dallas, TX, USA
e-mail: elizabeth.kurian2@utsouthwestern.edu



A. W. Park et al. (eds.), *Thyroid Radiofrequency Ablation*,
https://doi.org/10.1007/978-3-031-65288-2_4

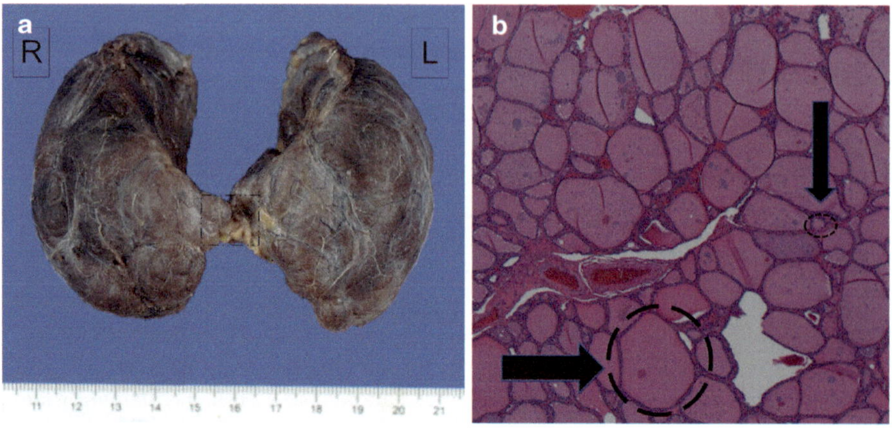


**Fig. 4.1** (**a**) Thyroid gland anterior surface: Right lobe (R), left lobe (L), and isthmus (dotted box), left panel. Photograph courtesy of Morgan Smith, PA. University of Texas Southwestern Pathology Department. (**b**, Right panel) Low magnification, H&E stain: Normal thyroid tissue composed of microfollicles (vertical arrow) and macrofollicles (horizontal arrow)

normal thyroid. Oncocytic cells exhibit abundant granular and eosinophilic cytoplasm, round to elongated nuclei with grooves, and prominent nucleoli. Oncocytes are more abundant in reactive processes (e.g., Hashimoto's thyroiditis and multinodular hyperplasia) or can be a neoplasm (adenoma or carcinoma). Another normal component of the thyroid includes calcitonin-secreting C-cells, or parafollicular cells. C-cells are scattered as indistinct single cells or groups between the follicular cells located predominantly in the upper poles of each lobe. These different cell types are the building blocks of normal thyroid tissue and subsequent pathogenesis.

## Classification of Thyroid Tumors

The World Health Organization (WHO) published a 2022 update of the classification of thyroid tumors, which divides tumors into benign, low-risk, and malignant categories (Table 4.1). For brevity, this chapter will cover only thyroid follicular nodular disease and discuss adenomas within the benign category. The former malignant 'noninvasive encapsulated follicular variant of papillary thyroid carcinoma (EFVPTC)' was renamed in 2016 as an indolent low-risk 'noninvasive follicular thyroid neoplasm with papillary-like nuclear features' (NIFTP); so we will discuss the delineation from true papillary thyroid carcinoma. Among the major malignant categories, the chapter will highlight papillary thyroid carcinoma (PTC), follicular thyroid carcinoma (FTC), high grade follicular-derived carcinoma (HGFDC), anaplastic/undifferentiated thyroid carcinoma (ATC), and medullary thyroid carcinoma (MTC). While additional thyroid malignancies originating from salivary and thymic origin exist, these are rare entities.

**Table 4.1** Modified from the WHO classification of thyroid tumors[a]

| Benign | Low risk | Malignant |
|---|---|---|
| Thyroid follicular nodular disease | Noninvasive follicular thyroid neoplasm with papillary-like nuclear features | Invasive encapsulated follicular variant papillary carcinoma |
| Follicular thyroid adenoma | Thyroid tumors of uncertain malignant potential | Papillary thyroid carcinoma |
| Follicular thyroid adenoma with papillary architecture | Hyalinizing trabecular tumor of thyroid | Follicular thyroid carcinoma |
| Oncocytic adenoma | | Oncocytic carcinoma of the thyroid |
| | | Medullary thyroid carcinoma |
| | | Follicular-derived carcinomas Non-anaplastic high grade |
| | | Anaplastic follicular cell-derived thyroid carcinoma |

[a] Note: Baloch ZW, Sobrino-Simoes M, Barletta J et al. Chapter 3: Thyroid gland. In: WHO Classification of Tumours Editorial Board. Endocrine and neuroendocrine tumours. Lyon (France): International Agency for Research on Cancer; 2022. (WHO classification of tumours series, 5th ed.; vol. 10). https://publications.iarc.fr [5]

The key features in defining a neoplasm are the presence of either capsule and/or vascular invasion. Most neoplasms are surrounded by a variably thick capsule. In slow expanding tumors, the capsule thickens gradually with deposition of collagen fibers separating the normal thyroid tissue from the growing tumor. Angioinvasion is defined as tumor invasion into an endothelial-lined vessel with attachment. The vessels must be within the tumor capsule or beyond [3, 4].

When tumor cells extend through the tumor capsule and/or are angioinvasive, the benign neoplasm is histologically considered malignant (e.g., follicular carcinoma, oncocytic carcinoma, invasive encapsulated papillary thyroid carcinoma).

A preoperative triage of nodules is often performed with fine needle aspiration (FNA). This technique uses a fine needle directed through the skin into the lesion for aspiration of cells. The cells are morphologically assessed for characteristic cytomorphologic features and in some cases can be concentrated to make a paraffin-embedded tissue block for subsequent staining or molecular assessment. It is important to recognize the limitation of cytologic specimens in triaging adenoma versus carcinoma, since neither capsule nor vascular invasion can be assessed by cytology.

## Benign Tumors

Clinically benign thyroid tumors encompass a variety of histologic entities which range from thyroiditis, diffuse or nodular hyperplasia, and benign neoplasms. Benign clonal-appearing neoplasms may be well-circumscribed (adenomatoid) or completely encapsulated (adenoma) and by definition cannot exhibit tumor capsule invasion or angioinvasion.

## *Thyroid Follicular Nodular Disease*

Per the WHO classification of thyroid tumors, follicular nodule disease (FND) is defined as a 'multifocal non-inflammatory benign proliferation of thyroid follicular cells that results in multiple clonal and non-clonal nodules with highly variable architecture' [5]. In pathology, diagnostic synonyms include adenomatous/adenomatoid nodule(s) and multinodular hyperplasia, while terms such as "colloid nodule" or "multinodular goiter" are limited to clinical terminology. Goiter is derived from the Latin word "guttur," which translates to "throat" and refers to enlargement of the thyroid gland [6].

Clinically, the mean age for diagnosis is 45–55 years old [6]. Nodular hyperplasia may be a single focus or multiple nodules that may distort and/or enlarge the gland. In 2–19% of cases, the thyroid nodule may extend through the thoracic inlet into the superior mediastinum, referred to as a retrosternal goiter [7]. The nodules may vary in clinical presentation. Some become autonomously functioning (toxic changes versus nontoxic), others may increase in size causing compressive symptoms (airway narrowing, odynophagia, dysphagia hoarseness), while many are asymptomatic. Multinodular hyperplasia may be due to iodine deficiency (endemic type) or less commonly sporadic. Risk factors for nodular hyperplasia include age, gender, smoking, environmental factors (e.g., nitrates, benzene, pesticides, etc.), insulin resistance, dietary deficiency in selenium, radiation (younger than 20 years old), and less than 10% are associated with mutations [6, 8, 9].

Gross examination shows a brown gelatinous surface composed of multiple nodules with variable amounts of fibrosis, hemorrhage, and cystic changes (Fig. 4.2a). The histologic sections show variably sized nodules composed of a mixture of microfollicles and macrofollicles containing abundant eosinophilic colloid

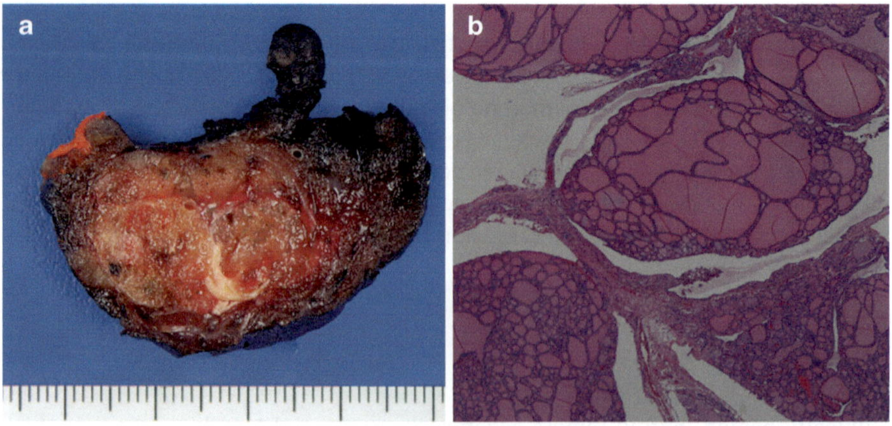


**Fig. 4.2** (**a**) Gross image, thyroid cross section with multinodular goiter. Courtesy of Morgan Smith, PA. University of Texas Southwestern Pathology Department. (**b**) Magnification 20×, H&E section. Several nodules composed of a mixture of microfollicles and macrofollicles distended with colloid, consistent with multinodular hyperplasia

(Fig. 4.2b). In long-standing lesions, there may be capsular thickening/fibrosis with calcifications, hemorrhage, and cystic changes (not pictured).

## Follicular Adenoma

Follicular adenoma is a benign encapsulated follicular-cell-derived clonal neoplasm. Histologically, the tumor is a clonal aggregate of microfollicles, macrofollicles, or a solid component that is contained within a capsule, without vascular invasion or papillary thyroid carcinoma nuclear features (Fig. 4.3a, b).

In cases where the clonal cell population is oncocytic, the tumor is called an oncocytic (Hurthle cell) adenoma (Fig. 4.4a–c).

These are usually painless, palpable lesions which may be symptomatic due to compressive symptoms. There is a high risk of follicular adenoma with exposure to radiation [10]. These may be sporadic or part of a tumor syndrome (e.g., Cowden syndrome and Carney complex) [11].

Most follicular adenomas are nonfunctional and harbor *RAS* mutations [12], but 1% may be functional [13], causing hyperthyroidism. In functional follicular adenomas, the follicles can have complex, organized papillary luminal folds which lack PTC nuclear features, and the colloid may have bubbles. According to the new WHO classification, the latter features can be diagnosed as 'follicular adenoma with papillary architecture' [12]. Functional adenomas are secondary to somatic, constitutively activating mutations in the thyrotropin receptor (TSHR) and guanine nucleotide-binding protein G subunit alpha (GNAS) [12, 14, 15]. These functional tumors may arise within multinodular hyperplasia, McCune Albright syndrome, Carney complex, and DICER syndrome [12].

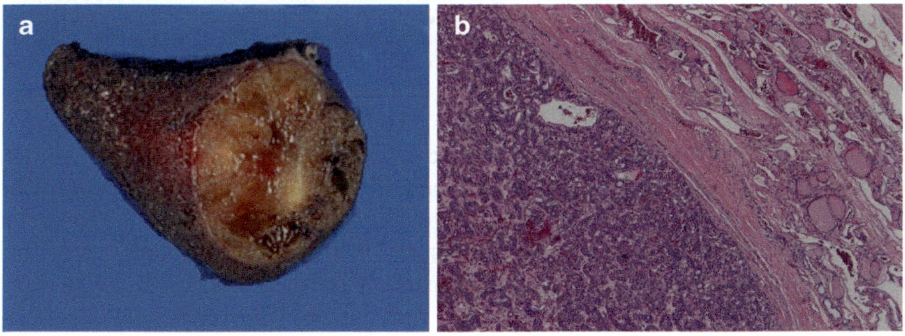


**Fig. 4.3** (**a**) Gross image: Follicular adenoma. Encapsulated yellow nodule within the thyroid tissue. (**b**) Magnification 40×, H&E stained section. There is a thick pink capsule containing a clonal proliferation of thyroid cells (lower left corner), which appear different from the histologically normal thyroid tissue (upper right corner)

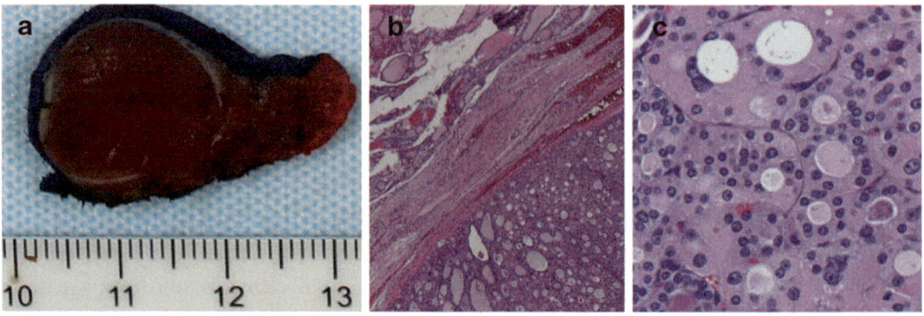


**Fig. 4.4** (**a**) Gross image: Oncocytic (Hurthle cell) adenoma. The red-mahogany lesion is surrounded by an intact circumferential white capsule (**b**) Magnification 40×, H&E stained section. The nodule has a thick, intact capsule (with intracapsular vessels) containing oncocytes (lower right). (**c**) Magnification 200×, H&E stained section. Hurthle cells (or oncocytes) are characterized by the abundant eosinophilic cytoplasm which is secondary to increased mitochondria

## Low-Risk Tumors

### *Noninvasive Follicular Thyroid Neoplasm with Papillary-Like Nuclear Features (NIFTP)*

NIFTP is the new name for the former malignant "encapsulated follicular variant of papillary thyroid carcinoma (EFVPTC)," which was formalized in the 2017 World Health Organization Classification of Tumors of Endocrine Organs [16]. It originated from malignant papillary thyroid carcinoma, which is subdivided into papillary or follicular pattern. Within the follicular pattern category, these nodules were then further subclassified as either unencapsulated/infiltrative (IFVPTC) or encapsulated (EFVPTC). These lesions were later noted to have different molecular profiles and corresponding behavior. The IFVPTC behaves like a papillary thyroid carcinoma and has BRAFV600E mutations, whereas the EFVPTC lacks the risk of recurrence or metastasis and has RAS mutations (similar to follicular neoplasms) [17].

Sonographic features are elusive and a cytologic diagnosis is limited; therefore, histologic evaluation of the excision is required for diagnosis. Evaluation of the resection specimen requires an intact, well-demarcated lesion (Fig. 4.5), a follicular pattern, and mild papillary thyroid carcinoma (PTC) nuclear features. Any true papillae formation, ≥3/10 mitotic activity, necrosis, psammoma bodies, >30% solid /trabecular/insular growth patterns, and/or invasive growth excludes the diagnosis of NIFTP [17, 18]. Considering this definition, the entire capsule and nodule must be histologically evaluated. The molecular profile is comparable to follicular adenoma, with expression of RAS mutations (NRAS, HRAS, KRAS), PAX8-PPARɣ less frequently PTEN, DICER1, THADA fusion, BRAFV601E, and EIF1AX [17, 18]. Any expression BRAFV600E is diagnostic for papillary thyroid carcinoma and excludes the diagnosis of NIFTP.

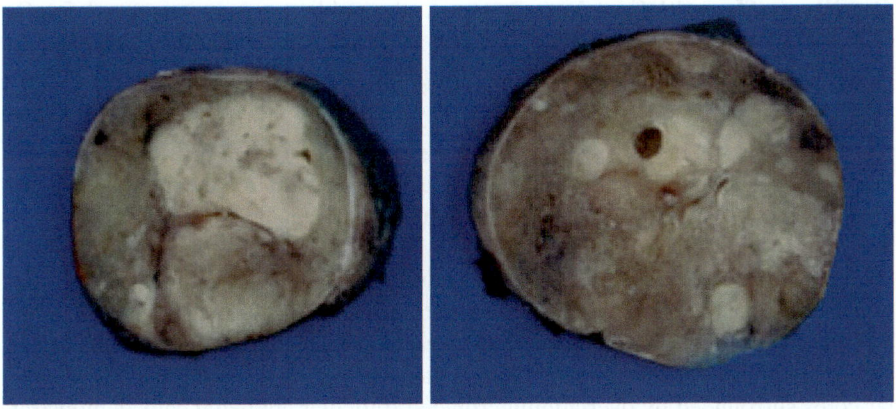

**Fig. 4.5** Gross image (serial sections) of thyroid with non-invasive follicular thyroid neoplasm with papillary-like nuclear features (NIFTP). Notice the circumferential and well-defined white capsule

## Malignant Tumors

Thyroid carcinomas can be broadly separated into follicular origin (the majority) and non-follicular origin (e.g., medullary thyroid carcinoma). The follicular cell-derived carcinomas are then categorized as well-differentiated (papillary thyroid carcinoma, follicular thyroid carcinoma, and oncocytic/Hurthle cell carcinoma), high-grade follicular-derived carcinomas (poorly differentiated thyroid carcinoma and differentiated high grade thyroid carcinomas), and anaplastic (undifferentiated) thyroid carcinoma.

Most well-differentiated thyroid carcinomas have a good prognosis. These carcinomas are generally treated with surgery and followed by radioactive iodine ablation (iodine-131) [19]. In contrast, undifferentiated thyroid carcinomas have a poor prognosis with associated rapid disease-associated mortality. High-grade follicular-derived carcinomas represent a prognosis intermediate to well-differentiated and anaplastic (undifferentiated) thyroid carcinoma [20].

In 2022, thyroid carcinoma was the 13th most common cancer and sixth most common cancer in women (threefold higher compared to men) [21]. The incidence of thyroid cancer has increased in higher-income countries [21]. The exact cause may be due to access to care, environmental exposure, and/or clinical practices [12, 21, 22]. There has been an increase in recognition of non-palpable nodules due to easy access of medical imaging since the 1980s. The increased identification resulted in increased sampling of small nodules and potential 'overdiagnosis' of lesions that would otherwise be unrecognized and insignificant. Clinical guidelines have been modified over the past 15 years to limit sampling of small lesions and the reclassification of an indolent malignancy to NIFTP [21]. The known risk factors for thyroid carcinoma include family history/genetics, radiation exposure, and iodine excess. Increased BMI is also associated with increased cancer incidence (of all types excluding medullary thyroid carcinoma) with increased mortality [23].

## *Papillary Thyroid Carcinoma*

Papillary thyroid carcinoma (PTC) accounts for 80% of all thyroid cancer [24]. The incidence is greater in women than in men. Risk factors for PTC include ionizing radiation, obesity, insulin resistance, and excess iodine [8, 24]. The relationship between obesity and thyroid cancer is unclear. In women, one theory suggests that physiologic variation in estrogen levels (due to pregnancy, abortion, menopause) may interrupt thyroid-stimulating hormone levels [22, 24]. The incidence of cancer changes for women based on age (or reproductive stages), with an increased female to male ratio at 15 years, which decreases in the early 50s [22].

Papillary thyroid carcinoma is diagnosed histologically by the combination of well-defined nuclear features and growth pattern. The classic pattern is fibrovascular cores surrounded by overlapping/crowded follicular epithelial cells demonstrating PTC nuclear features (Fig. 4.6a, b) PTC nuclear features refer to a combination of powdery chromatin, peripheral margination of chromatin, nuclear grooves, and cytoplasmic pseudonuclear inclusions. These features can be exploited for cytologic assessment through fine needle aspiration for diagnosis (Fig. 4.7a–c). When a nodule with these features measures less than 1.0 cm, it is called a papillary thyroid microcarcinoma.

There are many growth patterns, which are called subtypes (previously termed variants) [12]. The subtypes include: classic or conventional, encapsulated, follicular, diffuse sclerosis, tall cell, columnar cell, hobnail, PTC with fibromatosis/fascitis-like stroma, solid/trabecular, oncocytic, spindle cell, clear cell, and Warthin-like variant [25]. Conventional PTC is indolent with an associated good prognosis. In contrast, tall cell, columnar, and hobnail subtypes are aggressive with a poor prognosis [25].

- Briefly, the tall cell subtype must compose at least 30% of the overall tumor; and is defined by tumor cells with eosinophilic cytoplasm extending three times taller than the width of the nucleus. These cells have the nuclear features of PTC, but usually have an increased number of cells with pseudonuclear inclusions [25, 26]. Tall cell PTC is associated with increased recurrence and decreased survival compared to classic PTC [27]. Tall cell PTC commonly has *BRAFV600E* and telomer-

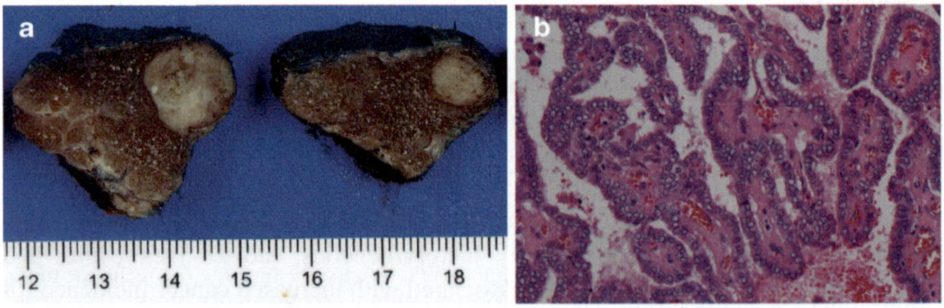


**Fig. 4.6** (**a**) Gross image of papillary thyroid carcinoma: Cross section of a thyroid with a white nodule. (**b**) Magnification 100×, H&E stained section. Papillary thyroid carcinoma composed of fibrovascular cores lined by epithelial cells with distinctive nuclear features

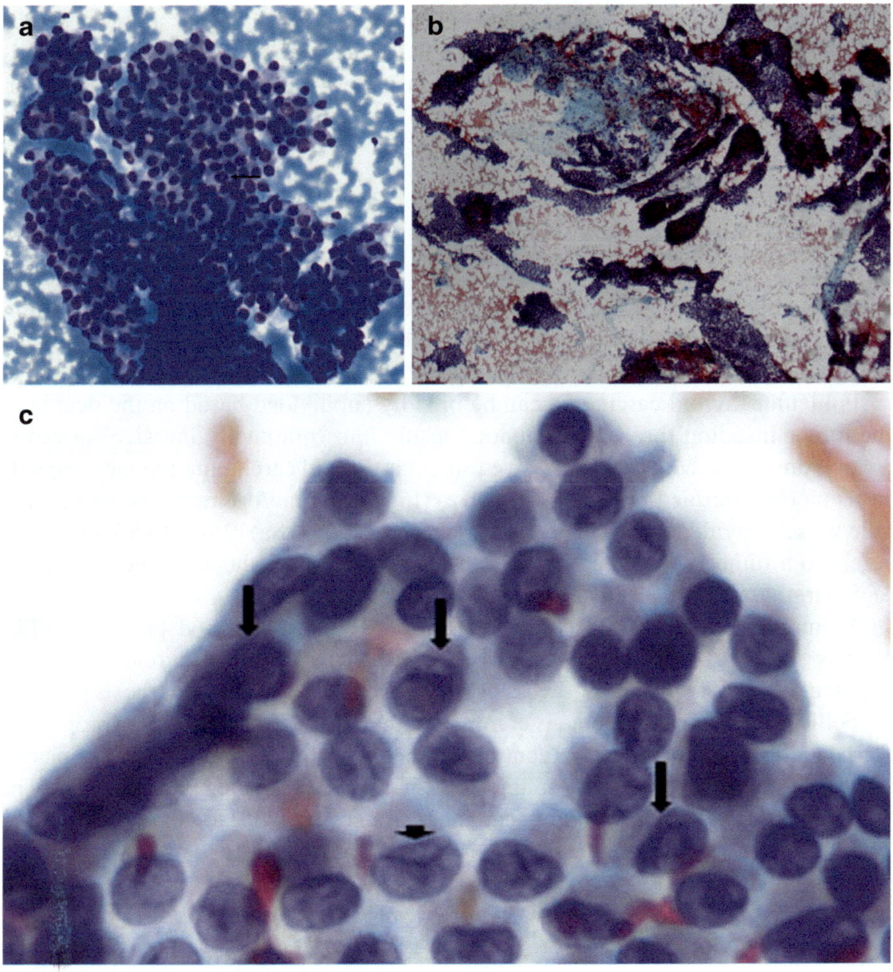


**Fig. 4.7** Fine needle aspiration cytology of PTC. (**a**) Upper left corner, Magnification 200×, Diff-Quick stain. Air-dried smear with a sheet of papillary thyroid carcinoma. (**b**) Upper right corner, Magnification 200×, Pap stain. Alcohol fixed papillary-configured groups of PTC. (**c**) Center bottom, Magnification 600×, Pap stain. Long arrows indicate pseudonuclear inclusions and short arrow shows nuclear grooves. All malignant cells demonstrate fine chromatin with nuclear crowding

ase reverse transcriptase (*TERT*) promoter mutations [28]. When present in PTC, the combined effect of *BRAFV600E* and *TERT* mutations lead to a worse prognosis due to distant metastasis and is usually refractory to radioactive iodine [12, 25].

- Columnar cell variant is composed of columnar cells with supranuclear cytoplasmic vacuoles and basal hyperchromatic nuclei with rare pseudonuclear inclusions, obscure nuclear grooves, and chromatin features [28]. In some cases, columnar PTC may mimic metastatic colon or endometrial carcinoma [28].
- Hobnail PTC is rare and characterized by a mix of papillary and micropapillary structures with discohesive cells with eosinophilic cytoplasm, apical nuclei with prominent nucleoli imparting a 'hobnail' appearance [26–28].

PTC can be multifocal in up to 20–30% of cases [29]. Multiple subtypes can be seen in one tumor, or multiple tumors, of the same patient. Lymphatic invasion is common with metastasis to regional lymph nodes. Vascular invasion can occur, although it is uncommon [12].

## *Follicular Thyroid Carcinoma*

Follicular carcinoma (FTC) is an encapsulated clonal neoplasm with tumor extension through or beyond the tumor capsule and/or vascular invasion. It is the second most common thyroid malignancy.

Follicular thyroid carcinoma can be broadly subdivided based on the degree of the tumor invading through the tumor capsule into 'minimally invasive' or rarely 'widely invasive.' Minimally invasive follicular thyroid carcinoma can have capsule invasion only (termed minimally invasive) (Fig. 4.8b) and/or invade the tumor capsule vessels (termed encapsulated angioinvasive) (Fig. 4.8a) [25]. 'Widely invasive' refers to a tumor with broad tumor capsule invasion into the surrounding thyroid and extrathyroidal tissue, usually multinodular.

Minimally invasive FTC is considered low risk with a good prognosis [12]. Widely invasive or any encapsulated angioinvasive follicular thyroid carcinoma (particularly involvement of ≥4 vessels) is associated with a poor prognosis [12, 25].

Follicular thyroid carcinoma is common in the fourth decade and has a propensity for hematogenous metastasis in contrast to PTC, which is predominantly lymphatic. Metastases are most frequently to the bones in the axial skeleton and lung [30]. The recurrence rate of follicular thyroid carcinoma ranges from 3% to 40% [30].

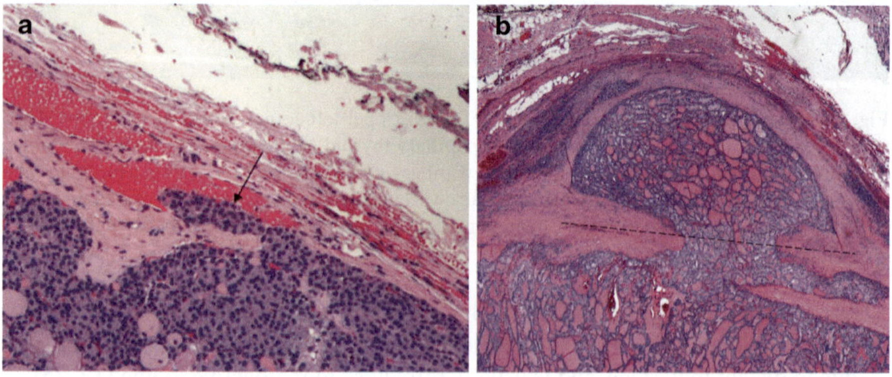


**Fig. 4.8** (**a**) Magnification 100×, H&E stained section. (Left) Encapsulated angioinvasive follicular carcinoma. Tumor cells are infiltrating into the adjacent vessel (see arrow). (**b**) (Right) Magnification 100×, H&E stained section. Encapsulated neoplasm with tumor extending through the capsule (dotted line) forming a 'mushroom' configuration

## *Oncocytic (Hurthle Cell) Carcinoma*

For the histologic diagnosis, oncocytes cells must compose at least 75% of the tumor population accompanied by either vascular invasion or invasion through the tumor capsule. Additionally, these cells should lack PTC nuclear features and not display high-grade characteristics [12]. Similar to FTC, oncocytic carcinoma is subclassified as minimally invasive, widely invasive, and/or angioinvasive. Cytologically, the tumor may show solid, trabecular, or papillary patterns. The cells are elongated with prominent nucleoli, nuclear grooves, and an eosinophilic cytoplasm.

The oncocytic phenotype is postulated to be due to a mitochondrial DNA mutation that impairs an electron transport chain and oxidative phosphorylation system, which results in the accumulation of tumor cell mitochondria [31].

Oncocytic carcinomas are only 5% of differentiated thyroid carcinomas in the US [12]. Oncocytic carcinomas tend to occur more commonly in men, at a late age, and are associated with a worse prognosis dependent on the extent of vascular invasion [12, 25]. The recurrence rate is 14–44% [30]. Metastasis is hematogenous; however, oncocytic carcinomas may have tumor deposits within the neck veins mimicking lymph node metastasis [12]. Oncocytic carcinomas are less likely to concentrate iodine-131 [19, 25].

## *Medullary Thyroid Carcinoma*

Medullary thyroid carcinoma (MTC) originates from the malignant proliferation of thyroid parafollicular C-cells and accounts for 2–4% of all thyroid carcinomas [32]. As a neuroendocrine tumor, it can produce calcitonin, carcinoembryonic antigen, procalcitonin, calcitonin gene-related peptide, and chromogranin A, which can be clinically tested in the serum [33, 34]. Some of these markers can be exploited histologically to stain the tumor cells (e.g., calcitonin and mCEA) for pathologic confirmation of diagnosis.

Medullary thyroid carcinoma can be sporadic (75% of cases [33, 35]) or hereditary. Sporadic MTC is generally diagnosed in the fifth or sixth decade, and locally aggressive with a disease-specific mortality rate ranging from 13.5% to 38% [33]. On presentation, 50% will have metastatic cervical lymphadenopathy and 5–10% will have distant metastasis to the lung or bones [19].

In hereditary *RET* proto-oncogene germline mutations, the multiple endocrine neoplasia type 2 (MEN2) has two subtypes. MEN2A presents in the third or fourth decade with MTC usually preceeding symptomatic presentation of pheochromocytoma and hyperparathyroidism [19, 25]. MEN2B is associated with infant onset MTC, pheochromocytoma, multiple mucosal neuromas, gastrointestinal ganglioneuromatosis, and megacolon [33]. These familial MTCs have early lymph node metastasis and local invasion [33] with a poor prognosis.

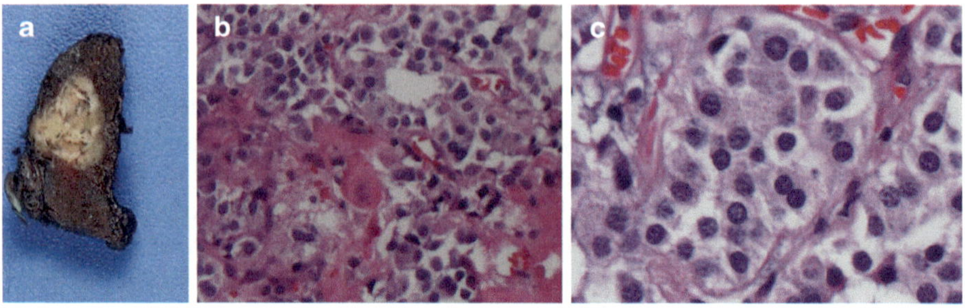

**Fig. 4.9** (**a**) Gross image medullary thyroid carcinoma: Cross section of a thyroid with a white nodule within the background of normal brown thyroid tissue (left panel). (**b**) (middle panel) Magnification 100×, H&E-stained sections. MTC with pink amyloid. (**c**) (right panel) Magnification 600×, H&E-stained sections. MTC cells with neuroendocrine salt-and-pepper nuclear chromatin in a nested pattern

Histologically, medullary thyroid carcinoma have nuclei have salt-and-pepper chromatin, which is a morphologic indication of neuroendocrine differentiation (Fig. 4.9a–c). The cytoplasm may be variable (spindled, epithelioid, plasmacytoid etc). These tumors can also have amyloid deposition, which is characterized by dense eosinophilic material derived from polypeptides of calcitonin [33]. In hereditary MTC, there may be a background of C-cell hyperplasia.

MTC is graded based on mitotic count, tumor necrosis, and Ki67 labeling index [12]. High-grade MTC has at least one of the following features: tumor necrosis, mitotic count of ≥5/2 mm$^2$, or Ki67 ≥5% [12]. This distinction is important, as high-grade medullary thyroid carcinomas are associated with a lower disease-specific survival and recurrence-free survival rates [26].

Pathologic indicators of poor outcome include large size, tumor necrosis, high mitotic index, and nodal disease [32]. In sporadic forms, somatic *RET* mutations are the most common. The second most common alteration is *RAS* mutation. These two mutations are mutually exclusive. Genomic alterations in *CDKN2C*, the *RB* tumor suppressor pathway, and mTOR pathway are associated with a worse prognosis [32].

## *High-Grade Follicular Cell-Derived Non-anaplastic Thyroid Carcinoma*

This category encompasses poorly differentiated thyroid carcinoma (PDTC) and differentiated high-grade thyroid carcinomas (DHGTC) and represents only 1–3% of all thyroid carcinomas [12, 20, 36]. The two entities are carcinomas of follicular cell origin with necrosis, high mitotic count, and without anaplastic features. The prognoses are intermediate between well-differentiated and anaplastic thyroid carcinoma [20].

Adults in the fifth and sixth decade are affected, and sometimes teenagers (frequently associated with *DICER1* mutations) [20, 37], with a higher male-to-female ratio [36]. Presentation with metastases can be seen in 20–50% of patients [20] and distant metastasis can occur up to 20 years later [37].

PDTC and DHGTC are usually highlighted by FDG-PET positive imaging and generally lack radioactive iodide uptake. Histologically, these tend to be large tumors with gross vascular invasion, extrathyroidal extension, perineural invasion, and often with lymph node metastases [12, 20].

Poorly differentiated thyroid carcinomas lose architectural and cytologic differentiation, but without anaplastic morphology. The Turin consensus criteria for diagnosis includes the: (1) presence of a solid/trabecular/insular pattern of growth, (2) absence of nuclear features of PTC, and (3) either convoluted nuclei, mitotic count $\geq$3 per 2 mm$^2$ or tumor necrosis [31, 38].

In contrast, DHGTC maintains the architecture and cytologic features of a well-differentiated thyroid carcinoma, but has necrosis and $\geq$5 mitosis per 2 mm$^2$ [31, 38].

## *Anaplastic Thyroid Carcinoma*

Anaplastic thyroid carcinoma is an undifferentiated carcinoma that may arise de novo, from, and/or coincide with a well-differentiated carcinoma; and accounts for only 1% of thyroid carcinomas [39, 40]. This is a rare high-grade malignancy with a poor clinical prognosis, usually leading to disease-specific mortality within 3–6 months [31, 41]. The survival rates may be improving with increased use of personalized molecular-based therapy (such as *BRAF*-directed targeted therapy) [41].

Older patients, 65–70 years old, present with enlarging neck mass, dyspnea, dysphagia, Horner syndrome, stroke, vocal cord paralysis, or hoarseness due to extensive local invasion. There is often local lymph node involvement and distant metastases [19, 40]. Common sites of metastasis include the lung/pleura, some in the bone, and fewer reports of metastasis to the brain, skin, liver, kidney, pancreas, heart, and adrenal glands [19, 40].

On the tissue section, the tumors cells may be sarcomatoid (spindled), epithelioid (squamoid), or pleomorphic and overall show a high mitotic activity, atypical mitosis, angiolymphatic invasion, necrosis, and frequent extrathyroidal extension [25, 39] (Fig. 4.10a, b). Pathologic diagnosis may be challenging as the tumor becomes undifferentiated. ATC frequently loses immunohistochemical staining markers (e.g., TTF-1 which is usually positive in thyroid). In some cases, these may arise from a well-differentiated carcinoma such as a PTC or FTC, in which case the tumor may express respective molecular *BRAFV600E* or *RAS* mutations. As the tumor becomes undifferentiated, it is thought that more mutations are acquired which conclude with *TERT* promoter mutations and the hallmark of ATC, inactivating *p53* mutations [31] (Table 4.2).

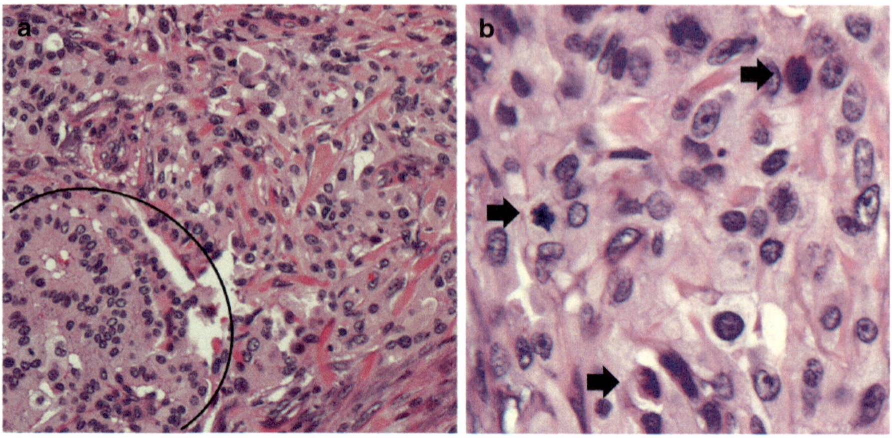


**Fig. 4.10** (**a**) Magnification 20×, H&E stain. Anaplastic thyroid carcinoma (upper right corner) arising within a papillary thyroid carcinoma (lower left corner). (**b**) Magnification 60×, H&E stain. Higher magnification of an anaplastic thyroid carcinoma composed of pleomorphic cells with spindled morphology and numerous mitotic figures

**Table 4.2** Common molecular associations with thyroid tumors

| | |
|---|---|
| **Benign** | |
| Follicular adenoma | *N-RAS, K-RAS* |
| **Intermediate-risk** | |
| Encapsulated FVPTC and NIFTP | *RAS* (30–52%); *PAX8-PPARɣ (0–38%)*; *THADA* fusion (0–22%) [31] |
| Hyalinizing trabecular tumors | *PAX8/GLIS* fusions [25] |
| **Malignant** | |
| Follicular thyroid carcinoma | *RAS (49%); PAX8-PPARɣ (30–58%); TERT* promoter mutation 17% [31] |
| Oncocytic (Hurthle cell) carcinoma | Recurrent mitochondrial mutations, whole chromosomal losses [31] and duplications of chromosomes 5 and 7; EZH1 mutation (small subset of tumors) [25] |
| Medullary thyroid carcinoma | |
| – Sporadic | *RET* mutation (50%) [25] or *RAS* (up to 20%) [31] mutually exclusive |
| – Familial | Germline *RET* mutation |
| Papillary thyroid carcinoma | *BRAFV600E (62%)* and *TERT (9%)* [31] |
| – Tall cell subtype | *BRAFV600E* and *TERT* |
| – Columnar cell subtypes | |
| – Hobnail subtypes | *BRAFV600E* (50–94%) [25]; *TP53* mutation |
| – Solid subtypes | *RET/PTC3* rearrangements (radiation associated); *RET/PTC1/3* and *ETV6/NTRK3* fusions (sporadic) [25] |
| – Diffuse sclerosing subtypes | *RET/PTC* rearrangement (initiation event); rarely BRAFV600E [25] |

(continued)

**Table 4.2** (continued)

| | |
|---|---|
| Poorly differentiated thyroid carcinoma | *TERT* promoter (40%), BRAFV600E (33%), RAS (45%), TP53 mutation (10%) [25, 31] |
| Anaplastic thyroid carcinoma | *TERT* promoter (30–75%), *PT53 (40–80%), BRAF (10–50%), RAS (10–50%), PIK3CA (5–25%), E1F1AX (5–15%), PTEN* mutations (10–25%) [25, 39]<br>(*TERT* promoter with *BRAF/RAS* mutations associated with worse outcome) [25] |

Note: BRAFV600E and RAS mutations are mutually exclusive
*NRAS:* neuroblastoma *RAS*; *THADA:* thyroid-associated adenoma; *PAX*8:* paired box gene 8; *PPARɣ:* peroxisome proliferator-activated receptor gamma; *RET:* rearranged during transfection, *BRAF:* v-raf murine sarcoma viral oncogene homolog B1: *TERT:* telomerase reverse transcriptase; *E1F1AX:* eukaryotic translation initiation factor 1A X-linked; *PTEN:* phosphatase and tensin homolog deleted on chromosome ten

## Concluding Remarks

As our understanding of molecular pathogenesis of thyroidal malignancies grows, the categorization of these tumors will improve. Use of molecular-based testing on fine needle aspirations is already widely used to triage patients based on the probability of malignancy. Continued progress to correlate imaging, molecular tests and histology will hopefully improve our accurate detection, limit over-testing, and expand patient-specific molecular targeted therapy.

## References


1. Braun EM, et al. The pyramidal lobe: clinical anatomy and its importance in thyroid surgery. Surg Radiol Anat. 2007;29(1):21–7.
2. Gurleyik E, et al. Pyramidal lobe of the thyroid gland: surgical anatomy in patients undergoing total thyroidectomy. Anat Res Int. 2015;2015:384148.
3. Nishino M, Jacob J. Invasion in thyroid cancer: controversies and best practices. Semin Diagn Pathol. 2020;37(5):219–27.
4. Jalaly JB, Baloch ZW. Hurthle-cell neoplasms of the thyroid: an algorithmic approach to pathologic diagnosis in light of molecular advances. Semin Diagn Pathol. 2020;37(5):234–42.
5. Barletta J, Mete O, Erickson L, et al. Thyroid tumors-benign tumours. WHO classification of tumours editorial board. Endocrine and neuroendocrine tumours. Baloch Z. and Sobrino-Simoes M, Editor. 2022, International Agency for Research on Cancer: Lyon.
6. Unlu MT, et al. Non-toxic multinodular goiter: from etiopathogenesis to treatment. Sisli Etfal Hastan Tip Bul. 2022;56(1):21–40.
7. Unlu MT, et al. Substernal goiter: from definitions to treatment. Sisli Etfal Hastan Tip Bul. 2022;56(2):167–76.
8. Yildirim Simsir I, Cetinkalp S, Kabalak T. Review of factors contributing to nodular goiter and thyroid carcinoma. Med Princ Pract. 2020;29(1):1–5.
9. Zheng R, et al. A contemporary analysis of goiters undergoing surgery in the United States. Am J Surg. 2020;220(2):341–8.
10. Ron E, Brenner A. Non-malignant thyroid diseases after a wide range of radiation exposures. Radiat Res. 2010;174(6):877–88.

11. Barletta J, Erickson L. et. al. Thyroid—follicular thyroid adenoma. In: Baloch ZW, editor. WHO classification of endocrine and neuroendocrine tumors online. International Agency for Research on Cancer; 2022.
12. Baloch ZW, et al. Overview of the 2022 WHO classification of thyroid neoplasms. Endocr Pathol. 2022;33(1):27–63.
13. McHenry CR, Phitayakorn R. Follicular adenoma and carcinoma of the thyroid gland. Oncologist. 2011;16(5):585–93.
14. Nishihara E, et al. Prevalence of TSH receptor and Gsalpha mutations in 45 autonomously functioning thyroid nodules in Japan. Endocr J. 2009;56(6):791–8.
15. Stephenson A, et al. Sensitive sequencing analysis suggests thyrotropin receptor and guanine nucleotide-binding protein G subunit alpha as sole driver mutations in hot thyroid nodules. Thyroid. 2020;30(10):1482–9.
16. Lloyd RV, Klöppel G, Rosai J. WHO classification of tumors of endocrine organs, vol. 4. Lyons: International Agency for Research on Cancer; 2017.
17. Chu YH, Sadow PM. Noninvasive follicular thyroid neoplasm with papillary-like nuclear features (NIFTP): diagnostic updates and molecular advances. Semin Diagn Pathol. 2020;37(5):213–8.
18. Xu B, Ghossein RA. Noninvasive follicular thyroid neoplasm with papillary-like nuclear features (NIFTP): an update. Head Neck Pathol. 2020;14(2):303–10.
19. Haddad RI, et al. Thyroid carcinoma, version 2.2022, NCCN clinical practice guidelines in oncology. J Natl Compr Cancer Netw. 2022;20(8):925–51.
20. Cracolici V, Cipriani NA. High-grade non-anaplastic thyroid carcinomas of follicular cell origin: a review of poorly differentiated and high-grade differentiated carcinomas. Endocr Pathol. 2023;34(1):34–47.
21. Kitahara CM, Schneider AB. Epidemiology of thyroid cancer. Cancer Epidemiol Biomarkers Prev. 2022;31(7):1284–97.
22. Suteau V, et al. Sex bias in differentiated thyroid cancer. Int J Mol Sci. 2021;22(23):12992.
23. Kitahara CM, et al. Impact of overweight and obesity on US papillary thyroid cancer incidence trends (1995-2015). J Natl Cancer Inst. 2020;112(8):810–7.
24. Hu MJ, et al. Body mass index and weight gain after middle adulthood are associated with risk of papillary thyroid cancer: a case-control study. Cancer Epidemiol. 2021;75:102039.
25. Bai Y, Kakudo K, Jung CK. Updates in the pathologic classification of thyroid neoplasms: a review of the world health organization classification. Endocrinol Metab (Seoul). 2020;35(4):696–715.
26. Jung CK, et al. New insights into classification and risk stratification of encapsulated thyroid tumors with a predominantly papillary architecture. J Pathol Transl Med. 2020;54(3):197–203.
27. Nath MC, Erickson LA. Aggressive variants of papillary thyroid carcinoma: hobnail, tall cell, columnar, and solid. Adv Anat Pathol. 2018;25(3):172–9.
28. Hernandez-Prera JC. The evolving concept of aggressive histological variants of differentiated thyroid cancer. Semin Diagn Pathol. 2020;37(5):228–33.
29. Harries V, et al. Should multifocality be an indication for completion thyroidectomy in papillary thyroid carcinoma? Surgery. 2020;167(1):10–7.
30. Grani G, et al. Follicular thyroid cancer and Hurthle cell carcinoma: challenges in diagnosis, treatment, and clinical management. Lancet Diabetes Endocrinol. 2018;6(6):500–14.
31. Haroon Al Rasheed MR, Xu B. Molecular alterations in thyroid carcinoma. Surg Pathol Clin. 2019;12(4):921–30.
32. Jaber T, Dadu R, Hu MI. Medullary thyroid carcinoma. Curr Opin Endocrinol Diabetes Obes. 2021;28(5):540–6.
33. Gambardella C, et al. Calcitonin negative medullary thyroid carcinoma: a challenging diagnosis or a medical dilemma? BMC Endocr Disord. 2019;19(Suppl 1):45.
34. Murphy DC, Johnson SJ, Aspinall S. Calcitonin-negative medullary thyroid carcinoma: the 'triple-negative' phenotype. Ann R Coll Surg Engl. 2020;102(3):e63–6.

35. Ceolin L, et al. Medullary thyroid carcinoma beyond surgery: advances, challenges, and perspectives. Endocr Relat Cancer. 2019;26(9):R499–518.
36. Xu B, Ghossein R. Poorly differentiated thyroid carcinoma. Semin Diagn Pathol. 2020;37(5):243–7.
37. Xu B, et al. Primary high-grade non-anaplastic thyroid carcinoma: a retrospective study of 364 cases. Histopathology. 2022;80(2):322–37.
38. Tallini G, Lam AK et al. Thyroid—high-grade follicular cell-derived non-anaplastic thyroid carcinoma. In: Ghossein R, Baloch A, and Erickson L, editors. WHO classification of endocrine and neuroendocrine tumours online. International Agency for Research on Cancer; 2022.
39. Erickson L, Nose V et al. Thyroid tumors—anaplastic thyroid carcinoma. In: Ghossein RA, editor. WHO classification of tumours online. International Agency for Research on Cancer; 2022.
40. Yang J, Barletta JA. Anaplastic thyroid carcinoma. Semin Diagn Pathol. 2020;37(5):248–56.
41. Maniakas A, et al. Evaluation of overall survival in patients with anaplastic thyroid carcinoma, 2000-2019. JAMA Oncol. 2020;6(9):1397–404.

# Chapter 5
# Surgical Management of Thyroid Neoplasms

**Ana Kashfia Islam and Emily Steen**

## Introduction

Surgery has historically been the mainstay of treatment of symptomatic benign or malignant lesions of the thyroid gland. Though radiofrequency ablation (RFA) has become a relevant option for many patients in the current era, surgery remains the standard of care in a number of clinical situations. In this chapter, we will first review the operative steps to thyroidectomy, including relevant anatomy. Next, we will review the indications for and rationale behind surgery for benign and malignant thyroid lesions. Finally, we will provide a brief review of surgery post-RFA.

## Thyroidectomy—Basic Operative Steps

The patient is first consented and apprised of the risks and benefits of surgery. General anesthesia is established with limited neuromuscular blockade (options include the use of short-acting succinylcholine or reversal), and the patient is intubated with an electromyographic endotracheal tube. A neck ultrasound may be performed to aid in incision and surgical planning. The patient is then prepped and draped with neck extended. A collar incision is made along the Langer lines and extended through the subcutaneous tissues and platysma, raising superior and inferior flaps. The strap muscles are then separated in the midline to reveal the thyroid

A. K. Islam (✉)
Department of Surgery, Division of Endocrine Surgery, University of Texas Southwestern Medical Center, Dallas, TX, USA
e-mail: Ana.Islam@UTSouthwestern.edu

E. Steen
Kelsey-Seybold, Fort Bend Medical and Diagnostic Center, Sugar Land, TX, USA


A. W. Park et al. (eds.), *Thyroid Radiofrequency Ablation*,
https://doi.org/10.1007/978-3-031-65288-2_5

gland. The middle thyroid vein is ligated on one side and the thyroid lobe is reflected anteriorly and medially for better identification of the recurrent laryngeal nerve in the tracheoesophageal groove, either visually, with a nerve monitoring device, or both. The cricopharyngeal space is then entered and the external branch of the superior laryngeal nerve is identified and preserved, if possible. With this space well defined, the superior pole vessels of the thyroid are then ligated to better mobilize the thyroid. Superior pole mobilization helps to identify the distal insertion of the recurrent laryngeal nerve. This nerve is then traced along its length to allow safe mobilization of the lateral and inferior attachments of the thyroid. Ultimately, the gland is elevated off the trachea with isolation and division of the ligament of Berry. If a thyroid lobectomy is being performed, the thyroid isthmus is divided at this point. If a total thyroidectomy is being performed, the aforementioned steps then proceed on the contralateral side. All steps are performed taking care to identify and preserve the parathyroid glands.

## Indications for and Extent of Thyroid Surgery in Benign Thyroid Disease

High-quality imaging and reliable biopsy is the most important first step in planning care for patients with thyroid pathology. The addition of molecular testing to biopsy results has further enhanced our ability to stratify and counsel patients about next steps. For any lack of biopsy concordance (e.g., concerning family history or lesion appearance on imaging), a fine needle aspiration (FNA) should be repeated.

For patients with benign thyroid disease, the choice of medical, surgical, or procedural management is often based on patient preference or individualized risk–benefit assessment. However, there are certain patient populations in whom surgery is preferred or strongly recommended, detailed in the next sections.

The choice of total thyroidectomy versus thyroid lobectomy is dependent upon the disease process and its extent in the gland. As a rule, if benign disease is confined to a single gland, lobectomy with or without isthmusectomy is appropriate. In contrast, patients with Graves' disease or large, multinodular goiter with bilateral lobe involvement should undergo total thyroidectomy.

Total thyroidectomy does necessitate lifelong thyroid hormone supplementation after surgery. Thyroid lobectomy generally does not result in permanent hypothyroidism; rates vary from 5% to 60% depending on the center, though most studies quote approximately 20–30% [1]. Need for hormone replacement can be difficult to predict preoperatively, with some studies showing preoperative thyroid stimulating hormone (TSH) >2–2.5 to be a risk factor for requiring hormone replacement [2]. Other risks to total thyroidectomy include parathyroid injury with possible permanent or temporary need for calcium supplementation; and recurrent laryngeal nerve injury, which can be temporary or permanent and can lead to weak, hoarse voice, and aspiration. Bilateral recurrent nerve injury results in respiratory distress as both vocal cords are paretic and can require tracheostomy. These risks are somewhat less prominent after lobectomy as the contralateral nerve and parathyroids can be considered untouched and intact.

## *Large, Compressive, or Substernal Goiter*

Surgery should be considered the first-line choice in patients with obstructive symptoms (dysphagia, dyspnea, globus or choking sensation, neck tethering) and large benign nodules (whether toxic or nontoxic), as it provides rapid symptomatic relief without the need for retreatment, as may be the case in RFA [3]. In addition, patients with substernal goiters should undergo surgical evaluation, as this lesion would likely be inaccessible to RFA.

## *Diffuse Thyroid Disease or Lack of Single-Lesion Disease*

Patients with diffuse thyroid disease (e.g., Graves' disease) generally do not have the desired response to a targeted therapy like RFA as there is not a frank lesion to point-ablate. Similarly, RFA may be less effective in toxic multinodular goiter as there may be multiple or bilateral toxic nodules to address, or the toxic nodule may be difficult to effectively access given the bulky, heterogeneous surrounds. There is active research into the use of RFA in relapsed or persistent Graves' after nonsurgical treatment, but more study is needed before high-quality recommendations can be made [4].

## *Concern for Malignancy or High-Risk Lesion*

With any concern for malignancy (atypia on cytology or suspicious findings on molecular testing) in the same or contralateral thyroid lobe, surgery can be considered both diagnostic and curative. Postoperative pathology and suspicious intraoperative findings (e.g., lymphadenopathy leading to node sampling or more extensive dissection) have been frequently shown to demonstrate the presence of occult malignancies undetectable on preoperative imaging [5]. This once again deeply underscores the importance of imaging and biopsy with molecular testing in patients with thyroid complaints.

## *Concurrent Hyperparathyroidism*

Hyperparathyroidism, whether single or multigland disease, is best managed with surgery, if possible. For that reason, one should attempt to address any synchronous thyroid pathology in the same operation as the parathyroid intervention in an attempt to avoid reoperation in the neck.

## *Need for Rapid Correction of Hyperthyroidism*

Patients in a thyroid storm or at high risk for devolution into a thyroid storm are not appropriate for RFA; in fact, surgery, too, should be delayed until the patient is resuscitated and their symptoms medically managed. Once this hyperdynamicity is treated, however, surgery has been shown to have superior and more rapid symptomatic results than RFA for toxic nodules [5, 6].

## *Proximity of Lesions to Critical Structures*

There are some patients whose lesions, while otherwise potentially RFA candidates, are too close to critical structures in the neck to perform the procedure safely. These structures include the recurrent laryngeal nerve, the vagus nerve, the vocal cords, the esophagus, and major blood vessels like the carotid artery and internal jugular vein. The posteromedial aspect of the thyroid near the tracheoesophageal groove is a particularly challenging location for RFA. A distance of 1 cm or more between the lesion and the critical structure is preferred in order to reduce the risk of thermal injury; some technicians will inject the region of interest with saline to create more distance between the two and for heat diffusion, but if this distance cannot be safely obtained, surgery should be recommended [7].

## *Extenuating Clinical Circumstances*

For some patients, the risk–benefit ratio inclines toward surgery because the actual RFA circuit presents a risk. Notable examples include pregnant patients, patients with significant history of cardiac arrhythmia, and those with cardiac pacemakers in place. In addition, if adequate peripheral or central access for electrode placement cannot be obtained or if the patient is unable to tolerate conscious sedation, they will be unlikely to undergo successful lesion ablation.

## Indications for Thyroid Surgery for Malignancy

### *Primary Thyroid Cancer*

The treatment—and, hopefully, cure—for patients with biopsy-proven, well-differentiated thyroid cancer is surgical removal of that cancer. Patients with very poor performance status or life-threatening cardiopulmonary disease that disallows general anesthesia may consider RFA a first-line management option, but certainly any patient who is amenable to surgery and can physiologically tolerate it should be offered one. Those with very large tumors, aggressive histologic or molecular features, bilateral lesions, or clinically/radiographically positive nodal disease should also undergo upfront surgery, even if staging has demonstrated distant metastatic disease [8]. RFA is not an option for medullary thyroid cancer at this time, nor is it recommended for follicular neoplasms, as one must demonstrate no capsular invasion to rule out carcinoma [9].

A notable exception is the case of papillary thyroid microcarcinoma (micro-PTC or -PTMC), defined as well-differentiated, strictly intrathyroidal PTC, which is $\leq$10 mm and without aggressive features or concern for local or distant invasion (classified as T1aN0M0). PTMC is very common, markedly indolent, and in general has an excellent clinical outcome whether it is surveilled or resected (generally via thyroid lobectomy) [10, 11]. For this reason, upfront RFA has been offered as a low morbidity alternative to these options, with proponents noting oncologic noninferiority to surgery with improved cosmesis and quality of life with fewer complications in small observational studies [7, 12, 13]. However, one does note that patients undergoing RFA for cancer treatment do not subsequently undergo postprocedural FT4 suppression with levothyroxine, which may have an adverse effect on tumor recurrence. There is also a concern that RFA may promote neoplastic cell progression or transformation, as has been shown in hepatocellular carcinoma—whether this is due to heat trauma or preexisting tumor biology is difficult to untangle [14, 15]. For these reasons, at the current time, there is no definitive role for RFA in healthy patients with thyroid cancer outside of the very low-risk condition of PTMC.

### *Recurrent Thyroid Cancer*

Current recommendations for recurrent thyroid cancer include reoperation with consideration for RAI and T4 suppression, with chemotherapy and radiation as adjuncts [16]. Reoperative neck surgery for thyroid cancer, however, is challenging and not without risk, as tissue plane/anatomic distortion from prior procedures increases the possibility of inadvertent injury and thus morbidity. At its most extreme, scar tissue can even disallow the identification of the recurrent disease in the surgical field, even if it has been detected on screening imaging. One can understand how critically important intraoperative nerve monitoring is in these circumstances, as well as high-quality imaging.

In light of these challenges, RFA has been used for early locoregional recurrence of PTC in the thyroid bed, as well as in recurrent or persistent nodal disease, with emerging data showing safe and reasonable outcomes in the right clinical scenarios [14, 17–21]. This may prove to be a particularly useful adjunct in patients with inaccessible or morbid tumor recurrence sites and, clearly, in those who are unfit for surgery or those that refuse further surgery. Overall, a personalized and multidisciplinary approach is the primary injunction for these patients.

## Consideration for Neck Surgery After RFA

Operative intervention after radiofrequency ablation of thyroid nodules is uncommon, and most reports of this are anecdotal. Most scenarios generally involve an RFA-treated Thyroid Imaging Reporting and Data Systems (TIRADS)-2 or 3 lesion with benign features that then recurs, was incompletely treated, or did not involute completely after ablation [22, 23]. Rapid regrowth, repeat biopsy, or clinically positive nodes then upstage the initial lesion and surgery is performed, however delayed. These anecdotal studies tend to agree that RFA does not seem to create excess scar tissue or make subsequent surgery more challenging—some assert that it may even make surgery easier in shrinking the initial nodule—though as above, nerve monitoring capability should be assured in these cases.

These studies also tend to internally agree that preoperative RFA does not seem to affect histology, though with the limited amount of data available it is probably more accurate to say that this is unknown [3, 24].

## References

1. Lee DY, Seok J, Jeong WJ, Ahn SH. Prediction of thyroid hormone supplementation after thyroid lobectomy. J Surg Res. 2015;193(1):273–8.
2. Cao Z, Liu R, Wu M, et al. Risk factors for thyroid hormone replacement therapy after hemithyroidectomy and development of a predictive nomogram. Endocrine. 2022;76:85–94.
3. Tufano RP, Pace-Asciak P, Russell JO, Suárez C, Randolph GW, López F, Shaha AR, Mäkitie A, Rodrigo JP, Kowalski LP, Zafereo M, Angelos P, Ferlito A. Update of radiofrequency ablation for treating benign and malignant thyroid nodules. Fut Front Endocrinol. 2021;12:698689.
4. Fung MHM, Lang BHH. Efficacy of single-session radiofrequency ablation (RFA) in rendering euthyroidism for persistent/relapsed graves' disease, a pilot study. Eur Radiol. 2023;33(9):6534–44.
5. Bernardi S, Dobrinja C, Fabris B, Bazzocchi G, Sabato N, Ulcigrai V, Giacca M, Barro E, De Manzini N, Stacul F. Radiofrequency ablation compared to surgery for the treatment of benign thyroid nodules. Int J Endocrinol. 2014;2014:934595.
6. Kim HJ, Cho SJ, Baek JH, Suh CH. Efficacy and safety of thermal ablation for autonomously functioning thyroid nodules: a systematic review and meta-analysis. Eur Radiol. 2021;31(2):605–15.

7. Zhang M, Tufano RP, Russell JO, Zhang Y, Zhang Y, Qiao Z, Luo Y. Ultrasound-guided radiofrequency ablation versus surgery for low-risk papillary thyroid microcarcinoma: results of over 5 years' follow-up. Thyroid. 2020;30(3):408–17.
8. Nixon IJ, Whitcher MM, Palmer FL, Tuttle RM, Shaha AR, Shah JP, Patel SG, Ganly I. The impact of distant metastases at presentation on prognosis in patients with differentiated carcinoma of the thyroid gland. Thyroid. 2012;22(9):884–9.
9. Biamonte E, Solbiati L, Ierace T, Colombo P, Lavezzi E, Mazziotti G, et al. Medullary thyroid carcinoma treated with percutaneous ultrasound-guided radiofrequency ablation. Endocrine. 2019;65(3):515–9.
10. Hay ID. Management of patients with low-risk papillary thyroid carcinoma. Endocr Pract. 2007;13(5):521–33.
11. Sugitani I, Toda K, Yamada K, Yamamoto N, Ikenaga M, Fujimoto Y. Three distinctly different kinds of papillary thyroid microcarcinoma should be recognized: our treatment strategies and outcomes. World J Surg. 2010;34(6):1222–31.
12. Teng D, Sui G, Liu C, Wang Y, Xia Y, Wang H. Long-term efficacy of ultrasound-guided low power microwave ablation for the treatment of primary papillary thyroid microcarcinoma: a 3-year follow-up study. J Cancer Res Clin Oncol. 2018;144(4):771–9.
13. Choi Y, Jung SL. Efficacy and safety of thermal ablation techniques for the treatment of primary papillary thyroid microcarcinoma: a systematic review and meta-analysis. Thyroid. 2020;30(5):720–31.
14. Park KW, Shin JH, Han BK, Ko EY, Chung JH. Inoperable symptomatic recurrent thyroid cancers: preliminary result of radiofrequency ablation. Ann Surg Oncol. 2011;18:2564–8.
15. von Breitenbuch P, Köhl G, Guba M, Geissler E, Jauch KW, Steinbauer M. Thermoablation of colorectal liver metastases promotes proliferation of residual intrahepatic neoplastic cells. Surgery. 2005;138(5):882–7.
16. Haugen BR, Alexander EK, Bible KC, Doherty GM, Mandel SJ, Nikiforov YE, et al. American thyroid association management guidelines for adult patients with thyroid nodules and differentiated thyroid cancer: the American thyroid association guidelines task force on thyroid nodules and differentiated thyroid cancer. Thyroid. 2016;26:1–133.
17. Dupuy DE, Monchik JM, Decrea C, Pisharodi L. Radiofrequency ablation of regional recurrence from well-differentiated thyroid malignancy. Surgery. 2001;130(6):971–7.
18. Lee SJ, Jung SL, Kim BS, Ahn KJ, Choi HS, Lim DJ, Kim MH, Bae JS, Kim MS, Jung CK, Chong SM. Radiofrequency ablation to treat loco-regional recurrence of well-differentiated thyroid carcinoma. Korean J Radiol. 2014;15(6):817–26.
19. Chung SR, Baek JH, Choi YJ, Lee JH. Longer-term outcomes of radiofrequency ablation for locally recurrent papillary thyroid cancer. Eur Radiol. 2019;Sep 29(9):4897–903.
20. Suh CH, Baek JH, Lee JH, Choi YJ, Lee JH. Efficacy and safety of radiofrequency ablation and ethanol ablation for treating locally recurrent thyroid cancer: a systematic review and meta-analysis. Thyroid. 2016;26(3):420–8.
21. Ding Z, Chen J, Chen Z, Zeng X, Zheng P, Wang X, Cui X, Sang L. Efficacy and safety of thermal ablation for treating lymph node metastasis from papillary thyroid carcinoma: a systematic review and meta-analysis. Front Oncol. 2022;12:738299.
22. Ma B, Wei W, Xu W, Wang Y, Guan H, Fan J, Zhao Z, Wen D, Yang S, Wang Y, Chang B, Ji Q. Surgical confirmation of incomplete treatment for primary papillary thyroid carcinoma by percutaneous thermal ablation: a retrospective case review and literature review. Thyroid. 2018;28(9):1134–42.
23. Monzani F, Caraccio N, Basolo F, Iacconi P, LiVolsi V, Miccoli P. Surgical and pathological changes after percutaneous ethanol injection therapy of thyroid nodules. Thyroid. 2000;10(12):1087–92.
24. Dobrinja C, Bernardi S, Fabris B, Eramo R, Makovac P, Bazzocchi G, Piscopello L, Barro E, Manzini N, Bonazza D, Pinamonti M, Zanconati F, Stacul F. Surgical and pathological changes after radiofrequency ablation of thyroid nodules. Int J Endocrinol. 2015;2015:1.

# Chapter 6
# Nuclear Medicine in the Diagnosis and Management of Thyroid Nodules and Cancer

**Nghi C. Nguyen, Satyanarayana Chekuri, and Orhan K. Öz**

Thyroid scintigraphy and radioactive iodine (RAI) therapy play a significant role in diagnosing and managing benign and malignant thyroid conditions. The history of nuclear medicine as a medical field began with the challenges presented by thyroid conditions. It was known before the era of radioactive iodine that the thyroid gland concentrates iodine. Dr. Plummer introduced the use of Lugol's iodine to block the release of thyroid hormone in preparation of thyrotoxic patients for surgery at the Mayo Clinic in the early 1920s reducing the post-surgical mortality from 11% to less than 1% [1, 2]. Then in the late 1930s it became possible to produce RAI with cyclotrons which were then used to study the iodine metabolism of the thyroid [3]. Thyroid scintigraphy is functional imaging and remains a valuable tool for guiding clinical decisions in patients with thyroid diseases despite the increasing utilization of US for diagnostic imaging and US-guided fine-needle aspiration (FNA) of thyroid nodules. RAI treatment is the oldest theragnostic procedure for patients with hyperthyroidism and well-differentiated thyroid cancer (DTC). Radioactive I-131 has been used to treat benign thyroid diseases for over 60 years. The therapeutic application of I-131 relies on the emission of β-particles to cause DNA damage to

N. C. Nguyen (✉) · S. Chekuri · O. K. Öz
Department of Radiology, Division of Nuclear Medicine, University of Texas Southwestern Medical Center, Dallas, TX, USA
e-mail: Nghi.Nguyen@UTSouthwestern.edu; Satyanarayana.Chekuri@UTSouthwestern.edu; Orhan.Oz@UTSouthwestern.edu


A. W. Park et al. (eds.), *Thyroid Radiofrequency Ablation*,
https://doi.org/10.1007/978-3-031-65288-2_6

cells that take up the radionuclide. The aim is to resolve the hyperthyroidism and to achieve euthyroidism or hypothyroidism. For the treatment of DTC the use of RAI therapy has seen a recent shift from a one-size-fits-all approach to an individualized risk-based approach.

## Radiopharmaceuticals

Thyroid scintigraphy is commonly used to determine the cause of a patient's hyperthyroidism (Graves' disease, toxic adenoma, toxic multinodular goiter, subacute, silent, and postpartum thyroiditis). The potential of iodine isotopes for diagnostic imaging has been established for more than 80 years [1]. Two radioiodine isotopes are used due to their suitable half-lives and radioactive emissions for diagnostic and therapeutic applications: Iodine-123 (I-123) and iodine-131 (I-131) [4, 5].

### *Iodine-123*

The sodium iodide symporter (NIS) is responsible for the RAI uptake within the thyroid tissue. This transmembrane protein transports iodide against an electrochemical gradient via a sodium-dependent active transport mechanism by which two sodium ions are transported along with one iodide ion [6]. Thyroid-stimulating hormone (TSH) is the primary regulator of NIS expression in thyroid glands through activation of the thyrotropin receptor [7]. I-123 has a half-life of 13.2 h and a principal gamma emission of 159 keV. The radiation dose to the patient is low, and the emission is well suited for gamma camera detection, which makes it ideal for diagnostic imaging of the thyroid. The benefit of I-123 is that it allows for both radioiodine uptake (RAIU) measurement and imaging of the thyroid gland. A dose of 7.4–14.8 MBq (0.2–0.4 mCi) is administered orally, followed by RAIU measurement at 4–6 h and 24 h, and thyroid scintigraphy during either time. Some imaging facilities obtain imaging and RAIU at 24 h only. Unfortunately, I-123 is less widely available for clinical use and is more expensive than alternatives such as I-131 or Technetium-99 m (Tc-99 m) pertechnetate [4, 8].

### *Iodine-131*

I-131 has a half-life of 8.04 days. It emits β-particles with an average energy of 192 keV, and gamma radiation with a dominant gamma ray of 364 keV [4, 5]. This higher energy photon requires thicker collimation to reduce scatter radiation and thicker scintillation crystals to achieve efficient detection. The main advantage of I-131 for diagnostic imaging is its inexpensive cost. In addition, its half-life is long enough so the radiopharmacy can have sufficient inventory to accommodate short-notice orders. The disadvantage is β emission, which does not provide imaging information and contributes significantly to patient radiation exposure. In clinical practice, an I-131 dose as little as 0.15 MBq (4 μCi) may be used for RAIU measurement at 4–6 h and 24 h, in combination with Tc-99 m pertechnetate for thyroid imaging [8]. The most common application of I-131 in clinical practice is whole-body scanning in suspected thyroid cancer recurrence.

## *Tc-99 M Pertechnetate*

Tc-99 m pertechnetate is an alternative to I-123 and I-131 for diagnostic imaging of thyroid disorders. It is a widely available and inexpensive radiopharmaceutical with a half-life of 6 h and a monoenergetic gamma emission of 140 keV. It has the advantage of low-cost, high-quality images, and lower radiation dose compared with I-131 and I-123 [8]. Tc-99 m pertechnetate mimics iodide uptake by follicular thyroid cells; however, it is not organified, and the radiotracer starts to wash out after 30 min of intravenous (IV) administration [4, 8]. Typically, 74–111 MBq (2–3 mCi) of Tc-99 m pertechnetate is administered IV, followed by uptake and scan of the thyroid 15–20 min later. In the United States, radioiodine is mainly used because of the concern of potential misdiagnosis with Tc-99 m pertechnetate. Notably, some malignant thyroid nodules may show decreased uptake (cold) on radioiodine scans but increased uptake (hot) on Tc-99 m pertechnetate scans [9–13]. But in many other countries, including Germany, Tc-99 m pertechnetate is preferred because of easy accessibility and low cost. Moreover, most patients have a good correlation between Tc-99 m pertechnetate and radioiodine scans. In a comparative study of 360 subjects with solitary or multinodular thyroid, discrepancies between I-123 and Tc-99 m pertechnetate were found in 8% of cases, twice as often in multinodular thyroid than single nodules. Cytologic examination, however, did not show a correlation between pathology and type of scan discrepancy. There were 12 thyroid carcinomas (4%), but none were associated with scan discrepancies. The readers preferred I-123 over Tc-99 m pertechnetate in terms of image quality because it showed slightly better contrast and sharper thyroid contours. Still, the slightly better image quality with I-123 was deemed not of diagnostic significance [14]. Besides I-123, the use of Tc-99 m pertechnetate for thyroid uptake and scan is endorsed by major professional societies [8, 15, 16]. However, the normal references are different between Tc-99 m pertechnetate and RAI (I-123 or I-131).

## *F-18 Fluorodeoxyglucose (FDG) PET*

F-18 is a positron emitter with a half-life of 110 min. The annihilation event with an electron results in the production of a pair photons with energy of 511 keV. FDG is utilized for diagnostic imaging in conjunction with positron-emission tomography (PET) [4, 5]. As a glucose analog, an FDG PET scan can identify glucose hypermetabolism in many types of neoplasm, including hyperfunctioning benign thyroid nodules and thyroid cancer. The uptake is mediated by an upregulation of transmembrane glucose transporter proteins and hexokinases, which results in the trapping of FDG within the cells which facilitates diagnostic imaging [17]. The role of FDG PET in evaluating thyroid nodules for potential primary malignancy or differentiating between benign and malignant thyroid nodules is less well-defined. However, it may be helpful in select cases [18–20]. According to the 2015 American Thyroid Association (ATA) guidelines, it is not routinely recommended to evaluate thyroid nodules with indeterminate cytology [19]. On the other hand, FDG PET is increasingly important for diagnostic imaging of thyroid cancer [17, 19]. In this regard, FDG is taken up by thyroid cancer lesions that do not concentrate radioiodine. The usefulness of FDG is thus in follow-up of patients with elevated serum thyroglobulin (Tg) and negative radioiodine scans [19].

### *Other Radiotracers*

I-123 or I-131 meta-iodobenzyl guanidine (MIBG), indium-111 (In-111) pentetreotide (Octreoscan®), Ga-68 or Cu-64 DOTA-somatostatin analogs, and Tc-99 m sestamibi are potential radiopharmaceuticals for staging and restaging medullary carcinomas. They have relatively low sensitivity but may be considered when other imaging approaches have proven unsuccessful [21–25].

## Methodology for Thyroid Uptake and Scan

Thyroid scintigraphy provides a functional evaluation of the thyroid and complements the clinical examination. The nuclear medicine physician or radiologist should be familiar with the clinical setting in which the exam is being requested, including presenting complaints, relevant clinical history, and prior thyroid function test results. For example, a positive family history will increase the pre-test probability for multinodular goiter and Graves' disease. A complaint of neck pain predisposes to subacute thyroiditis [26]. A history of radiation exposure in a patient with a thyroidal mass increases the probability of thyroid malignancy. A history of Hashimoto's thyroiditis is frequently associated with thyroid lymphoma and other forms of thyroid cancer. Patients with a history of Hashimoto's thyroiditis and rapidly enlarging neck mass deserve expedited work-up. The thyroid gland should be palpated for size and nodules during the clinic visit. Available thyroid US should be reviewed to allow for an optimal interpretation of the thyroid scintigraphy.

Patients may self-medicate with vitamins and other iodine substances and be exposed to iodine-containing medicines and agents. Therefore, they should be withdrawn before the thyroid uptake and scan (RAI or Tc-99 m pertechnetate), Table 6.1 [8].

**Table 6.1** List of factors influencing thyroid uptake and scan and their respective withdrawal times

| **Iodinated substances** | **Duration of withdrawal** |
|---|---|
| Amiodarone | 3–6 months |
| Oil-based iodinated contrast media | 3–6 months |
| IV contrast media | 1–2 months |
| Iodine solutions (Lugol's or SSKI) | 4–6 weeks |
| Iodine-containing medicines and preparations | 4 weeks |
| Iodine-containing antiseptics | 4 weeks |
| Kelp | 4 weeks |
| **Thyroid medications** | |
| Levothyroxine (LT4) | 4 weeks |
| Liothyronine (LT3) | 2 weeks |
| Perchlorate | 1 week |
| Methimazole, carbimazole, propylthiouracil | 3–7 days |

Thyroid imaging is best performed on a gamma camera fitted with a pinhole collimator to achieve the highest possible spatial resolution. The disadvantages of pinhole gamma cameras are image distortion and low sensitivity. There is also the risk of image distortion, especially when the neck/thyroid is off-centered [5]. Imaging with a standard gamma camera with a parallel collimator is also an option.

The assessment of thyroid uptake (in %) can be obtained using a non-imaging gamma probe or a gamma camera; however, a gamma probe is preferred because of its higher sensitivity for count statistics. The uptake measurements are obtained at 4–6 h and 24 h after oral radiopharmaceutical administration of I-123 or I-131. Some imaging facilities acquire only the 24 h uptake measurement to save time and for patient convenience. There are various approaches to thyroid RAIU calculation. The following method involves the measurements of thyroid counts, mid-thigh counts, and phantom counts. The formula for the RAUI calculation is as follows [8]:

$$\text{RAIU} = \frac{\text{Patient neck counts} - \text{Thigh counts}}{\text{Phantom counts} - \text{Background counts}} \times 100$$

Normal references for RAIU vary in different geographic regions depending on dietary iodine intake and need to be determined locally by each nuclear medicine laboratory. In most subjects, the thyroid RAI uptake increases over time and reaches a plateau at approximately 24 h. A normal RAIU is between 6–18% at 4-h and 10–35% at 24-h [27]. A 24-h RAIU greater than 25–35%, dependent on local laboratory normal references and regional dietary iodine intake, is compatible with hyperfunctioning thyroid in the setting of clinical hyperthyroidism [8, 27]. In North America and iodine-sufficient regions, a 24-h RAIU >25% may be considered abnormal [8] though it is not clear how many centers are using this.

As with RAIU, Tc-99 m pertechnetate uptake depends on iodine uptake and patient-related factors, such as thyroid size and degree of hyperthyroidism. A local normal reference should be established, which may range from 0.2 to 4.0% at 15–20 min [8, 28]. The uptake patterns commonly seen in specific disease entities

**Table 6.2** The various medical conditions and clinical situations are outlined for the differential diagnosis of hyperthyroidism

| | Elevated thyroid uptake | Reduced thyroid uptake |
|---|---|---|
| Common | Graves' disease<br>Toxic multinodular goiter<br>Toxic adenoma | Primary hypothyroidism<br>Destructive thyroiditis<br>Subacute thyroiditis<br>Silent thyroiditis<br>Postpartum thyroiditis<br>Amiodarone |
| Uncommon | Marine-Lenhart syndrome<br>TSH-secreting pituitary adenoma<br>Hashimoto thyroiditis<br>Lithium carbonate therapy<br>Trophoblastic tumors | Exogenous iodine (factitious)<br>Iodine-induced (CT contrast)<br>Previous I-131 treatment<br>External neck radiation |

are highlighted in Table 6.2 [26]. In addition, thyroid RAIU is also used for calculating the therapeutic radioiodine dose to treat hyperthyroidism and euthyroid multinodular goiter.

## Indications for Thyroid Uptake and Scintigraphy

The most common indications for thyroid scintigraphy in adults are as follows [8]:

- Abnormal thyroid function consistent with overt or subclinical hyperthyroidism.
- Differentiation of hypoechogenic thyroids according to low and high thyroid uptake.
- Suspected focal masses or diffuse thyroid disease.
- Evaluation of thyroid nodules detected on clinical examination and/or other imaging examinations.
- Evaluation of multinodular goiter to identify suspicious hypofunctional (cold) areas that require further evaluation with FNA-biopsy.
- Evaluation of multinodular goiter for hyperfunctioning (hot) thyroid nodules prior to radioiodine ablation.
- Evaluation of thyroid nodules with indeterminate FNA-biopsy results to identify autonomously functioning thyroid nodules.
- Evaluation of thyroid nodules with indeterminate FNA-biopsy results to identify those at higher risk of malignancy.

## Scintigraphy of Thyroid Nodules

Goiters are endemic in regions characterized by iodine deficiency and sporadically in all populations. Several factors can stimulate the growth of new follicles contributing to the development of thyroid nodules and goiter. The process is usually slow, requiring years or decades. In addition, the nodules may display heterogeneous growth patterns, which can give rise to the presence of hot, warm, and cold nodules coexisting in the same goiter. Secondary events, such as central necrosis in a rapidly growing nodule or loss of functional capacity over time, may also contribute to the transition from functioning adenomas to hypofunctioning (cold) nodules [26, 29–32].

Thyroid scintigraphy helps determine the functional status of a nodule and thus guide clinical management. On scintigrams, thyroid nodules may appear as hypofunctioning compared to surrounding thyroid tissue ("cold"), hyperfunctioning with suppression of the normal thyroid tissue ("hot"), increased uptake compared with surrounding thyroid tissue, which shows preserved uptake ("warm"), or indeterminate (not visible relative to the surrounding thyroid tissue). Most thyroid nodules (>90%) are either indeterminate or cold on thyroid scintigram. Most cold nodules are benign, for example, colloid nodules, degenerating nodules with necrosis or hemorrhage, and simple cysts. The incidence of cancer in a cold thyroid nodule is between 5% and 15% [15, 33–36]. The risk of malignancy is lower in a multinodular goiter (approximately 5%) and higher in a gland with a single nodule (approximately 15%). Cold nodules may be considered for FNA; however, the predictive value for thyroid primary is low [8, 15, 37]. It is recommended that cold thyroid nodules be further evaluated with thyroid US and managed according to sonographic features according to TI-RADS classification [8, 19, 37].

Ultrasound is the imaging modality of choice to characterize goiter and thyroid nodules. Its use permits a confident determination of whether the gland is diffusely enlarged or contains one or more nodules. Thyroid RAIU and scan have added value in determining the functional status of goiters and thyroid nodules (Fig. 6.1). Nuclear medicine studies, however, no longer play the major role in goiter or thyroid nodule evaluation as they did before the availability of high-resolution

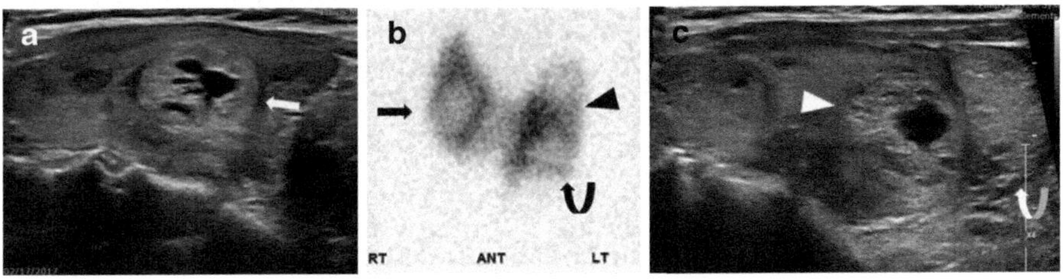


**Fig. 6.1** (**a**) US, right thyroid, longitudinal; (**b**) Thyroid scintigram, anterior image; (**c**) US, left thyroid, longitudinal. A 59-year-old female with a history of subclinical hyperthyroidism—TSH <0.1 mIU/mL, and normal free triiodothyronine (fT3) and free thyroxin (fT4)—underwent thyroid RAIU and scan after oral administration of 0.22 mCi I-123. The 24-h RAIU was 43%. A cold right thyroid nodule (**b**, arrow) corresponded to a 1.5 × 1.7 cm echogenic nodule with a cystic component on US (**a**, arrow). Subsequent total thyroidectomy showed papillary thyroid carcinoma, tall cell variant (0.9 cm), right side, in the background of nodular hyperplasia, with one right level VI node (0/1) negative for tumor (pT1aN0Mx). There was no lymphovascular invasion or extrathyroidal extension; resection margins negative for tumor. Scintigram also showed a cold nodule in the left inferior lobe (**b**, curved arrow) and adjacent hyperfunctioning nodule (**b**, arrowhead), corresponding to echogenic nodules, partially with a cystic component at US (**c**, curved arrow and arrowhead). They were hyperplastic nodules at surgery

**Table 6.3** Recommendation for thyroid scintigraphy based on thyroid nodule size an TSH levels. American Thyroid Association (ATA), 2015 [19]; American Association of Endocrine Surgeons (AAES), 2020 [43]; American Association of Clinical Endocrinologists (AACE), Associazione Medici Endocrinologi (AME), and European Thyroid Association (ETA) [15]

| ATA 2015 | AAES 2020 | AACE, AME, ETA 2016 |
|---|---|---|
| Nodules ≥10 mm | Nodules—No specific size provided | Nodules—No specific size provided |
| TSH—Subnormal | TSH—Subnormal | TSH—Subnormal or low-normal in iodine-deficient regions |

US. High-resolution US provides an accurate assessment of thyroid nodules using the standardized thyroid imaging and data reporting system (TI-RADS) [8, 37]. However, the TI-RADS criteria do not address the functional status of thyroid nodules, as a scintigraphically hyperfunctioning (i.e., "hot") thyroid nodule has a 96–99% negative predictive value for malignancy [8, 20, 38]. Thyroid scintigraphy is the only exam demonstrating the presence of autonomously functioning thyroid nodules (AFTNs). While AFTNs rarely harbor malignancy, indeterminate cytology (e.g., Bethesda classes III and IV) is frequently reported in these cases. In a study of 615 AFTNs (size, 23.2 ± 10 mm), analyzed prospectively with TI-RADS based on US features, more than 80% of AFTNs were classified as TI-RADS ≥4 (i.e., moderately suspicious, requiring FNA for nodules ≥1.5 cm), only 16% of AFTNs were classified as TI-RADS ≤3, and <0.1% of AFTNs were classified as TI-RADS 5. Therefore, the integration of thyroid scintigraphy into TI-RADS model helps prevent unnecessary FNA biopsies for nodules that demonstrate autonomy [39]. Current professional guidelines recommend diagnostic work-up of thyroid nodules to avoid unnecessary invasive procedures, including surgical resection [8]. The recommendations for using thyroid scintigraphy vary according to TSH levels, as the detectability of AFTNs is affected by the TSH levels and regional dietary iodine sufficiency [19, 40–42]. The indications for thyroid scintigraphy to assess thyroid nodules issued by the various medical societies are listed in Table 6.3 [8].

## *Toxic Adenoma*

AFTNs are benign adenomas that operate independently of the thyroid-pituitary feedback control mechanisms. Thyrotoxicosis may occur when the hormone production from such a nodule exceeds the body's hormone requirements. The initial work-up begins with a thyroid function test. The etiology of subclinical or clinical hyperthyroidism should be determined in the presence of a suppressed TSH. Diagnostic imaging with US and thyroid scintigraphy complements each other when the diagnosis is not apparent based on the clinical presentation and

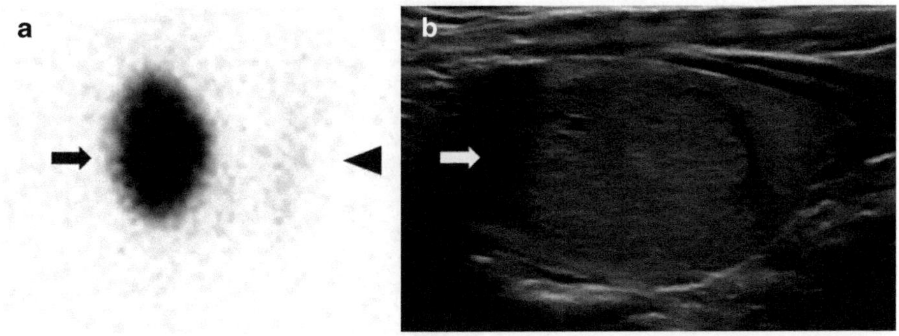

**Fig. 6.2** (**a**) Scintigram, anterior; (**b**) thyroid US, right lobe. A 50-year-old female with heart palpitations was found to have subacute thyroiditis (TSH 0.03, normal fT3 and fT4). RAIU and scan showed a hot nodule in the right lobe (**a**, arrow), suppressed uptake in the left thyroid lobe (**a**, arrowhead), and 24-h uptake of 37% (normal 15–35%). On US, the right thyroid nodule was slightly echogenic relative to the surrounding thyroid tissue (**b**, arrow)

initial laboratory assessment. In particular, when there is a clinical suspicion of AFTN or multinodular goiter, thyroid scintigraphy with RAIU should be performed to confirm the presence of hot nodules (Fig. 6.2) [8, 16, 44]

## *Toxic Multinodular Goiter (TMNG)*

TMNG, also known as Plummer's disease, is primarily a disease of older people who may have a longstanding nodular goiter. The clinical onset is often insidious and, in the elderly age group, may be superimposed on other chronic pathologies [16, 45]. Congestive heart failure, atrial fibrillation or other arrhythmias, weight loss, or an apparent psychiatric illness may be seen. The appearance of an unexpected illness and the presence of a goiter require the exclusion of thyrotoxicosis.

The thyroid scan in a TMNG reveals an irregular distribution of "hot" and "cold" regions, and the RAIU may be normal or only mildly elevated (Fig. 6.3) [8, 30, 46]. In patients with iodine-induced thyrotoxicosis, the uptake may be low initially but will increase on serial uptakes once the source of iodine is eliminated. With sufficient RAI uptake, subsequent RAI therapy provides an effective treatment mode for TMNG [16, 47, 48].

A variant of Graves' disease with coexisting nodular goiter may be seen in 1–4% of patients, which is referred to as Marine-Lenhart syndrome [49–51]. Scintigraphy findings of high RAI uptake and one or several cold thyroid nodules are characteristics. During the course of medical treatment, these nodules may become hot on the scintigram.

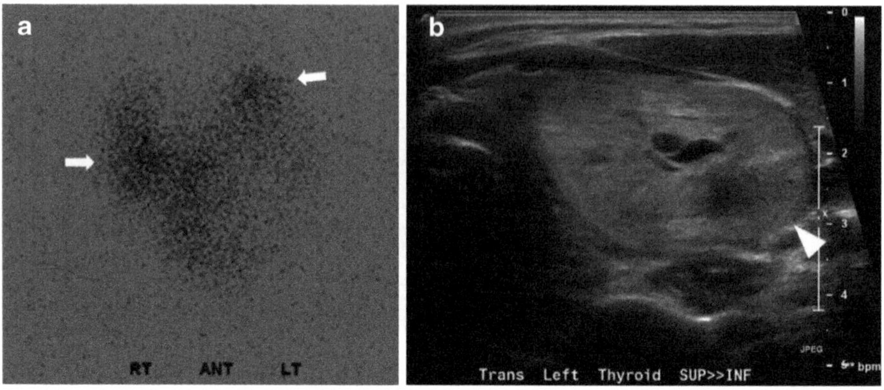


**Fig. 6.3** (**a**) Thyroid scintigram, anterior image; (**b**) Thyroid US, longitudinal. A 54-year-old female with subclinical hyperthyroidism (TSH 0.11 mIU/mL, normal fT3 and fT4) underwent thyroid RAIU and scan after oral administration of 0.23 mCi of I-123. There was a cold nodule occupying much of the left thyroid lobe (**a**, arrowhead) and foci with subtly increased uptake elsewhere in both thyroid lobes (**a**, arrow). The left thyroid nodule measured 4 × 6 cm with central areas of cystic degeneration (**b**). FNA of the lesion showed benign follicular cells

## Radioiodine Therapy for Benign Thyroid Disorders

For diagnostic imaging, a small radioiodine dose of I-123, I-131, or Tc-99 m pertechnetate is administered to patients, so the gamma emission from the thyroid tissue can be imaged with a gamma camera. In therapy applications, however, the intent is to deposit high energy in a target tissue to destroy those cells. Thus, the administration of radionuclides with a short path length in tissues and high energy is used to damage cell deoxyribonucleic acid (DNA). Therefore, RAI treatment with I-131, a β-emitter with path lengths of an average of 0.8 mm in soft tissue, is ideal for various thyroid conditions with hyperthyroidism, even though it is associated with gamma emissions, representing a challenge in radiation protection [52].

Radioactive iodines have been used to treat benign thyroid diseases for over 80 years, most commonly in a capsule or oral solution [3]. The therapeutic application of I-131 relies on the emission of β-particles to cause damage to thyroid gland tissue. I-131 has a physical half-life of 8.1 days and a β-emission with an average energy of 192 keV and a tissue range of 0.8 mm [4, 5]. RAI is rapidly taken up in the thyroid tissue and induces extensive tissue inflammation and damage, resulting in a size reduction of the hyperfunctioning thyroid nodules and a reduction in hormone synthesis within 6–18 weeks [53–56]. Some thyroid conditions associated with hyperthyroidism can be treated with RAI, including Graves' disease, AFTN, and TMNG. The aim is to resolve hyperthyroidism and to achieve euthyroidism or hypothyroidism, substituted by daily thyroid hormone. RAI may also benefit patients with subclinical hyperthyroidism, particularly those at risk for cardiac or systemic complications. However, RAI is not indicated for treating euthyroid nodules and goiters [16, 57, 58].

## *Indication for RAI Therapy*

Although antithyroid medication can alleviate symptoms and ameliorate hyperthyroidism, definitive treatment is more commonly accomplished with surgery or RAI therapy. The recommendations for either RAI therapy versus surgery are not always straightforward. Each treatment option has its advantages and disadvantages, which should be discussed with patients, and ideally in a multidisciplinary effort. RAI therapy is often considered in patients with AFTNs (<4 cm) and TMNG (<80 g) when there is increased nonnodular uptake on thyroid RAIU and scan. Particularly, RAI therapy is beneficial to patients with advanced age, existing comorbidities, increased surgical risk (e.g., pulmonary hypertension, congestive heart failure, COPD), previously treated with thyroid surgery or neck radiation, and lack of access to experienced thyroid surgeons [16, 43].

On the other hand, surgery should be strongly favored in patients with symptomatic compressive or large goiters (>80 g tissue); large thyroid nodules, particularly those with cold (hypofunctioning) appearance on thyroid scintigram; relatively low uptake on thyroid RAIU and scan; nodules with increased risk of thyroid malignancy (e.g., suspicious or indeterminate thyroid cytology); coexisting hyperparathyroidism requiring surgery; and young women planning a pregnancy in less than 6 months [16, 43]. Treatment decisions should be made in consultation with an endocrinologist, a surgeon with expertise in thyroid surgery, and nuclear medicine physicians/radiologists. Other treatment approaches, such as radiofrequency ablation, high-intensity focused US, and percutaneous ethanol injection, are also used [16, 43, 59].

The use of RAI therapy for treating hyperthyroidism, for example, Graves' disease, may vary in different countries. In a survey by the American Thyroid Association, European Thyroid Association, and Japanese Thyroid Association, published in 1991, 69%, 22%, and 11% of respondents with Graves' disease chose RAI as the therapy of choice, respectively [60]. These differences were related to the perceived risks of RAI therapy, local requirements for inpatient therapy, patient compliance, and procedural cost, among others. Although RAI is a first-line treatment option for many patients with hyperthyroidism, its use is declining in the United States [61]. On the other hand, therapy with thionamides has increased over the years [62].

Most countries have specific regulations for the possession and use of unsealed sources, including I-131 for diagnostic and therapeutic applications. In the United States, authorized physicians who use radioisotopes must be knowledgeable and in compliance with all Nuclear Regulatory Commission (NRC) laws and requirements. Therapeutic decisions should always be made in accordance with professional guidelines and local practice standards. The criteria for admitting patients for RAI therapy vary across countries. In many European countries, admission is required for even low-dose RAI therapy. In Germany, for example, admission is required for doses equal to or greater than 75 MBq (2.0 mCi) [63]. In the United States, outpatient administration of I-131 doses up to 1221 MBq (33.0 mCi) is considered safe, with radiation exposure to the public unlikely to exceed 5 mSv (0.5 rem). For higher doses, patient-specific calculation and radiation safety requirements must be met. However, instructions regarding radiation safety must be provided to the patient if a dose of more than 259 MBq (7 mCi) is administered [64].

## *Contraindications to Radioiodine-133 Therapy*

- RAI therapy is not a suitable therapy option for individuals unable to comply with radiation safety guidelines, especially after home release. RAI is not indicated in hyperthyroid conditions that are self-limiting. These conditions include silent, subacute, postpartum thyroiditis, and factitious hyperthyroidism.
- RAI therapy is contraindicated in pregnant patients. RAI crosses freely into the placenta, and the fetal thyroid tissue accumulates radioiodine after the 12th week of gestation, which may result in severe neonatal hypothyroidism. Fetal and neonatal I-131 radiation exposure may also increase the risk of developing thyroid cancer. Retained activity in the maternal bladder may also increase the risk of malignancy by direct radiation exposure to the fetus [16, 58, 65]. Females of childbearing age must be tested for a pregnancy test (urine or serum human chorionic gonadotropin (hCG), within 24–72 h of RAI treatment. The treating physician should be aware of the limitations of the pregnancy test. In patients who have had unprotected intercourse within 10 days of the therapy appointment, a delay of the RAI therapy until the beginning of the next menstruation cycle may be considered [58]. Women who are actively lactating or nursing also should not undergo RAI therapy. RAI is taken up and excreted in breast milk, resulting in significant radiation exposure to the breast and infant. Nursing should be stopped for at least 4–6 weeks before RAI administration [58]. Breastfeeding mothers considering RAI therapy can be counseled on the value of archiving their breast milk prior to therapy and the availability of human breast milk banks.
- Uncontrolled hyperthyroidism with high total T3, fT3, or fT4 is a relative contraindication for RAI administration. In these cases, a short-term antithyroid medication should be considered to achieve less severe hyperthyroidism before the RAI administration [16, 58].

## *Patient Preparation*

Patient evaluation before RAI should include the following:

- Clinical history with an emphasis on symptoms (e.g., increased sweating, weight loss, heart palpitation, anxiety); past medical history (e.g., chronic heart failure, COPD); previous treatments (e.g., antithyroid medication, RAI therapy, neck radiation); and exposure to high-dose iodine agents (e.g., contrast media), in which case the indication for RAI treatment should be revisited or delayed dependent on the type and amount of iodine exposure.

- Laboratory tests focusing on thyroid function test (e.g., TSH, fT4, fT3, antithyroid antibodies).
- Obtain thyroid Tc-99 m pertechnetate or RAI uptake and scan to confirm the presence of hyperfunctioning nodules and to exclude cold nodules. The latter may need further evaluation with US and FNA before RAI treatment. When RAI is used, the 24-h RAUI should be >20% to avoid potential RAI treatment failure [57]. A 4–6 h RAIU, in addition to the standard 24-h RAIU, helps identify patients with fast RAI clearance, which may be encountered in 5–23% of Graves' disease patients [66, 67]. In these cases, the prescribed RAI dose should be adjusted higher to allow for a sufficient absorbed dose to the thyroid tissue [57, 58].
- Review of previous FNA results and correlation with thyroid scintigraphy to ensure there are no cold thyroid nodules that may represent thyroid cancer. If there is a cold (hypofunctioning) thyroid nodule, an FNA should precede the RAI, if not already performed, to rule out a thyroid primary according to professional guidelines [16, 57, 68].
- Assessment of thyroid volume by clinical exam or better by US, especially when intrathoracic extension of the thyroid may be present.
- A negative pregnancy test should be performed within 24–72 h before the RAI treatment in females of childbearing age unless the clinical history indicates that the patient cannot conceive a child permanently (e.g., hysterectomy) [16].
- Additional local institutional guidelines are to be followed, such as requirements regarding pregnancy tests (e.g., serum vs. urine test; 24-h vs. 72-h prior to RAI therapy).

## *RAI Dose Determination*

### Toxic Adenoma

Recommended absorbed dose ranges from 200 to 300 gray (Gy) for Graves' disease and 300–400 Gy for autonomously functioning nodules [57, 69]. Dosimetry is required for specific calculations of the absorbed dose to the tissue (in Gy) [69]. Dosimetry is a preferred method in many European countries. Still, it is rarely used in the United States because its outcome has not been shown to be better than the fixed approach or simplified dose calculation, adjusted for 24-h RAIU [57, 70]. For the fixed-dose method, the amount of radioactivity is empirically chosen based on the size of the thyroid gland or nodule, RAIU value, and severity of hyperthyroidism, typically between 370 and 740 MBq (10–20 mCi) (Fig. 6.4). Administered doses of less than 370 MBq (10 mCi) are associated with higher treatment failure rates and should be avoided [71]. In the hands of an experienced nuclear medicine physician/radiologist, a fixed dosage works equally well compared to a dose

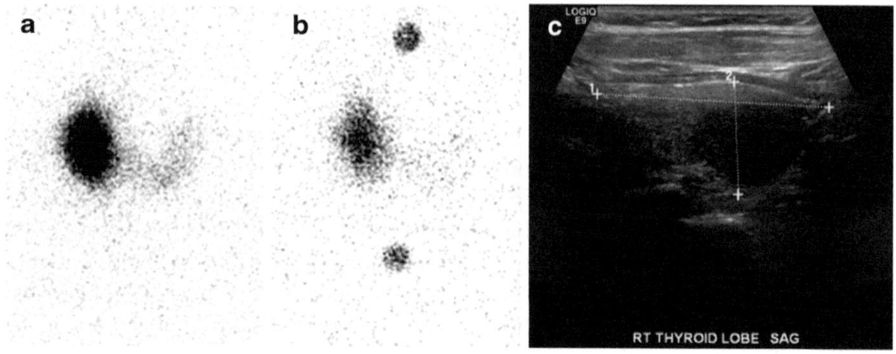


**Fig. 6.4** (**a**) anterior image of thyroid scintigram; (**b**), anterior scintigram with skin markers above and below the thyroid; (**c**)US, longitudinal. A 68-year-old female with a history of subclinical hyperthyroidism (TSH of 0.21 mIU/mL and normal fT3 and fT4 values. RAIU and scan after the oral administration of 8.1 MBq (0.220 mCi) of I-123 showed a focus of increased uptake in the inferior right thyroid lobe and almost complete suppression of normal thyroid uptake (**a**, **b**). The RAIU was 6.2% at 4-h and 15.9% at 24-h (normal 5–15% and 10–30%, respectively). On the US, a hypoechoic thyroid nodule measured 2.2 × 2.4 × 2.2 cm, with a thyroid volume of 21 mL on the right and 15 mL on the left. FNA of the nodule 4 weeks earlier showed benign thyroid tissue (consisting of colloid and follicular cells). Subsequently, the patient was treated with 533 MBq (14.4 mCi) I-131 and was euthyroid at the 12-month follow-up

calculation, achieving the same clinical outcome [16]. A simplified dose calculation (without dosimetry) based on nodule or thyroid size, corrected for 24-h RAIU, is preferred, as it is an objective way for prescribing the radioactivity. This approach requires two visits to the nuclear medicine facility, one for dosing the RAI and the other for the 24-h RAIU and scan, with subsequent RAI treatment within the same day. The simplified dose calculation has been shown to provide a greater success rate than the fixed dosage. It can help avoid undertreatment, particularly in patients with large goiters and low RAI uptake [16, 72, 73].

AFTN and TMNG are usually more radioresistant than diffuse goiters or Graves' disease. The radioactivity for autonomously functioning nodules is between 5.5 and 8.1 MBq (150–220 μCi) per gram tissue, based on nodule size and corrected for 24-h RAIU [16, 58, 74]. A dose calculation based on thyroid size, instead of nodule size, may be considered when there is some degree of RAI uptake within the normal tissue besides the hot uptake of the AFNN. The radiotracer dose is calculated as follows, where the RAI uptake is expressed as the decimal to the percentage value (e.g., 0.4 for a 40% uptake at 24 h) [58]:

$$\text{RAI activity} = \frac{\text{Thyroid tissue mass}\,(\text{g}) \times \text{Radioactivity per g tissue}}{\text{RAI uptake at 24 h}}$$

For example, an RAI dose of 200 μCi/g tissue is prescribed to a patient with an AFTN of 15 g with a 24-h uptake of 40%, where there is no discernible RAI uptake within the normal thyroid tissue. In this patient, the administered dose would be:

$$\text{Dose} = \left(15\,\text{g} \times 200\,\mu Ci / \text{g}\right) \div 0.40 = 7.5\,\text{mCi}\left(278\,\text{MBq}\right)$$

Following the RAI treatment, a response rate of approximately 75% is seen at 3 months and about 89% at 1 year, and patients become hypothyroid over time [56, 75, 76]. There is, however, a 6–18% risk for persistent hyperthyroidism and recurrent hyperthyroidism [56, 75]. Therefore, a dosage toward the upper end of the dose range, for example, 7.4 MBq (200 μCi) per gram tissue, shall be used if a high success rate is desired; in patients with larger thyroid adenomas; repeated RAI treatment or fast RAI turnover [58, 77]. In addition, in patients with incomplete suppression of normal thyroid parenchyma, typically associated with subclinical hyperthyroidism, characterized by suppressed TSH and normal thyroid hormone levels, there is a higher rate of hypothyroidism following the RAI treatment [74, 78].

## Toxic Multinodular Goiter

For the treatment of TMNGs, the dose prescription is based on the goiter size with a dosage of 5.5–8.1 MBq (150–220 μCi) per gram of tissue, corrected for 24-h RAIU [16, 58, 74]. In some instances, such as for elderly patients with comorbidities, a dosage toward the lower end of the dose range, for example, 5.5 MBq (150 μCi) per gram tissue, may be prescribed to achieve euthyroid status and spare them from the need to take daily hormone replacement [44]. For example, an RAI dose of 150 μCi/g tissue is prescribed to a patient with TNMG whose thyroid size is 50 g and has a 24-h uptake of 40%. In this patient, the administered dose would be:

$$\text{Dose} = \left(50\,\text{g} \times 150\,\mu Ci / \text{g}\right) \div 0.40 = 18.8\,\text{mCi}\left(694\,\text{MBq}\right)$$

Because the thyroid size is more prominent in TMNG than in AFTN, the dose administered to TMNG is generally higher than in AFTN (Fig. 6.5). With the administration of a higher RAI dose, the treatment success is higher at the expense of a greater risk of hypothyroidism. The goal of functional status after RAI treatment (euthyroidism vs. hypothyroidism) and the risks of persistent or recurrent hyperthyroidism should be discussed with the patients. The response rate is 50–60% by 3 months and 80% by 6 months [55, 79, 80]. The prevalence of hypothyroidism is 3–4% at 1 year and 16% at 5 years [81, 82].

## Graves' Disease

RAI therapy is considered a suitable therapeutic option for Graves' disease patients without ophthalmopathy, who have developed major adverse reactions to antithyroid medication, have comorbidities with increased surgical risk, or an aversion to surgery due to potential surgical and anesthetic risks as well as cosmetic reasons [16]. RAI for Graves' disease is outside the scope of this book chapter, and the readers are referred to other literature [16, 57, 58].

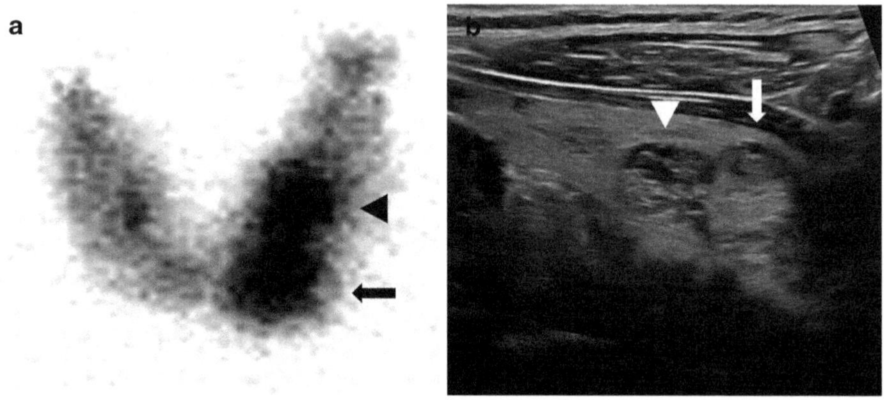


**Fig. 6.5** (**a**) anterior image of thyroid scintigram; (**b**) US, longitudinal. A 39-year-old female with a history of subclinical hyperthyroidism (TSH of 0.19 mIU/mL and normal fT3 and fT4 values. RAIU and scan after the oral administration of 10.3 MBq (0.278 mCi) of I-123 showed two adjacent foci of increased uptake in the inferior left thyroid lobe (**a**, arrow, and arrowhead) without significant suppression of normal thyroid uptake. The RAIU was 31% at 4-h and 48% at 24-h (normal 5–15% and 10–30%, respectively). There was no cold thyroid nodule on the scintigram. On the US, there were two heterogeneously echogenic nodules in the left inferior lobe measuring 2.1 × 2.2 × 2.3 cm (**b**, arrowhead) and 2.4 × 2.7 × 3.0 cm (**b**, arrow), with thyroid volume of 26 mL on the left and 23 mL on the right. Subsequently, the patient was treated with 670 MBq (18.1 mCi) I-131, became euthyroid at 3-month follow-up, and hypothyroid at 12-month follow-up

## *Adverse Effects*

Side effects of RAI given at doses to treat benign thyroid disease are generally mild, infrequent, and self-limiting. These include mild thyroid tenderness, salivary gland discomfort, and nausea [83–85].

In addition to permanent hypothyroidism, transient hyperthyroidism may also occur. A temporary rise in the serum T3, fT3, and fT4 about 5–10 days following the RAI administration can exacerbate symptoms, including heart palpitations and arrhythmia, which can be controlled with β-blocker medication. Thyroid storm is uncommon with concurrent β-blocker medication [86]. In patients with large goiters, the radiation-induced inflammation and swelling of the thyroid may cause dyspnea in some patients, which can be treated with corticosteroids [83]. Vocal cord paresis has also been reported, but it is an extremely rare event [87].

Several published Cooperative Thyrotoxicosis Therapy Follow-up Study Group studies, mainly consisting of clinic sites within the United States, have shown either no increase in cancer mortality or a slight increase in thyroid cancer risk, particularly for those receiving RAI for toxic nodular goiter [88, 89]. Other studies have also shown an increased risk of breast cancer, stomach cancer, small bowel cancer, and renal cancer [90–92]. Thus far, these studies compared cancer risks in hyperthyroid patients treated with RAI to the normal populations, and there were no comparisons across treatment groups (i.e., hyperthyroid patients treated with RAI vs.

antithyroid medication). Therefore, it cannot be ruled out that some excess deaths noted in these studies are associated with underlying thyroid disorders [88–90]. Other studies also indicate a slight but significant increase in overall mortality, which could be related to the patient's history of hyperthyroidism or persistent subclinical hyperthyroidism rather than the RAI effect per se [92–95]. A recent study compared patients who received RAI ($n = 2829$) vs. antithyroid drugs ($n = 13{,}808$) and found no difference in cancer incidence between the two groups over a mean of 7.3 years of follow-up [96]. Similarly, a 2020 study of 31,363 patients with hyperthyroidism showed no association between treatment groups (RAI therapy, antithyroid medication, and/or surgery) and risk of solid cancer mortality. But among patients receiving RAI treatment, solid cancer mortality increased with the total administered activity [97]. Despite some concerns regarding cancer risk and mortality risk, RAI treatment is widely accepted and considered safe and effective for treating patients with hyperthyroidism [44, 98]. Nonetheless, the potential risk of secondary malignancies following RAI treatment needs to be discussed with the patients as part of the informed consent process.

### *Post-Treatment Precautions*

Patients undergoing RAI therapy can potentially expose their family members and the public via saliva, urine, or radiation from their bodies. Although there is little evidence to suggest that small amounts of RAI from treating hyperthyroid patients can cause significant health problems to others, patients are required to follow simple instructions to reduce unnecessary radiation exposure, especially to pregnant women, infants, and children. In the United States, the NRC requires verbal and written instructions to patients before treatment with RAI [99, 100]. Some precautions involve sleeping in a separate bedroom, keeping distance from other people (at least 3 ft.), sexual contact, and close contact with children and pregnant women. Fluid intake and frequent voiding should be encouraged for at least the first 24 h following the RAI administration. Sharing food and eating utensils is not allowed. The toilet should be flushed twice or more after each usage. Handwashing should be performed routinely and frequently. The duration of post-treatment precautions may vary based on local requirements. In the United States, most local institutions require 3 days following RAI treatment for benign thyroid conditions. The period is extended for infants, young children, and pregnant women [64, 100].

## Radioiodine Therapy for Thyroid Cancer

Thyroid cancer is one of the most common endocrine malignancies. It has an increasing incidence of 1.2% as of 2022 in the United States, with a three-fold higher incidence in women than men [101, 102]. Most cases are DTC, consisting of papillary and follicular histology, which are slow-growing tumors. Most patients have an indolent clinical course (90–95%), but subgroups of patients (5–10%) may have an aggressive clinical course or an elevated risk of developing recurrence [19, 103, 104]. Papillary thyroid carcinoma typically spreads to regional lymph nodes and metastasizes to the lungs. Small central lymph node involvement has a negligible effect on the prognosis as these are typically easy to treat by resection. However, lateral cervical or mediastinal nodal metastasis may adversely affect the prognosis. Hematogenous dissemination to the lungs represents a considerable risk for disease persistence and recurrence. Metastases to bone and brain are less common but are associated with an unfavorable prognosis. Follicular carcinoma tends to metastasize more often via the hematogenous route with the involvement of bones, lungs, brain, and other visceral organs [105, 106]. The ATA has defined three groups of DTC with different risks of recurrence: ATA low risk (<5%), ATA intermediate risk (5–20%), and ATA high risk (>20%) [19]. The disease-specific 5-year survival rate is 99.9% for localized disease, 98.3% for regional metastatic disease, and 54.9% for distant metastatic disease [102].

Surgery is the first-line therapy for DTC thyroid cancer. Standard-of-care post-surgical management includes RAI therapy and thyroid hormone therapy. In cases of RAI refractory tumors, additional treatment may involve reoperation of the neck, external radiotherapy, and interventional radiology for the treatment of locoregional metastases and combinations of BRAF and MEK inhibitors [19, 107–111].

## *Indications for RAI Therapy*

Iodine-131 therapy has been used for over 50 years to treat DTC. The goal is to destroy both thyroid remnant cells and cancer cells postoperatively [3]. RAI therapy of DTC is based on the ability of tumor cells to accumulate iodine, albeit less than normal thyroid cells, leading to selective and tumoricidal irradiation [112–114]. The recommendations for RAI therapy focus on the risk factors for disease recurrence following total thyroidectomy. The postoperative Tumor-Node-Metastasis (pTNM) system is most commonly used for classifying and staging DTC. Histology and patient age are also incorporated to classify disease stages further. Other clinical schemes for evaluating the risk of disease recurrence exist, such as MACIS (metastasis, age, completeness of resection, invasion, size), AMES (age, metastasis, extent, size), and AGES (age, grade, metastasis, and size) [115–118]. These risk assessments help evaluate the post-surgical risk and guide the decision for post-surgical RAI treatment [19].

"RAI therapy" is a broad term that encompasses all aspects of the RAI administrations for remnant ablation, adjuvant therapy, and therapy of known or suspected metastatic or residual structural disease [119]. Nowadays, only select cases of DTC warrant RAI treatment, typically performed for remnant ablation, adjuvant therapy, or treatment of known persistent disease [19, 120, 121]. According to the 2015 ATA guidelines, RAI adjuvant therapy is recommended after total thyroidectomy for patients with high-risk disease and should be considered for intermediate-risk disease. RAI treatment is, however, not routinely recommended for the following clinical scenarios in the absence of other adverse features: low-risk disease, unifocal papillary microcarcinoma, and multi-focal papillary microcarcinoma [19, 119–122]. A 2019 joint statement issued by the ATA, European Association of Nuclear Medicine (EANM), Society of Nuclear Medicine and Molecular Imaging (SNMMI), and European Thyroid Association (ETA), acknowledged the absence of high-quality evidence either for or against RAI treatment in low-risk patients [119].

The decision for postoperative RAI therapy should be based on initial prognostic indicators for thyroid cancer-related death and recurrence, including the surgical and pathological findings, postoperative serum Tg level, and the result of neck US obtained after surgery. Regardless of the risk category, the results of neck US, serum Tg level, and diagnostic RAI scan play an essential role in patient selection for RAI therapy [19, 121]. The sensitivity of neck US is high for cervical metastases, except for the central compartment [119]. Tg measurements are helpful as a screening tool, but they are affected by concurrent TSH levels and the presence of potential Tg antibodies. There are no established Tg values that can be used to justify an adjuvant vs. high-risk RAI therapy [19, 59, 121, 123]. The role of diagnostic RAI scans prior to RAI therapy is discussed in the following section. The indications for RAI treatment concur among the pertinent professional guidelines of ATA, ETA, and SNMMI/EANM. Depending on the individual risk stratification, the goal of RAI treatment is as follows [19, 120, 121, 124]:

1. Ablation of thyroid remnant: Remnant ablation refers to the use of RAI to destroy the presumably benign thyroid tissue left after thyroidectomy to facilitate optimal follow-up studies (e.g., monitoring of Tg levels and neck US) [19, 59, 119, 121]. While the main goal is to ablate the normal thyroid tissue, the provided RAI dose can also have a tumoricidal effect.
2. Adjuvant therapy: The RAI therapy is for suspected but unproven residual disease with curative intent to destroy potential microscopic tumor deposits. It is most beneficial for patients with advanced age, aggressive histologies, an increasing volume of nodal disease, extra-nodal extension of the tumor, and multiple locoregional cervical nodes (N1). In these patients, the RAI therapy is administered as an adjuvant treatment, which has been shown to improve overall survival, both for younger (<45 years) and older patients (≥65 years) [120]. Adjuvant RAI therapy is associated with a 29% reduction in the risk of death for all patients [125].
3. Treatment of known or suspected metastasis, residual or recurrent disease with curative or palliative intent. RAI is used to destroy known persistent or recurrent tumor lesions to improve survival. Patients with biochemical, structural, or functional evidence of persistent disease are suitable candidates for RAI treatment of known disease [119]. There is evidence from retrospective or non-controlled prospective studies that overall survival and disease-free survival are improved with post-surgical RAI therapy [120, 121, 126].

## *Pre-Therapy Diagnostic RAI Imaging*

Diagnostic RAI scan in conjunction with RAI treatment for thyroid cancer is the oldest theragnostic application in nuclear medicine. Diagnostic RAI imaging, as a whole-body scan combined with single-photon emission computed tomography/computed tomography (SPECT/CT) technique, is the mainstay in nuclear imaging for DTC patients. It provides the opportunity to identify the thyroid remnant, locoregional nodal disease, and distant metastasis [121]. Pre-treatment diagnostic RAI scan is a valuable tool for staging and risk stratification, especially by detecting unsuspected nodal and distant metastases [105, 127–131]. Imaging results have been shown to alter the prescribed RAI dose in 26–58% of patients, especially with the inclusion of tomographic SPECT/CT in addition to whole-body planar imaging [128]. The diagnostic accuracy of RAI scans, commonly performed with either I-123 or I-131, may vary dependent on the method of patient preparation (i.e., thyroid hormone withdrawal (THW) vs. recombinant human TSH (rhTSH; Thyrogen® injections) and acquisition protocol (planar vs. SPECT/CT) [127, 132, 133]. However, pre-treatment diagnostic RAI scans may or may not be offered at local institutions, dependent on local factors, such as procedure logistics and collaborative efforts between referring network and nuclear medicine facility, clinician's perception of the need for pre-therapy diagnostic RAI scan, and availability of adequate gamma camera equipment.

When a diagnostic RAI scan is performed based on a THW protocol, a small dose of 37–74 MBq (1–3 mCi) I-123 or I-131 is administered orally, followed by imaging at 24 h (next day) [121]. The RAI therapy should be completed within 72 h after the completion of the diagnostic scan [134, 135]. When using an rhTSH protocol, 110–148 MBq (3–4 mCi) of I-123 or I-131 is administered orally, with a delay of 2 h, after the second rhTSH injection (day 2). An RAI scan is obtained 24 h later (day 3), followed by RAI therapy administration within the same day.

## *RAI Dose Determination*

### Empiric Approach Based on Standard Dosage

An empiric, standard dosage of RAI is most used for treating patients with DTC. A standard RAI dose is chosen based on the risk assessment of tumor recurrence in individual patients, among others. The dose recommendations differ slightly among professional societies (Table 6.4). For remnant ablation, most professional societies recommend a dose of 1.11–1.85 GBq (30–50 mCi) I-131, and a higher dosage is not warranted [19, 120, 121, 136]. Only the 2019 ACR–ACNM–ASTRO–SNMMI–SPR practice parameters endorse the use of 1.11–3.7 GBq (30–100 mCi) I-131 for remnant ablation [137]. It is anticipated that their upcoming update on RAI dose recommendations, Resolution 12 to be released in October 2024, will be similar to those recently published by the SNMMI/EANM in 2022 [121].

**Table 6.4** Summary of RAI dose recommendations for DTC from major professional societies ATA (American Thyroid Association) [19]; ETA (European Thyroid Association) [120]; SNMMI/EANM (Society of Nuclear Medicine and Molecular Imaging/European Association of Nuclear Medicine) [121]; NCCN (National Comprehensive Cancer Network) [136]; ACR–ACNM–ASTRO–SNMMI–SPR (American College of Radiology [ACR], American College of Nuclear Medicine [ACNM], American Society for Radiation Oncology [ASTRO], Society of Nuclear Medicine and Molecular Imaging [SNMMI], Society for Pediatric Radiology [SPR] [137]

| Professional guideline | Thyroid remnant ablation | Adjuvant therapy | Known or suspected metastatic disease | Comments |
|---|---|---|---|---|
| 2015 ATA | 1.11 GBq (30 mCi) | 1.15–5.6 GBq (30–150 mCi) | 3.7–7.4 GBq (100–200 mCi)<br>Empiric dose >5.6 GBq (150 mCi) should be avoided in patients >70 years old | For thyroid ablation, higher radioactivity should be considered in patients with less than a total or near total thyroidectomy in which a larger remnant is suspected or in which adjuvant therapy is intended. It is uncertain whether routine use of higher administered activities >5.6 GBq (150 mCi) will reduce structural disease recurrence for T3 and N1 disease |
| 2022 ETA | 1.11 GBq (30 mCi) | • 1.15–3.7 GBq (30–100 mCi)<br>• >3.7 GBq (100 mCi), if high risk | >3.7 GBq (100 mCi) | For intermediate-risk category, greatest benefit of RAI is in patients with: Advanced age; aggressive histologies; increasing volume of nodal disease; extra-nodal extension of the tumor; multiple N1; and/or lymph node metastases outside the central neck. There is no evidence that >3.7 GBq (100 mCi) improves prognosis for adjuvant treatment |

(continued)

**Table 6.4** (continued)

| Professional guideline | Thyroid remnant ablation | Adjuvant therapy | Known or suspected metastatic disease | Comments |
|---|---|---|---|---|
| 2022 SNMMI/EANM | 1.11–1.85 GBq (30–50 mCi) | 1.85–3.7 GBq (50–100 mCi) | 3.7–5.6 GBq (100–150 mCi)—For small volume locoregional disease<br>5.6–7.4 GBq (150–200 mCi)—For advanced locoregional disease and/or small volume distant metastasis<br>>7.4 GBq (200 mCi) or maximum tolerable based on dosimetry calculation—For diffuse distant metastasis | Some committee members recommend up to 5.6 GBq (150 mCi) for adjuvant treatment |
| 2024 NCCN | 1.11 GBq (30 mCi) | 2.78–5.6 GBq (75–150 mCi) | 3.7–7.4 GBq (100–200 mCi) | Consider 30–50 mCi with T1b/T2 (1–4 cm) with small volume N1a disease (fewer than 5 lymph node metastases <2 mm) and for patients with primary <4 cm, clinical M0 with minor extrathyroidal extension. Consider 5.6–7.4 GBq (150–200 mCi) for tumor extrathyroidal growth, incompletely resected |
| 2019 ACR–ACNM–ASTRO–SNMMI–SPR[a] | 1.11–3.7 GBq (30–100 mCi) | 3.7–5.6 GBq (100–150 mCi) | 5.6–7.4 GBq (150–200 mCi) | 5.6 Gbq (150 mCi) for nodal disease; 6.5 Gbq (175 mCi) for pulmonary metastasis; and 7.4 Gbq (200 mCi) for skeletal metastasis |

[a] Revised Resolution 12 of the ACR practice parameter is expected to be released in October 2014, suggesting 1.11–1.85 GBq (30–50 mCi) for remnant ablation. RAI dose recommendations for adjuvant therapy and metastatic disease would remain unchanged

Dose recommendations for adjuvant therapy are challenging as the optimal RAI dose cannot be accurately determined based on published reports. Consequently, the RAI recommendations vary between 1.11 GBq and 5.55 GBq (30–150 mCi). Prescribed RAI doses most likely range from 1.85 to 3.7 GBq (50–100 mCi), but institutions may opt to extend this range to 5.55 GBq (150 mCi) [19, 120, 121, 136, 137]. The updated National Comprehensive Cancer Network (NCCN) guidelines for thyroid cancer, March 2024, recommend 1.11 GBq (30 mCi) for remnant ablation and 2.78–5.55 GBq (75–150 mCi) for adjuvant therapy based on surgical pathology or pre-therapy RAI scan results. For proven unresectable or metastatic disease, a dose of 3.7–7.4 GBq (100–200 mCi) is recommended [136]. However, there are no published reports on the effectiveness of 3.7 GBq (100 mCi) vs. 5.6 GBq (150 mCi) for adjuvant treatment. An empiric dose of 7.4 MBq (200 mCi) is usually preserved for high-risk patients with known residual tumors especially bone metastases. Current guidelines emphasize the use of RAI dose >3.7 GBq (100 mCi) is associated with the increased risk of xerostomia and sialadenitis risk, which should be related to the patient [138]. The recommendations for RAI dosage continue to be investigated and updated by professional societies. It is important that the RAI dose selection be discussed in a multidisciplinary expert setting.

## RAI Dosimetry

The I-131 therapy is performed by either empirically administering a standard dose or dosimetry calculations. Dosimetry is a quantitative method to determine a patient-specific RAI activity based on individual pharmacokinetics. There are two dosimetry methods—blood/whole-body dosimetry and lesion-based dosimetry [139–141].

The blood/whole-body method is commonly used in the US, which involves a 3-to-5-day procedure dependent on the institutional protocol. A small RAI dose is administered orally, followed by daily radioactivity measurements from the body and blood samples. Dosimetry uses blood measurements as a surrogate for the bone marrow. It aims to determine the radioactivity as-high-as-safely-administrable (AHASA). In contrast, the absorbed dose to the radiosensitive bone marrow is limited to 2 Gy, and the whole body to 2.96 Gbq (80 mCi) at 48 h after the RAI administration, which is considered the threshold for the risk for pulmonary fibrosis in patients with extensive pulmonary metastases [121, 136, 139, 142, 143]. This approach helps avoid severe hematopoietic side effects, pulmonary fibrosis, and pneumonitis. A diagnostic RAI scan is also obtained during the dosimetry procedure. For RAI treatment of known disease, there are different opinions on the use of dosimetry vs. empiric dosage. However, the largest study of 353 patients with metastatic DTC did not show the benefit of dosimetry over empirically administered dose >3700 MBq (100 mCi) [144]. There was no statistical difference in overall survival after correction for sex, age at the diagnosis of distant metastases, metastases site, and metastases extension ($P = 0.16$). Overall survival at 5 years was 96%

and 96% for patients younger than 40 years with micrometastases, and 70% and 65% for patients older than 40 years with macrometastases or multiple metastases, respectively [144]. However, the study's design and results have been criticized by various rebuttals [145–147]. Moreover, it is well recognized from a radiobiological standpoint that there is a correlation between the administered absorbed dose and treatment response, as well as toxicity. This indicates that dosimetry-based RAI therapy may improve clinical outcomes and survival compared to standard doses [142, 148].

The lesion-based dosimetry is most suitable for macroscopic and measurable lesions, so specific absorbed doses for these lesions can be calculated [141]. It aims to determine the radioactivity as-low-as-reasonable-achievable (ALARA) while delivering the desired radioactivity dose to the target tissue. Generally, an absorbed dose of 40–80 Gy and 300–500 Gy should be delivered to tumor lesions and thyroid remnants, respectively [113, 141]. This approach is frequently used in Europe but infrequently in the United States.

Contrary to the standard-dose approach, dosimetry accounts for patient-to-patient variability in the rate of iodine clearance and allows for administering a maximum tolerable RAI dose [121]. Thus, administered RAI doses with dosimetry are mostly ≥7.4 GBq (200 mCi) I-131. Current guidelines do not provide specific recommendations for dosimetry vs. standard dose in treating advanced DTC [19, 59, 121]. Dosimetry-guided RAI therapy may, however, be considered in patients with distant metastatic disease when technical and medical expertise is available, and the RAI treatment can be performed safely regarding adverse effects and radiation safety requirements. When dosimetry is used, a THW protocol is preferred over the rhTSH protocol to achieve a higher radiation-absorbed dose, even though there are currently no published results comparing the clinical outcome between THW vs. rhTSH protocol [127, 149, 150].

## *Patient Preparation for RAI Therapy*

The nuclear medicine physician/radiologist should ideally meet the patient in a consultation before the RAI therapy. The physician will discuss the purpose of RAI therapy, procedure steps, side effects, and aspects of radiation safety with the patients. An RAI therapy at 4–6 weeks post-surgery works well in most cases. The typical patient preparation is as follows [121]:

- The eligibility for outpatient vs. inpatient RAI administration is determined based on the intended RAI dose and the patient's ability to comply with radiation safety requirements after discharge. These requirements vary among countries, and patients may be treated as an outpatient or admitted for inpatient administration, dependent on national regulations and patients' home environment and personal circumstances. In the United States, the rules regarding RAI administrations ≤8.14 GBq (220 mCi) are as follows, in accordance with the Nuclear Regulatory Commission (NRC) regulatory guide 8.39 [151]:

- If a patient can comply with the required radiation safety measures, he/she can be treated as an outpatient. Most patients with DTC fall into this category. The patient is discharged immediately following the RAI administration, but the radioactivity dosage and instructions for radiation safety must be documented.
- If a patient cannot meet any of the following criteria, he/she will require hospitalization if the administered dose exceeds 1221 MBq (33 mCi) I-131 [64, 152].

  Patient will sleep alone in a room for at least the first night.
  Patient will not travel by airplane or mass transportation for at least the first day.
  Patient will have sole use of a bathroom for at least the first 2 days.
  Patient can maintain a prudent distance from others for at least the first 2 days.
  Patient will not travel on a prolonged automobile trip with others for at least the first 2 days.
  Patient will drink plenty of fluids for the first 2 days.

- Most patients receiving >8.14 GBq (220 mCi) of I-131 require admission to a dedicated patient room with appropriate radiation safety personnel and protection, including a separate bathroom and lead lining of the treatment room. Per NRC guide, patients can be discharged when their radioactivity decreases to below 1221 MBq (33 mCi) or when the dose rate is <0.07 mSv/h (7.0 mrem/h) at 1 m. It is important to note that local regulations may differ and required dose rates may be lower for discharge. Dependent on the amount of administered radioactivity, the typical hospital stay is 2–5 days.

• 1–2 weeks of a low-iodine diet is recommended for optimal RAI uptake. A dietary iodine restriction (< 50 μg/days) is essential to help avoid interfering with the RAI uptake in thyroid remnant and cancer cells. Helpful suggestions about low-iodine diets are available on the American Thyroid Association website (https://www.thyroid.org/low-iodine-diet).
• Achieving TSH stimulation ≥30 mIU/L measured 1–3 days before RAI therapy. A lower TSH level may be sufficient for thyroid remnant treatment [153]. The goal of TSH stimulation is to increase the NIS expression and uptake of RAI, which can be achieved in two ways:

  - Endogenous TSH stimulation based on THW: The patient is instructed to stop the T4 replacement for 4 weeks. An alternative THW protocol based on T3 and T4 intake may also be used [121].
  - Exogenous TSH stimulation based on rhTSH (Thyrogen®) administration. The use of rhTSH administrations is convenient for patients because they continue to take their thyroid hormone during the entire procedure. It is also associated with better renal clearance. Patients receive 0.9 mg rhTSH intramuscularly on two consecutive days (day 1 and 2), followed by RAI therapy administration at 48 h (day 3) [150]. The selection of THW vs. rhTSH

is individualized for patients. However, in patients with low-risk or intermediate-risk DTC without lateral cervical nodal involvement (i.e., pN1a), preparation with rhTSH is an acceptable alternative to THW, as normal thyroid tissue is expected to have high NIS expression resulting in adequate RAI uptake within a short period after rhTSH stimulation [19, 120, 121, 127]. For high-risk patients with known metastases, the THW protocol is favored because it allows for a more prolonged TSH stimulation compared with the short-term TSH stimulation with rhTSH, which enhances RAI uptake and retention in metastatic lesions. There is a risk that the use of rhTSH can lead to missed diagnosis and suboptimal treatment of metastatic lesions [154–156].

- For females of childbearing age, a negative pregnancy test is required within 24–72 h of RAI administration unless the patient is status post hysterectomy or postmenopausal.

## *Radiation Safety*

Patients who receive RAI therapy constitute a source of radiation exposure to their family members and the general public. Patients are provided specific instructions regarding radiation safety at release, for both inpatient and outpatient therapies, to keep radiation exposures at the lowest possible levels, according to the principle of ALARA. The key measure is to avoid prolonged and close contact with others and the general public during this period. The instructions regarding radiation safety are similar to those given to patients treated with RAI for benign thyroid conditions [64, 100].

## *Adverse Effects*

The β-particles emitted by I-131 can cause cellular damage to normal tissue, which can be irreversible if the radiation dose is high enough. Patients treated with I-131 may develop acute and chronic side effects and carry a small risk of secondary malignancies. Therefore, it is prudent that the RAI therapy is offered only to select patients with DTC after carefully considering therapy indication and dose determination by a multidisciplinary team with expertise in DTC management. The importance of copious fluid intake (at least 4.5 L/day or 1 US gal/day) following the RAI needs to be emphasized during patient education and the consent process. Increased fluid intake aims to reduce radiation exposure to non-target organs, such as by increasing salivation and flushing of the oropharynx, diluting the radioiodine concentration within the stomach, and accelerating the RAI clearance from the body brought by increased renal clearance and frequency of bladder emptying.

### Acute Adverse Events

RAI therapy is considered safe and well-tolerated for treating DTC patients, but there are some risks of adverse events [19, 121, 157]. Besides the thyroid gland, several other organs exhibit NIS, leading to RAI uptake with potential side effects, most frequently affecting the salivary and nasolacrimal glands. Acute side effects of RAI therapy concerning the salivary and lacrimal glands are common but usually mild and short term. Symptoms may manifest as sialadenitis, radiation thyroiditis, neck edema, dysgeusia (taste dysfunction), nausea, and gastritis [138, 158, 159]. Symptomatic radiation thyroiditis and neck edema may be treated with nonsteroidal anti-inflammatory drugs. Gastrointestinal symptoms may be treated with antiemetics (nausea) and antacids (gastritis).

In general, acute side effects to the salivary glands may be seen in up to 14% of patients receiving RAI doses between 1.11 and 1.85 GB1 (30–50 mCi) [158–163]. Acute sialadenitis occurs in 10–41% of patients with radioactivity <22.2 GBq (600 mCi) I-131 [159, 162, 164, 165]. Patients may experience pain, tenderness, and swelling of the salivary glands. Chronic symptoms of sialadenitis may be seen in 3–25% of patients at 1-year post-therapy [159–162, 164, 165]. Acute symptoms of xerostomia range between 10% and 43% with administered radioactivity <18.500 GBq (500 mCi) I-131 [158, 159, 161, 166]. The severity of dry mouth decreases over time in these patients, but up to 15% of patients may still be symptomatic 3 years after the RAI therapy. The risk of sialadenitis and xerostomia is dose-dependent and increases with cumulative RAI doses. The RAI threshold is estimated at 3.7 GBq (100 mCi) for xerostomia and 5.55 GBq (150 mCi) for sialadenitis [138, 159, 161, 165, 167].

Using lemon juice or sour candies and abundant fluid intake can reduce the absorbed dose to the salivary glands and decrease the incidence and severity of sialadenitis. However, the optimal time to start taking the lemon juice and sour candies (24 h vs. sooner) following the RAI administration remains controversial [168, 169]. Although less frequently, patients may also experience dry eyes due to lacrimal dysfunction [138].

### Infertility Risk

Late adverse effects of therapy RAI may occur months or even years post-therapy. In females, the primordial oocytes in the ovaries are relatively resistant to the radiation effect emitted from the excreted urine within the bladder. Generally, RAI therapy may not affect fertility in women [170]. However, more recent data indicate a potential negative impact of RAI therapy on ovarian reserve and the potential risk of reduced birth rate in women aged 35–39 [171–173]. Future studies are warranted to elucidate these potential risks further.

In men, on the other hand, there is a clear risk of infertility because the sperms are highly radiosensitive. The testis is exposed to radiation not only from the nearby urinary activity within the bladder but also because the germinal and

Leydig cells of the testis express the NIS resulting in radioiodine uptake [174]. Reduced male fertility is a concern; however, the long-term impact on fertility is minimal when receiving a single dose of RAI or cumulative doses <14.8 GBq (400 mCi). Men and teenagers should consider sperm banking before the RAI therapy when cumulative RAI doses exceeding 14.8 GBq (400 mCi) are anticipated [175, 176].

## Hematopoietic Side Effects

Bone marrow suppression is a significant concern following RAI therapy [177–181]. The 2015 ATA guidelines recommend that empirically administered activities >5.55 GBq (150 mCi) of I-131 should be avoided in patients >70 years of age, based on calculated bone marrow dosimetry estimates [19]. In a subsequent study of 122 patients with age >70 years old and mean RAI activity of 5.06 ± 1.78 GBq (136.8 ± 48 mCi), with 82% of patients receiving ≥3.7 GBq (100 mCi) and 66% receiving ≥5.55 GBq (150 mCi), mild myelosuppression was noted which was not of clinical significance. There was mild platelet suppression with administered activity ≥3.7 GBq (100 mCi) and mild suppression of white blood cells and hemoglobin with activities ≥5.55 GBq (150 mCi), with mean values remaining within references. No clinically significant cytopenia was noted during the follow-up [180]. Other studies with cumulative administered activities ≥9.25 GBq (250 mCi) under dosimetry guidance also showed a small but statistically insignificant decrease in blood counts [182, 183]. Other studies also indicate that bone marrow suppression in the elderly is similar to that in younger patients [181–185]. Nonetheless, there should be a careful risk-benefit assessment for repeated RAI therapies. The current 2022 NCCN guidelines recommend that patients with high cumulative dose administrations >37 GBq (1000 mCi) should be monitored for myelosuppression and potential long-term toxicities [136].

## Risk of Lung Fibrosis

The risk of pulmonary fibrosis is rare when using dosimetry to limit the whole-body retention to 2.96 Gbq (80 mCi) at 48 h or empiric radioactivity ≤200 mCi I-131 [19, 136, 143]. This risk was seen in 7–25% of pediatric patients with diffuse, RAI avid pulmonary metastases who had undergone multiple courses of high-dose RAI therapies, resulting in cumulative activities of 21–71 GBq (568–1919 mCi) I-131 [186, 187]. A pulmonary function test should be considered before RAI therapy when there is evidence of widespread pulmonary metastasis, particularly for patients with underlying parenchymal lung conditions such as emphysema and fibrotic lung disease.

### Cancer Risk

There is an ongoing debate about the risk of developing secondary malignancies due to RAI therapy for DTC. The incidence of RAI-associated secondary malignancies may vary according to the study design and detection method. Several studies showed no increased incidence, and no specific cancer or cancer group was linked to RAI exposures [188–191]. These include a 2022 study of 24,318 patients in South Korea which showed no significant difference in secondary cancer risk between DTC patients treated and not treated with RAI, according to the propensity score analysis [192]. In other studies, however, there appears to be a correlation between RAI dose and the risk of secondary malignancies [193–199]. Several studies have shown that patients exposed to RAI risk developing leukemia [194, 198–202]. In the most recent study using the US Surveillance, Epidemiology, and End Results (SEER) data (1975–2017) of 27,050 pediatric DTC patients, the risk of secondary neoplasms was elevated for both hematologic malignancies (RR = 1.51; 95% CI: 1.08–2.01), including leukemia (RR = 1.92; 95%:1.04–3.56); and solid cancers (RR = 1.47; 95% CI: 1.24–1.74), including breast cancer (RR = 1.46; 95% CI: 1.10–1.95). They estimated 6%, 5%, and 14% of second solid, breast, and hematologic malignancies, respectively, might be attributable to RAI therapy. But given the modest relative risks and relatively rare incidence of solid malignancies in DTC survivors, the absolute lifetime excess risks associated with RAI are thought to be small [199]. Another SEER-based study indicated a higher rate of secondary breast cancer in younger DTC patients who received RAI therapy compared with both non-RAI treated patients (HR 1.65; 95% CI: 1.33–2.05) and the general population (HR 1.21; 95% CI: 1.02–1.44) [203]. However, RAI-associated breast cancer risk remains controversial. A meta-analysis of 200,247 DTC patients indicated that DTC patients treated with RAI do not have a higher risk of primary breast cancer compared to those not treated with RAI [204]. Although the risk of developing secondary hematologic malignancies is higher than primary solid malignancies following RAI therapy, the quality of evidence is considered low, particularly for secondary solid malignancies [205].

According to some reports, cumulative RAI doses greater than 150–200 mCi I-131 pose a statistically significant risk for developing secondary malignancies [194, 195]. However, the current literature does not provide a clearly defined dose threshold. Therefore, caution must be exercised while administering repeated RAI therapies for persistent metastatic PTC, especially when the cumulative dose exceeds 1000 mCi, due to the risk of developing SPM and long-term toxicity, such as myelosuppression [136, 196, 206].

Published reports often have limitations in terms of study design and execution. Although most studies adjusted for gender and age at the time of DTC diagnosis, potential biases, such as inappropriate control groups, prior cancer treatment, and familial disposition to malignancies, were not always assessed and adjusted for during data analyses. This may have contributed to conflicting results among published reports, including a variable range of low to moderate of absolute excess risk of SPM [195, 199, 207]. Further research is warranted to understand better the relationship between RAI dose and the risk of secondary malignancy.

## *Post-Therapy Imaging*

Due to the higher administered RAI activity for therapy, the post-therapy scan provides greater sensitivity for detecting radioiodine avid lesions than a pre-treatment scan. Therefore, within 2–7 days after RAI administration, it is vital to obtain a post-therapy scan, typically as a whole-body scan, to confirm RAI avid thyroid remnant. If clinically indicated, a regional SPECT/CT may be added to enhance lesion detection and characterization, especially for locoregional and distant metastases [121]. Several clinical scenarios may emerge from the post-therapy scan result:

- If the scan shows only focal uptake within the thyroidectomy and no suspicious local regional lymphadenopathy or distant metastases, the prognosis is excellent, particularly when Tg level is undetectable. If Tg is minimally elevated (Fig. 6.6), findings are cautiously reassuring but a diagnostic RAI scan in 6–12 months should be considered to confirm successful remnant ablation and that the Tg has become undetectable.
- On the other hand, if the scan reveals remnant uptake and no suspicious metastases, but the Tg level is high, findings may suggest RAI-negative, poorly differentiated metastases. Additional imaging is warranted for further staging and clinical management, including US of the neck, CT of the neck and chest, and FDG PET/CT.
- If the scan indicates the presence of nodal and/or distant metastasis, a diagnostic RAI scan in 6–12 months is required, and an RAI retreatment may be warranted (Figs. 6.7 and 6.8).

## *Role of FDG PET in DTC Imaging*

A diagnostic RAI scan, either as a whole-body scan or combined with SPECT/CT technique, is the nuclear imaging of choice for following up DTC patients with suspected locoregional or distant metastases [121, 208]. Rising Tg levels with a negative diagnostic RAI scan typically indicate the presence of refractory metastatic disease, which may prompt further evaluation with FDG PET/CT, often in conjunction with US neck and CT neck and chest [121]. A mismatched uptake pattern of metastatic lesions, seen as a negative RAI scan but positive FDG PET/CT, indicates tumor dedifferentiation, in which case repeated RAI treatments are not beneficial [209]. Surgical resection is the preferred therapeutic option if FDG avid metastatic disease is limited to the neck. Otherwise, if multiple FDG avid lesions within the body are not amenable to surgical resection, systemic therapy with multikinase tyrosine kinase inhibitors (TKI) is the current standard of care [19, 109].

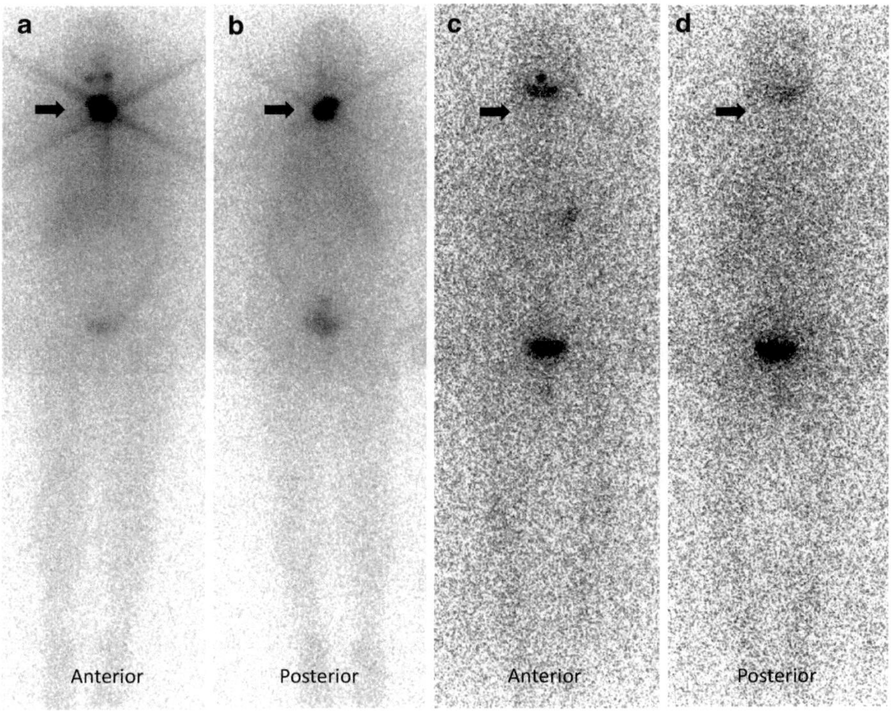


**Fig. 6.6** A 53-year-old female with a history of right lobe DTC, status post right lobectomy followed by completion left thyroidectomy 4 weeks earlier (2.3 cm, left thyroid; classical papillary carcinoma; negative for extrathyroidal extension, lymphatic invasion, or angioinvasion; 3 of 8 level VI nodes positive for metastases, largest 0.4 cm, pT2N1aNx, AJCC stage I). The patient was treated with 1.89 Gbq (51 mCi) I-131 for remnant ablation, using an rhTSH protocol (TSH 100.3 mIU/L, Tg 2.1 ng/mL, Tg antibody <20 IU/mL). Five days later, a post-therapy whole-body scan demonstrated an area of intense RAI uptake within the thyroidectomy bed (**a** and **b**, arrow) but no evidence of local regional adenopathy or distant metastasis. The patient underwent a diagnostic RAI scan 12 months later using an rhTSH protocol (**c** and **d**). Whole-body imaging obtained 24-h after the oral administration of 41 MBq (1.1 mCi) I-131 showed resolution of previous RAI uptake in the thyroidectomy bed (**c** and **d**, arrow). There was no evidence of local regional or distant metastasis (Tg < 0.1 ng/mL, and Tg antibody < 20 IU/mL). The follow-up exam documented the successful remnant ablation and the absence of metastatic disease. The patient remained disease-free on subsequent tumor surveillance with clinical exam, serum Tg, and neck US

## *Retreatment with RAI*

Metastatic disease is encountered in approximately 10% of DTC patients, with the most frequent sites involving the lungs, bone, brain, and liver [108]. Patients with solitary metastasis, lower Tg values at their first RAI treatment, and those of younger age (<45 years) have the best clinical outcome [105, 210–215]. High-risk patients undergoing RAI therapy may require retreatment due to persistent metastatic disease. When a standard dose is used, the RAI dose is usually between 5.5 and 7.4 GBq (150–200 mCi), provided renal function is normal [121]. There is,

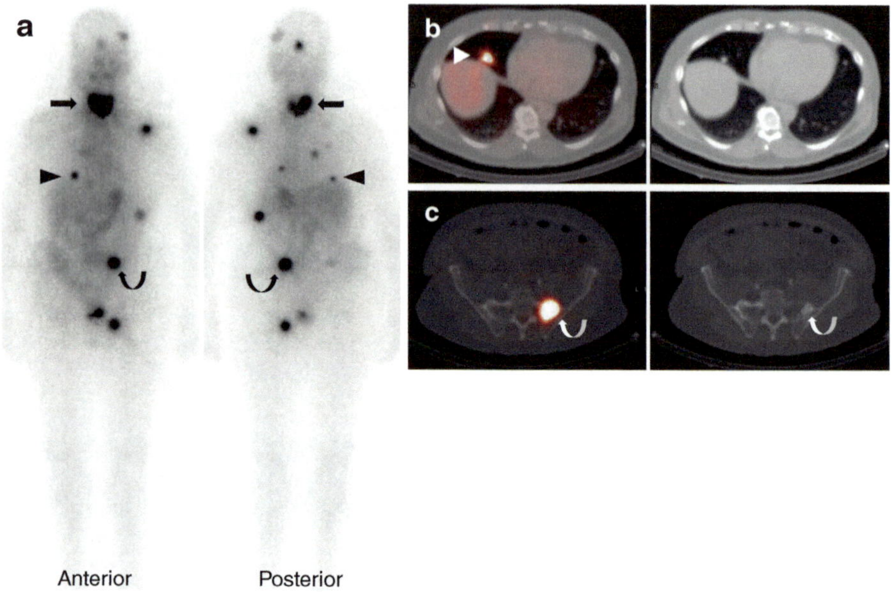


**Fig. 6.7** (**a**) Whole-body post-RAI scan; (**b** and **c**) fused SPECT/CT and CT. A 56-year-old female with papillary thyroid carcinoma, tall cell variant, right lobe (2.6 cm), with macroscopic extrathyroidal extension invading the strap muscles, surgical margin positive for tumor, 10 of 23 level IV nodes positive for metastasis (larges 2.1 cm), pT3bN1b. Post-thyroidectomy lab results showed Tg 265 ng/mL, Tg antibody <20 IU/mL, and TSH 60.4 mIU/L upon THW. The patient was treated with 7.59 GB1 (205 mCi) I-131, given suspected cervical lymphadenopathy and pulmonary metastases at CT, histopathology, and laboratory results. A post-therapy scan 5 days later showed RAI avid lesions in the thyroidectomy bed (**a**, arrow), pulmonary metastases, including a 1 cm right lower lobe pulmonary lesion (**a** and **b**, arrowhead), and multiple avid bone lesions, including a lucent lesion involving left S1 (**a** and **c**, curved arrow)

however, an advantage to dosimetry calculation in these cases, which will allow the administration of doses AHASA. If multiple treatments are required, there should be a 6–12-month interval between RAI therapies depending upon the clinical urgency. Repeated RAI therapies may be administered until a complete response is achieved or refractory disease occurs, but severe adverse effects due to cumulative RAI exposure needs to be considered [216, 217]. The 10-year disease-specific survival is 92% for patients who show RAI uptake and response to the treatment. It may decrease to 30% and 10% in patients who do not achieve a complete response despite evidence of RAI uptake and those who do not show RAI uptake, respectively [105]. In some patients, the disease progresses even in the presence of avid RAI uptake indicating refractory disease, typically observed in patients with follicular thyroid carcinoma and those with BRAF V600E, telomerase reverse transcriptase (TERT) promoter, and RAS mutations [218, 219]. Due to their ineffectiveness, patients who develop RAI refractory disease should not undergo

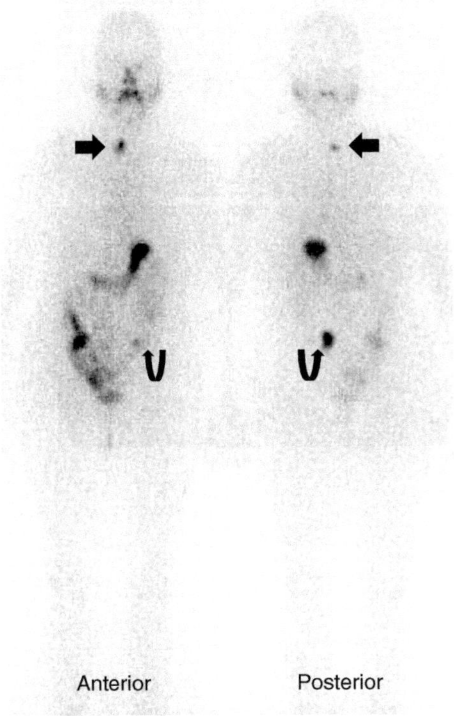


**Fig. 6.8** A diagnostic whole-body scan was performed 6 months later, the same patient as in Fig. 6.7, after the oral administration of 159 MBq (4.3 mCi) I-123, using a THW protocol (TSH 45 mIU/L, Tg 32 ng/mL, Tg antibody <20 IU/mL). The scan showed resolution of most previously RAI avid lesions, except for two small foci of mild uptake in the right thyroid bed (arrow) and left S1 (curved arrow). The patient was then treated with 5.33 Gbq (144 mCi) I-131. The patient achieved a complete response at 6-month follow-up, with a negative diagnostic RAI scan and lab work (undetectable Tg with TSH stimulation)

further RAI treatments [19]. The therapy may be offered in select patients after carefully considering potential clinical benefits and risk assessment of significant adverse events.

## *Strategies to Overcome RAI—Refractory Thyroid Cancer*

RAI refractory DTC implies the loss of cellular proteins involved in iodine uptake and metabolism (Fig. 6.9). More recently, research has been paying attention to the molecular phenotype of refractory tumors, identifying mitogen-activated protein kinase (MAPK) signaling as the most frequent pathway for the RAI refractory process. The major hallmark of the MAPK pathway is represented by the BRAF V600E mutation, which leads to the activation of extracellular signal-regulated kinase (ERK). The mutation results in a downregulation of genes in the iodine metabolism pathway, such as NIS and thyroid peroxidase (TPO) [110, 220–224]. Research attempts have evolved around these molecular pathways, aiming to induce the redifferentiation process through selective BRAF and MEK inhibitors for therapeutic

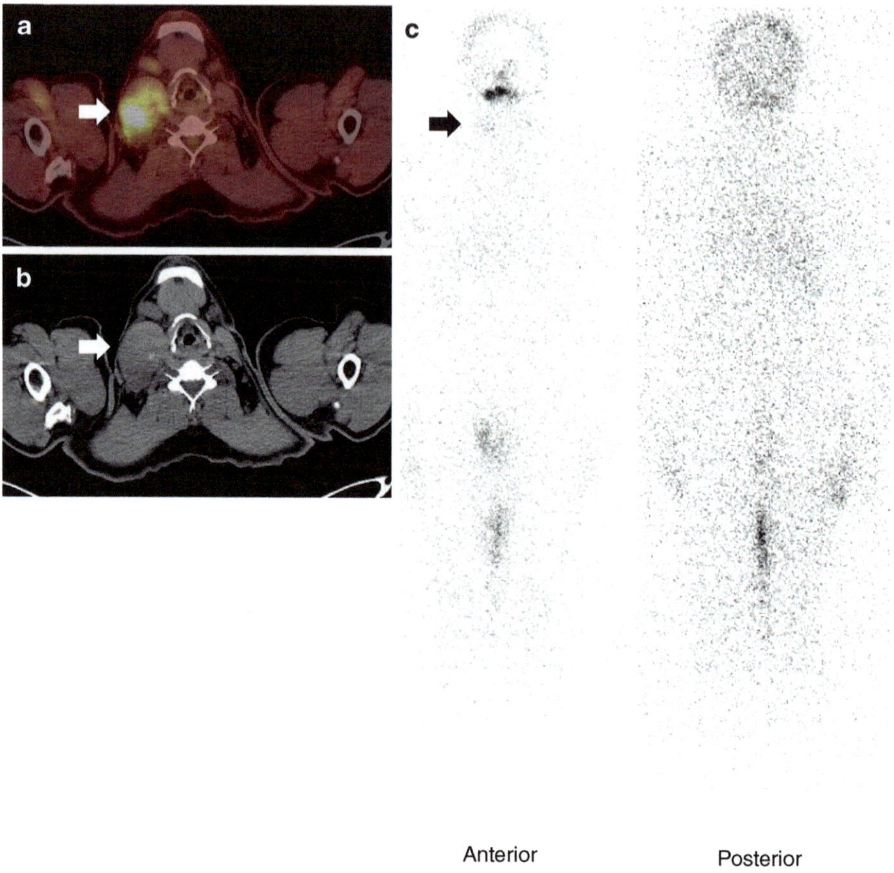


**Fig. 6.9** A 48-year-old man was diagnosed with multi-focal papillary thyroid carcinoma, greatest diameter 0.8 cm, at thyroidectomy and bilateral neck dissection, pT1aN1b. There was no extracapsular extension or angioinvasion; however, surgical margins were positive for tumor, and lymphatic invasion was present. 46 of 130 cervical nodes (level I-VI) were involved, largest 8.0 cm. The tumor was positive for thyroid transcription factor-1 (TTF-1) and BRAF(V600E) but negative for CDX2, a nuclear transcription factor. Presurgical FDG PET/CT demonstrated an FDG avid nodal conglomerate in the right neck, 4.5 × 6.7 cm, with a maximum standard uptake value (SUV) of 9.1 (arrow—**a**, fused PET/CT; **b**, CT). There were no FDG avid thyroid lesions, and two bilateral pulmonary nodules measuring up to 0.5 cm were not FDG avid. The patient underwent RAI therapy 3 months later with 4.66 GBq (126 mCi) I-131. Post-therapy whole-body scan 7 days later showed no significant RAI activity within the neck (**c**, arrow) or the remainder of the body. TSH and Tg levels were unavailable at that time because the patient was noncomplying with appointments. However, 1 year after the initial RAI therapy, lab results showed Tg 26.2 ng/mL, Tg Ab <0.9 IU/mL, and TSH 15.49 mIU/L. A subsequent biopsy of a right cervical node and a pulmonary nodule confirmed metastatic PTC. A redo lateral neck dissection (level V and bilateral level IA) was performed. The patient was deemed RAI refractory at this point and put on a 2-month course of dabrafenib (BRAF inhibitor) and trametinib (MEK inhibitor)

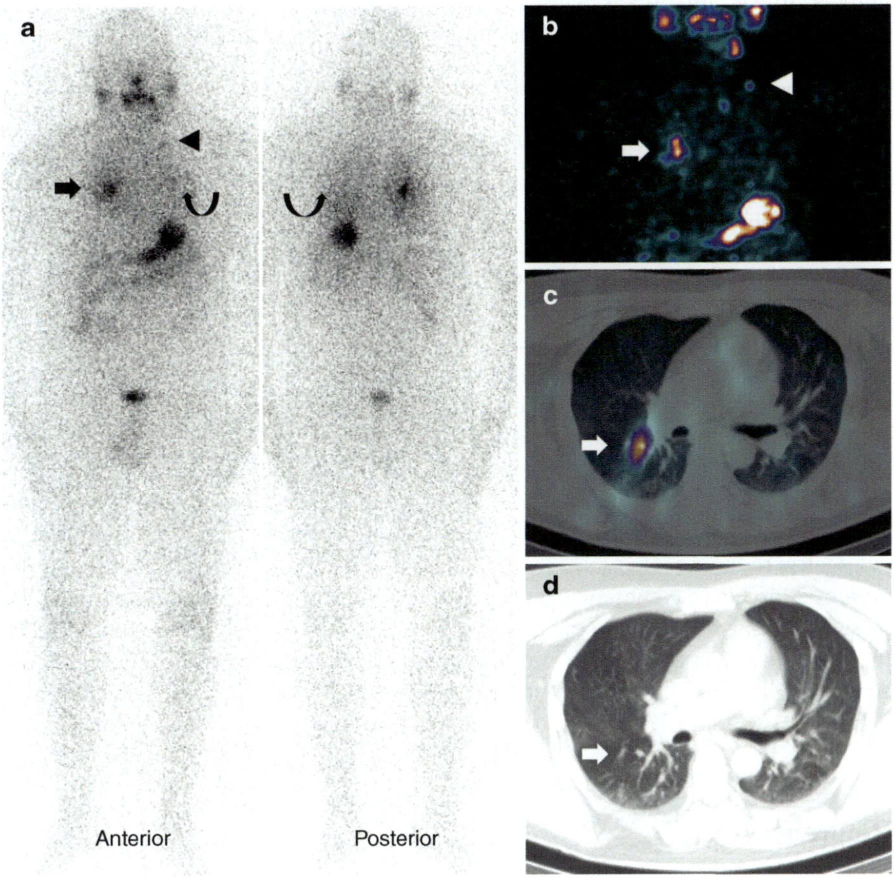


**Fig. 6.10** Radioiodine scans after redifferentiation therapy. (**a**) whole-body scan; (**b**) maximum intensity projection (MIP); (**c**) fused SPECT/CT; (**d**) CT. A diagnostic RAI scan was obtained following the 2-month intake of dabrafenib and trametinib, using a THW protocol and after the oral administration of 167 MBq (4.5 mCi) I-123. The scan showed an area of increased RAI activity in the right lung, corresponding to two adjacent right lower lobe pulmonary nodules of 0.5 cm (arrow), besides diffusely increased RAI activity in both longs (curved arrow). In addition, focal uptake in the left neck (arrowhead) corresponded to a 0.3 cm supraclavicular node. Tg rose to 93.6 ng/mL, with Tg Ab <0.9 IU/mL and TSH 23 mIU/L. Imaging findings indicated redifferentiation of cervical lymphadenopathy and pulmonary metastases. As a result, the patient underwent a second RAI therapy with 7.4 GBq (200 mCi) I-131

applications (Figs. 6.10 and 6.11) [110, 224]. Selumetinib was the first anti-MEK agent used in clinical practice. Five of the 20 evaluable subjects had a partial RECIST response, and three had stable disease, with RAS-mutated patients being better responders [225]. Subsequent clinical trials using BRAF and MEK inhibitors show promising results, with response rates ranging from 20 to 50% [226–228].

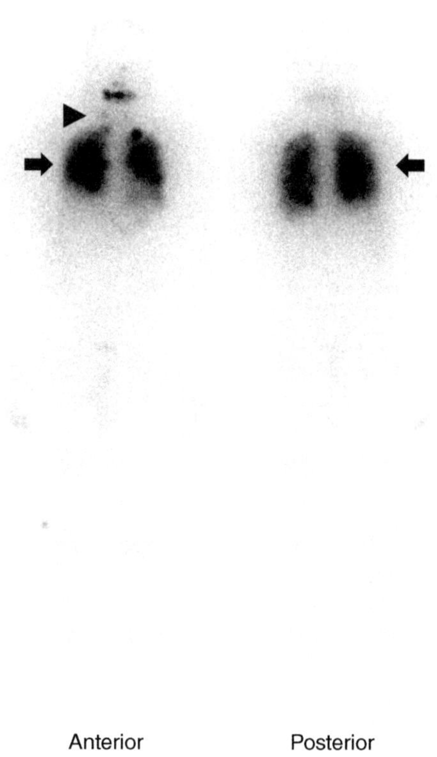


**Fig. 6.11** Post-therapy whole-body scan 7 days later demonstrated diffusely increased radioactivity in both lungs (arrow), along with increased uptake in cervical nodes (arrowhead). Tg was down trending 7 months later, at 21.3 ng/mL, with Tg Ab <0.9 IU/mL and TSH 0.14 mIU/L. CT neck and chest showed resolution or diminished size of previous cervical nodes and pulmonary nodules. The patient showed no clinical symptoms of pneumonitis or pulmonary fibrosis at this time

# References


1. Mayo CH. Pre-iodine and post-iodine days: a review of 37,228 cases of goiter at the Mayo Clinic. Western J Surg. 1935;9:477–820.
2. Lahey FH. The decisions for surgery and the management of the patient with hypertension. Surg Clin N Am. 1933;13:731–4.
3. Becker DV, Sawin CT. Radioiodine and thyroid disease: the beginning. Semin Nucl Med. 1996;26(3):155–64.
4. Saha GB. Fundamentals of nuclear pharmacy. 7th ed; 2018.
5. Cherry SR, Sorenson JA, Phelps ME. Physics in nuclear medicine. 4th ed. Saunders Elsevier; 2012.
6. Spitzweg C, Heufelder AE, Morris JC. Thyroid iodine transport. Thyroid. 2000;10(4):321–30.
7. Saito T, Endo T, Kawaguchi A, Ikeda M, Nakazato M, Kogai T, et al. Increased expression of the Na+/I- symporter in cultured human thyroid cells exposed to thyrotropin and in Graves' thyroid tissue. J Clin Endocrinol Metab. 1997;82(10):3331–6.
8. Giovanella L, Avram AM, Iakovou I, Kwak J, Lawson SA, Lulaj E, et al. EANM practice guideline/SNMMI procedure standard for RAIU and thyroid scintigraphy. Eur J Nucl Med Mol Imaging. 2019;46(12):2514–25.
9. Shapiro B, Britton K, Fountos A, Granowska M, Hawkins L, Kiriaki P, et al. A multiobserver comparison of 99mTcO4 and 123I thyroid imaging. Eur J Nucl Med. 1981;6(4):135–8.
10. Arnold JE, Pinsky S. Comparison of 99mTc and 123I for thyroid imaging. J Nucl Med. 1976;17(4):261–7.

11. Ryo UY, Vaidya PV, Schneider AB, Bekerman C, Pinsky SM. Thyroid imaging agents: a comparison of I-123 and Tc-99m pertechnetate. Radiology. 1983;148(3):819–22.
12. Shambaugh GE 3rd, Quinn JL, Oyasu R, Freinkel N. Disparate thyroid imaging. Combined studies with sodium pertechnetate Tc 99m and radioactive iodine. JAMA. 1974;228(7):866–9.
13. Szonyi G, Bowers P, Allwright S, Ellis G, Wiseman J, Cooper R, et al. A comparative study of 99mTc and 131I in thyroid scanning. Eur J Nucl Med. 1982;7(10):444–6.
14. Kusic Z, Becker DV, Saenger EL, Paras P, Gartside P, Wessler T, et al. Comparison of technetium-99m and iodine-123 imaging of thyroid nodules: correlation with pathologic findings. J Nucl Med. 1990;31(4):393–9.
15. Gharib H, Papini E, Garber JR, Duick DS, Harrell RM, Hegedus L, et al. American association of clinical endocrinologists, American college of endocrinology, and associazione medici endocrinologi medical guidelines for clinical practice for the diagnosis and management of thyroid nodules—2016 update. Endocr Pract. 2016;22(5):622–39.
16. Ross DS, Burch HB, Cooper DS, Greenlee MC, Laurberg P, Maia AL, et al. 2016 American thyroid association guidelines for diagnosis and management of hyperthyroidism and other causes of thyrotoxicosis. Thyroid. 2016;26(10):1343–421.
17. Treglia G, Annunziata S, Muoio B, Salvatori M, Ceriani L, Giovanella L. The role of fluorine-18-fluorodeoxyglucose positron emission tomography in aggressive histological subtypes of thyroid cancer: an overview. Int J Endocrinol. 2013;2013:856189.
18. Deandreis D, Al Ghuzlan A, Auperin A, Vielh P, Caillou B, Chami L, et al. Is (18) F-fluorodeoxyglucose-PET/CT useful for the presurgical characterization of thyroid nodules with indeterminate fine needle aspiration cytology? Thyroid. 2012;22(2):165–72.
19. Haugen BR, Alexander EK, Bible KC, Doherty GM, Mandel SJ, Nikiforov YE, et al. 2015 American thyroid association management guidelines for adult patients with thyroid nodules and differentiated thyroid cancer: the American thyroid association guidelines task force on thyroid nodules and differentiated thyroid cancer. Thyroid. 2016;26(1):1–133.
20. Giovanella L, Ceriani L, Treglia G. Role of isotope scan, including positron emission tomography/computed tomography, in nodular goitre. Best Pract Res Clin Endocrinol Metab. 2014;28(4):507–18.
21. Hayes AR, Crawford A, Al Riyami K, Tang C, Bomanji J, Baldeweg SE, et al. Metastatic medullary thyroid cancer: the role of 68Gallium-DOTA-somatostatin analogue PET/CT and peptide receptor radionuclide therapy. J Clin Endocrinol Metab. 2021;106(12):e4903–e16.
22. Tuncel M, Kilickap S, Suslu N. Clinical impact of (68)Ga-DOTATATE PET-CT imaging in patients with medullary thyroid cancer. Ann Nucl Med. 2020;34(9):663–74.
23. Pajak C, Cadili L, Nabata K, Wiseman SM. (68)Ga-DOTATATE-PET shows promise for diagnosis of recurrent or persistent medullary thyroid cancer: a systematic review. Am J Surg. 2022;224(2):670–5.
24. De Luca S, Fonti R, Camera L, Salvatore B, Faggiano A, Ciarmiello A, et al. Multimodal imaging with (18)F-FDG-PET/CT and (111)in-octreotide SPECT in patients with metastatic medullary thyroid carcinoma. Ann Nucl Med. 2016;30(3):234–41.
25. Ilias I, Divgi C, Pacak K. Current role of metaiodobenzylguanidine in the diagnosis of pheochromocytoma and medullary thyroid cancer. Semin Nucl Med. 2011;41(5):364–8.
26. Braverman LE. Werner & Ingbar's the thyroid. Wolters Kluwer: 11th Edition; 2020.
27. Balon HS; Meier, D.A; Charkes, N.D.; Royal, H.D.; Sarkar, S.D. Society of nuclear medicine procedure guideline for thyroid uptake measurement. Version 3.0, approved September 5, 2006. 2006.
28. Macauley M, Shawgi M, Ali T, Curry A, Howe K, Howell E, et al. Assessment of normal reference values for thyroid uptake of technetium-99m pertechnetate in a single centre UK population. Nucl Med Commun. 2018;39(9):834–8.
29. Giuffrida D, Gharib H. Controversies in the management of cold, hot, and occult thyroid nodules. Am J Med. 1995;99(6):642–50.
30. Mizukami Y, Michigishi T, Nonomura A, Yokoyama K, Noguchi M, Hashimoto T, et al. Autonomously functioning (hot) nodule of the thyroid gland. A clinical and histopathologic study of 17 cases. Am J Clin Pathol. 1994;101(1):29–35.

31. Aeschimann S, Kopp PA, Kimura ET, Zbaeren J, Tobler A, Fey MF, et al. Morphological and functional polymorphism within clonal thyroid nodules. J Clin Endocrinol Metab. 1993;77(3):846–51.
32. Apel RL, Ezzat S, Bapat BV, Pan N, LiVolsi VA, Asa SL. Clonality of thyroid nodules in sporadic goiter. Diagn Mol Pathol. 1995;4(2):113–21.
33. La Rosa GL, Belfiore A, Giuffrida D, Sicurella C, Ippolito O, Russo G, et al. Evaluation of the fine needle aspiration biopsy in the preoperative selection of cold thyroid nodules. Cancer. 1991;67(8):2137–41.
34. Belfiore A, La Rosa GL, La Porta GA, Giuffrida D, Milazzo G, Lupo L, et al. Cancer risk in patients with cold thyroid nodules: relevance of iodine intake, sex, age, and multinodularity. Am J Med. 1992;93(4):363–9.
35. Gharib H, Goellner JR, Zinsmeister AR, Grant CS, Van Heerden JA. Fine-needle aspiration biopsy of the thyroid. The problem of suspicious cytologic findings. Ann Intern Med. 1984;101(1):25–8.
36. Gharib H, Papini E. Thyroid nodules: clinical importance, assessment, and treatment. Endocrinol Metab Clin N Am. 2007;36(3):707–35. vi
37. Tessler FN, Middleton WD, Grant EG, Hoang JK, Berland LL, Teefey SA, et al. ACR thyroid imaging, reporting and data system (TI-RADS): white paper of the ACR TI-RADS Committee. J Am Coll Radiol. 2017;14(5):587–95.
38. Schroder S, Marthaler B. Autonomy and malignancy of thyroid glad tumors. A critical analysis of the literature on the existence of hyperfunctioning follicular and papillary thyroid gland carcinomas. Pathologe. 1996;17(5):349–57.
39. Schenke S, Seifert P, Zimny M, Winkens T, Binse I, Gorges R. Risk stratification of thyroid nodules using the thyroid imaging reporting and data system (TIRADS): the omission of thyroid scintigraphy increases the rate of falsely suspected lesions. J Nucl Med. 2019;60(3):342–7.
40. Giovanella L, D'Aurizio F, Campenni A, Ruggeri RM, Baldari S, Verburg FA, et al. Searching for the most effective thyrotropin (TSH) threshold to rule-out autonomously functioning thyroid nodules in iodine deficient regions. Endocrine. 2016;54(3):757–61.
41. Musholt TJ, Clerici T, Dralle H, Frilling A, Goretzki PE, Hermann MM, et al. German Association of Endocrine Surgeons practice guidelines for the surgical treatment of benign thyroid disease. Langenbeck's Arch Surg. 2011;396(5):639–49.
42. Gharib H, Papini E, Paschke R, Duick DS, Valcavi R, Hegedus L, et al. American association of clinical endocrinologists, associazione medici endocrinologi, and European thyroid association medical guidelines for clinical practice for the diagnosis and management of thyroid nodules. Endocr Pract. 2010;16(Suppl 1):1–43.
43. Patel KN, Yip L, Lubitz CC, Grubbs EG, Miller BS, Shen W, et al. The American association of endocrine surgeons guidelines for the definitive surgical management of thyroid disease in adults. Ann Surg. 2020;271(3):e21–93.
44. Mariani G, Tonacchera M, Grosso M, Orsolini F, Vitti P, Strauss HW. The role of nuclear medicine in the clinical management of benign thyroid disorders, part 1: hyperthyroidism. J Nucl Med. 2021;62(3):304–12.
45. Wiener JD. Long-term follow-up in untreated Plummer's disease (autonomous goiter). Clin Nucl Med. 1987;12(3):198–203.
46. Campbell WL, Santiago HE, Perzin KH, Johnson PM. The autonamous thyroid nodule: correlation of scan appearance and histopathology. Radiology. 1973;107(1):133–8.
47. Martino E, Bartalena L, Mariotti S, Aghini-Lombardi F, Ceccarelli C, Lippi F, et al. Radioactive iodine thyroid uptake in patients with amiodarone-iodine-induced thyroid dysfunction. Acta Endocrinol. 1988;119(2):167–73.
48. Stanbury JB, Ermans AE, Bourdoux P, Todd C, Oken E, Tonglet R, et al. Iodine-induced hyperthyroidism: occurrence and epidemiology. Thyroid. 1998;8(1):83–100.
49. Intenzo CM, dePapp AE, Jabbour S, Miller JL, Kim SM, Capuzzi DM. Scintigraphic manifestations of thyrotoxicosis. Radiographics. 2003;23(4):857–69.
50. Carnell NE, Valente WA. Thyroid nodules in Graves' disease: classification, characterization, and response to treatment. Thyroid. 1998;8(8):647–52.

51. Charkes ND. Graves' disease with functioning nodules (marine-Lenhart syndrome). J Nucl Med. 1972;13(12):885–92.
52. Meier DA, Brill DR, Becker DV, Clarke SE, Silberstein EB, Royal HD, et al. Procedure guideline for therapy of thyroid disease with (131)iodine. J Nucl Med. 2002;43(6):856–61.
53. Curran RC, Eckert H, Wilson GM. The thyroid gland after treatment of hyperthyroidism by partial thyroidectomy or iodine 131. J Pathol Bacteriol. 1958;76(2):541–60.
54. Dobyns BM, Vickery AL, Maloof F, Chapman EM. Functional and histologic effects of therapeutic doses of radioactive iodine on the thyroid of man. J Clin Endocrinol Metab. 1953;13(5):548–67.
55. Nygaard B, Hegedus L, Ulriksen P, Nielsen KG, Hansen JM. Radioiodine therapy for multinodular toxic goiter. Arch Intern Med. 1999;159(12):1364–8.
56. Nygaard B, Hegedus L, Nielsen KG, Ulriksen P, Hansen JM. Long-term effect of radioactive iodine on thyroid function and size in patients with solitary autonomously functioning toxic thyroid nodules. Clin Endocrinol. 1999;50(2):197–202.
57. Stokkel MP, Handkiewicz Junak D, Lassmann M, Dietlein M, Luster M. EANM procedure guidelines for therapy of benign thyroid disease. Eur J Nucl Med Mol Imaging. 2010;37(11):2218–28.
58. Silberstein EB, Alavi A, Balon HR, Clarke SE, Divgi C, Gelfand MJ, et al. The SNMMI practice guideline for therapy of thyroid disease with 131I 3.0. J Nucl Med. 2012;53(10):1633–51.
59. Papini E, Monpeyssen H, Frasoldati A, Hegedus L. 2020 European thyroid association clinical practice guideline for the use of image-guided ablation in benign thyroid nodules. Eur Thyroid J. 2020;9(4):172–85.
60. Wartofsky L, Glinoer D, Solomon B, Nagataki S, Lagasse R, Nagayama Y, et al. Differences and similarities in the diagnosis and treatment of Graves' disease in Europe, Japan, and the United States. Thyroid. 1991;1(2):129–35.
61. Brito JP, Schilz S, Singh Ospina N, Rodriguez-Gutierrez R, Maraka S, Sangaralingham LR, et al. Antithyroid drugs-the Most common treatment for Graves' disease in the United States: a Nationwide population-based study. Thyroid. 2016;26(8):1144–5.
62. Brito JP, Payne S, Singh Ospina N, Rodriguez-Gutierrez R, Maraka S, Sangaralingham LR, et al. Patterns of use, efficacy, and safety of treatment options for patients with Graves' disease: a Nationwide population-based study. Thyroid. 2020;30(3):357–64.
63. de Klerk JM. 131I therapy: inpatient or outpatient? J Nucl Med. 2000;41(11):1876–8.
64. Tuttle WK 3rd, Brown PH. Applying nuclear regulatory commission guidelines to the release of patients treated with sodium iodine-131. J Nucl Med Technol. 2000;28(4):275–9.
65. Stoffer SS, Hamburger JI. Inadvertent 131I therapy for hyperthyroidism in the first trimester of pregnancy. J Nucl Med. 1976;17(02):146–9.
66. Aktay R, Rezai K, Seabold JE, Bar RS, Kirchner PT. Four- to twenty-four-hour uptake ratio: an index of rapid iodine-131 turnover in hyperthyroidism. J Nucl Med. 1996;37(11): 1815–9.
67. Zhang R, Tan J, Wang R, Zhang G, Jia Q, Meng Z, et al. Analysis of risk factors of rapid thyroidal radioiodine-131 turnover in Graves' disease patients. Sci Rep. 2017;7(1):8301.
68. Mariani G, Tonacchera M, Grosso M, Fiore E, Falcetta P, Montanelli L, et al. The role of nuclear medicine in the clinical Management of Benign Thyroid Disorders, part 2: nodular goiter, hypothyroidism, and subacute thyroiditis. J Nucl Med. 2021;62(7):886–95.
69. Hanscheid H, Canzi C, Eschner W, Flux G, Luster M, Strigari L, et al. EANM dosimetry committee series on standard operational procedures for pre-therapeutic dosimetry II. Dosimetry prior to radioiodine therapy of benign thyroid diseases. Eur J Nucl Med Mol Imaging. 2013;40(7):1126–34.
70. Salvatori M, Luster M. Radioiodine therapy dosimetry in benign thyroid disease and differentiated thyroid carcinoma. Eur J Nucl Med Mol Imaging. 2010;37(4):821–8.
71. Estour B, Millot L, Vergely N, Clavier A, Dhondt O, Caillot A, et al. Efficacy of low doses of radioiodine in the treatment of autonomous thyroid nodules: importance of dose/area ratio. Thyroid. 1997;7(3):357–61.
72. Zakavi SR, Mousavi Z, Davachi B. Comparison of four different protocols of I-131 therapy for treating single toxic thyroid nodule. Nucl Med Commun. 2009;30(2):169–75.

73. Rokni H, Sadeghi R, Moossavi Z, Treglia G, Zakavi SR. Efficacy of different protocols of radioiodine therapy for treatment of toxic nodular goiter: systematic review and meta-analysis of the literature. Int J Endocrinol Metab. 2014;12(2):e14424.
74. Ferrari C, Reschini E, Paracchi A. Treatment of the autonomous thyroid nodule: a review. Eur J Endocrinol. 1996;135(4):383–90.
75. Vidal-Trecan GM, Stahl JE, Eckman MH. Radioiodine or surgery for toxic thyroid adenoma: dissecting an important decision. A cost-effectiveness analysis. Thyroid. 2004;14(11):933–45.
76. Szumowski P, Rogowski F, Abdelrazek S, Kociura-Sawicka A, Sokolik-Ostasz A. Iodine isotope (1)(3)(1)I therapy for toxic nodular goitre: treatment efficacy parameters. Nucl Med Rev Cent East Eur. 2012;15(1):7–13.
77. Hermus AR, Huysmans DA. Treatment of benign nodular thyroid disease. N Engl J Med. 1998;338(20):1438–47.
78. Pedersen-Bjergaard U, Kirkegaard C. Relationship between serum TSH and the responsiveness of toxic solitary autonomous thyroid nodules to radioiodine therapy. Eur J Endocrinol. 1998;139(6):587–90.
79. Erkan ME, Demirin H, Asik M, Celbek G, Yildirim M, Aydin Y, et al. Efficiency of radioactive I-131 therapy in geriatric patients with toxic nodular goiter. Aging Clin Exp Res. 2012;24(6):714–7.
80. Erickson D, Gharib H, Li H, van Heerden JA. Treatment of patients with toxic multinodular goiter. Thyroid. 1998;8(4):277–82.
81. Holm LE, Lundell G, Israelsson A, Dahlqvist I. Incidence of hypothyroidism occurring long after iodine-131 therapy for hyperthyroidism. J Nucl Med. 1982;23(2):103–7.
82. Yano Y, Sugino K, Akaishi J, Uruno T, Okuwa K, Shibuya H, et al. Treatment of autonomously functioning thyroid nodules at a single institution: radioiodine therapy, surgery, and ethanol injection therapy. Ann Nucl Med. 2011;25(10):749–54.
83. Becker DV, Hurley JR. Complications of radioiodine treatment of hyperthyroidism. Semin Nucl Med. 1971;1(4):442–60.
84. Ross DS. Radioiodine therapy for hyperthyroidism. N Engl J Med. 2011;364(6):542–50.
85. Clark JD, Gelfand MJ, Elgazzar AH. Iodine-131 therapy of hyperthyroidism in pediatric patients. J Nucl Med. 1995;36(3):442–5.
86. McDermott MT, Kidd GS, Dodson LE Jr, Hofeldt FD. Radioiodine-induced thyroid storm. Case report and literature review. Am J Med. 1983;75(2):353–9.
87. Snyder S. Vocal cord paralysis after radioiodine therapy. J Nucl Med. 1978;19(8):975–6.
88. Ron E, Doody MM, Becker DV, Brill AB, Curtis RE, Goldman MB, et al. Cancer mortality following treatment for adult hyperthyroidism. Cooperative thyrotoxicosis therapy follow-up study group. JAMA. 1998;280(4):347–55.
89. Dobyns BM, Sheline GE, Workman JB, Tompkins EA, McConahey WM, Becker DV. Malignant and benign neoplasms of the thyroid in patients treated for hyperthyroidism: a report of the cooperative thyrotoxicosis therapy follow-up study. J Clin Endocrinol Metab. 1974;38(6):976–98.
90. Kitahara CM, Berrington de Gonzalez A, Bouville A, Brill AB, Doody MM, Melo DR, et al. Association of radioactive iodine treatment with cancer mortality in patients with hyperthyroidism. JAMA Intern Med. 2019;179(8):1034–42.
91. Franklyn JA, Maisonneuve P, Sheppard M, Betteridge J, Boyle P. Cancer incidence and mortality after radioiodine treatment for hyperthyroidism: a population-based cohort study. Lancet. 1999;353(9170):2111–5.
92. Metso S, Auvinen A, Huhtala H, Salmi J, Oksala H, Jaatinen P. Increased cancer incidence after radioiodine treatment for hyperthyroidism. Cancer. 2007;109(10):1972–9.
93. Franklyn JA, Maisonneuve P, Sheppard MC, Betteridge J, Boyle P. Mortality after the treatment of hyperthyroidism with radioactive iodine. N Engl J Med. 1998;338(11):712–8.
94. Franklyn JA, Sheppard MC, Maisonneuve P. Thyroid function and mortality in patients treated for hyperthyroidism. JAMA. 2005;294(1):71–80.
95. Boelaert K, Maisonneuve P, Torlinska B, Franklyn JA. Comparison of mortality in hyperthyroidism during periods of treatment with thionamides and after radioiodine. J Clin Endocrinol Metab. 2013;98(5):1869–82.

96. Gronich N, Lavi I, Rennert G, Saliba W. Cancer risk after radioactive iodine treatment for hyperthyroidism: a cohort study. Thyroid. 2020;30(2):243–50.
97. Kitahara CM, Preston DL, Sosa JA, Berrington de Gonzalez A. Association of radioactive iodine, antithyroid drug, and surgical treatments with solid cancer mortality in patients with hyperthyroidism. JAMA Netw Open. 2020;3(7):e209660.
98. Thyroid Disease: Assessment and Management. U.K. National Institute for health and care excellence. Published 20 November 2019.
99. Tuttle RM, Becker DV. The Chernobyl accident and its consequences: update at the millennium. Semin Nucl Med. 2000;30(2):133–40.
100. Sisson JC, Freitas J, McDougall IR, Dauer LT, Hurley JR, Brierley JD, et al. Radiation safety in the treatment of patients with thyroid diseases by radioiodine 131I : practice recommendations of the American Thyroid Association. American Thyroid Association taskforce on Radioiodine, safety. Thyroid. 2011;21(4):335–46.
101. Siegel RL, Miller KD, Jemal A. Cancer statistics, 2017. CA Cancer J Clin. 2017;67(1):7–30.
102. Cancer Stat Facts: Thyroid Cancer. National Cancer Institute. Surveillance, epidemiology, and end result program. https://seer.cancer.gov/statfacts/html/thyro.html. Accessed 1 Oct 2022.
103. Orosco RK, Hussain T, Noel JE, Chang DC, Dosiou C, Mittra E, et al. Radioactive iodine in differentiated thyroid cancer: a national database perspective. Endocr Relat Cancer. 2019;26(10):795–802.
104. Amin MB, Edge SB, Greene FL, Byrd DR, Brookland RK, Washington MK, et al. AJCC cancer staging manual. 8th ed. Springer; 2017. ISBN: 978-3-319-40617-6
105. Durante C, Haddy N, Baudin E, Leboulleux S, Hartl D, Travagli JP, et al. Long-term outcome of 444 patients with distant metastases from papillary and follicular thyroid carcinoma: benefits and limits of radioiodine therapy. J Clin Endocrinol Metab. 2006;91(8):2892–9.
106. Lamartina L, Deandreis D, Durante C, Filetti S. ENDOCRINE TUMOURS: imaging in the follow-up of differentiated thyroid cancer: current evidence and future perspectives for a risk-adapted approach. Eur J Endocrinol. 2016;175(5):R185–202.
107. Sabra MM, Sherman EJ, Tuttle RM. Tumor volume doubling time of pulmonary metastases predicts overall survival and can guide the initiation of multikinase inhibitor therapy in patients with metastatic, follicular cell-derived thyroid carcinoma. Cancer. 2017;123(15):2955–64.
108. Cabanillas ME, McFadden DG, Durante C. Thyroid cancer. Lancet. 2016;388(10061):2783–95.
109. Porter A, Wong DJ. Perspectives on the treatment of advanced thyroid cancer: approved therapies, resistance mechanisms, and future directions. Front Oncol. 2020;10:592202.
110. Buffet C, Wassermann J, Hecht F, Leenhardt L, Dupuy C, Groussin L, et al. Redifferentiation of radioiodine-refractory thyroid cancers. Endocr Relat Cancer. 2020;27(5):R113–R32.
111. Sparano C, Moog S, Hadoux J, Dupuy C, Al Ghuzlan A, Breuskin I, et al. Strategies for radioiodine treatment: what's new. Cancers (Basel). 2022;14(15):3800.
112. Filetti S, Bidart JM, Arturi F, Caillou B, Russo D, Schlumberger M. Sodium/iodide symporter: a key transport system in thyroid cancer cell metabolism. Eur J Endocrinol. 1999;141(5):443–57.
113. Maxon HR 3rd, Smith HS. Radioiodine-131 in the diagnosis and treatment of metastatic well differentiated thyroid cancer. Endocrinol Metab Clin N Am. 1990;19(3):685–718.
114. Klain M, Ricard M, Leboulleux S, Baudin E, Schlumberger M. Radioiodine therapy for papillary and follicular thyroid carcinoma. Eur J Nucl Med Mol Imaging. 2002;29(Suppl 2):S479–85.
115. Hay ID, Bergstralh EJ, Goellner JR, Ebersold JR, Grant CS. Predicting outcome in papillary thyroid carcinoma: development of a reliable prognostic scoring system in a cohort of 1779 patients surgically treated at one institution during 1940 through 1989. Surgery. 1993;114(6):1050–7. discussion 7-8.
116. Hay ID, Grant CS, Taylor WF, McConahey WM. Ipsilateral lobectomy versus bilateral lobar resection in papillary thyroid carcinoma: a retrospective analysis of surgical outcome using a novel prognostic scoring system. Surgery. 1987;102(6):1088–95.
117. Cady B, Rossi R. An expanded view of risk-group definition in differentiated thyroid carcinoma. Surgery. 1988;104(6):947–53.

118. Dean DS, Hay ID. Prognostic indicators in differentiated thyroid carcinoma. Cancer Control. 2000;7(3):229–39.
119. Tuttle RM, Ahuja S, Avram AM, Bernet VJ, Bourguet P, Daniels GH, et al. Controversies, consensus, and collaboration in the use of (131)I therapy in differentiated thyroid cancer: a joint statement from the American thyroid association, the European association of nuclear medicine, the society of nuclear medicine and molecular imaging, and the European thyroid association. Thyroid. 2019;29(4):461–70.
120. Pacini F, Fuhrer D, Elisei R, Handkiewicz-Junak D, Leboulleux S, Luster M, et al. ETA consensus statement: what are the indications for post-surgical radioiodine therapy in differentiated thyroid cancer? Eur Thyroid J. 2022;2022:11(1).
121. Avram AM, Giovanella L, Greenspan B, Lawson SA, Luster M, Van Nostrand D, et al. SNMMI procedure standard/EANM practice guideline for nuclear medicine evaluation and therapy of differentiated thyroid cancer: abbreviated version. J Nucl Med. 2022;63(6):15N–35N.
122. Leboulleux S, Bournaud C, Chougnet CN, Zerdoud S, Al Ghuzlan A, Catargi B, et al. Thyroidectomy without Radioiodine in patients with low-risk thyroid cancer. N Engl J Med. 2022;386(10):923–32.
123. Lamartina L, Grani G, Biffoni M, Giacomelli L, Costante G, Lupo S, et al. Risk stratification of neck lesions detected Sonographically during the follow-up of differentiated thyroid cancer. J Clin Endocrinol Metab. 2016;101(8):3036–44.
124. Dizdarevic S, Tulchinsky M, McCready VR, Mihailovic J, Vinjamuri S, Buscombe JR, et al. The world association of radiopharmaceutical and molecular therapy position statement on the initial radioiodine therapy for differentiated thyroid carcinoma. World J Nucl Med. 2019;18(2):123–6.
125. Ruel E, Thomas S, Dinan M, Perkins JM, Roman SA, Sosa JA. Adjuvant radioactive iodine therapy is associated with improved survival for patients with intermediate-risk papillary thyroid cancer. J Clin Endocrinol Metab. 2015;100(4):1529–36.
126. Jonklaas J, Sarlis NJ, Litofsky D, Ain KB, Bigos ST, Brierley JD, et al. Outcomes of patients with differentiated thyroid carcinoma following initial therapy. Thyroid. 2006;16(12):1229–42.
127. Avram AM, Esfandiari NH, Wong KK. Preablation 131-I scans with SPECT/CT contribute to thyroid cancer risk stratification and 131-I therapy planning. J Clin Endocrinol Metab. 2015;100(5):1895–902.
128. Schmidt D, Szikszai A, Linke R, Bautz W, Kuwert T. Impact of 131I SPECT/spiral CT on nodal staging of differentiated thyroid carcinoma at the first radioablation. J Nucl Med. 2009;50(1):18–23.
129. Van Nostrand D, Aiken M, Atkins F, Moreau S, Garcia C, Acio E, et al. The utility of radioiodine scans prior to iodine 131 ablation in patients with well-differentiated thyroid cancer. Thyroid. 2009;19(8):849–55.
130. Chen MK, Yasrebi M, Samii J, Staib LH, Doddamane I, Cheng DW. The utility of I-123 pretherapy scan in I-131 radioiodine therapy for thyroid cancer. Thyroid. 2012;22(3):304–9.
131. Song H, Mosci C, Akatsu H, Basina M, Dosiou C, Iagaru A. Diagnostic 123I whole body scan prior to ablation of thyroid remnant in patients with papillary thyroid cancer: implications for clinical management. Clin Nucl Med. 2018;43(10):705–9.
132. Lee SW. SPECT/CT in the treatment of differentiated thyroid cancer. Nucl Med Mol Imaging. 2017;51(4):297–303.
133. Lind P, Kohlfurst S. Respective roles of thyroglobulin, radioiodine imaging, and positron emission tomography in the assessment of thyroid cancer. Semin Nucl Med. 2006;36(3):194–205.
134. Sisson JC, Avram AM, Lawson SA, Gauger PG, Doherty GM. The so-called stunning of thyroid tissue. J Nucl Med. 2006;47(9):1406–12.
135. McDougall IR, Iagaru A. Thyroid stunning: fact or fiction? Semin Nucl Med. 2011;41(2):105–12.
136. Thyroid Carcinoma. NCCN Clinical Practice Guidelines in Oncology. Version 2.2024—March 2024. Assessed 1 Apr 2024.

137. ACR–ACNM–ASTRO–SNMMI–SPR Pratice Parameter For Treatment of Benign and Malignant Thyroid Disease With I-131 Sodium Iodide. Adopted 2019 (Resolution 37).
138. Singer MC, Marchal F, Angelos P, Bernet V, Boucai L, Buchholzer S, et al. Salivary and lacrimal dysfunction after radioactive iodine for differentiated thyroid cancer: American head and neck society endocrine surgery section and salivary gland section joint multidisciplinary clinical consensus statement of otolaryngology, ophthalmology, nuclear medicine and endocrinology. Head Neck. 2020;42(11):3446–59.
139. Benua RS, Cicale NR, Sonenberg M, Rawson RW. The relation of radioiodine dosimetry to results and complications in the treatment of metastatic thyroid cancer. Am J Roentgenol Radium Therapy Nucl Med. 1962;87:171–82.
140. Maxon HR, Thomas SR, Hertzberg VS, Kereiakes JG, Chen IW, Sperling MI, et al. Relation between effective radiation dose and outcome of radioiodine therapy for thyroid cancer. N Engl J Med. 1983;309(16):937–41.
141. Maxon HR 3rd, Englaro EE, Thomas SR, Hertzberg VS, Hinnefeld JD, Chen LS, et al. Radioiodine-131 therapy for well-differentiated thyroid cancer--a quantitative radiation dosimetric approach: outcome and validation in 85 patients. J Nucl Med. 1992;33(6):1132–6.
142. Klubo-Gwiezdzinska J, Van Nostrand D, Atkins F, Burman K, Jonklaas J, Mete M, et al. Efficacy of dosimetric versus empiric prescribed activity of 131I for therapy of differentiated thyroid cancer. J Clin Endocrinol Metab. 2011;96(10):3217–25.
143. Sgouros G, Song H, Ladenson PW, Wahl RL. Lung toxicity in radioiodine therapy of thyroid carcinoma: development of a dose-rate method and dosimetric implications of the 80-mCi rule. J Nucl Med. 2006;47(12):1977–84.
144. Deandreis D, Rubino C, Tala H, Leboulleux S, Terroir M, Baudin E, et al. Comparison of empiric versus whole-body/-blood clearance dosimetry-based approach to radioactive iodine treatment in patients with metastases from differentiated thyroid cancer. J Nucl Med. 2017;58(5):717–22.
145. Jentzen W, Nahum AE, Bockisch A, Binse I, Tulchinsky M. Fixed 3.7-GBq (131)I activity for metastatic thyroid cancer therapy ignores science and history. J Nucl Med. 2017;58(9):1530.
146. Tulchinsky M, Gross LJ. Comparison of empiric versus dosimetry-guided Radioiodine therapy: the devil is in the details. J Nucl Med. 2017;58(5):863.
147. Flux GD, Verburg FA, Chiesa C, Bardies M, Gleisner KS, Hertz B, et al. Comparison of empiric versus dosimetry-guided Radioiodine therapy: the devil is in the details. J Nucl Med. 2017;58(5):862.
148. Strigari L, Konijnenberg M, Chiesa C, Bardies M, Du Y, Gleisner KS, et al. The evidence base for the use of internal dosimetry in the clinical practice of molecular radiotherapy. Eur J Nucl Med Mol Imaging. 2014;41(10):1976–88.
149. Plyku D, Hobbs RF, Huang K, Atkins F, Garcia C, Sgouros G, et al. Recombinant human thyroid-stimulating hormone versus thyroid hormone withdrawal in (124)I PET/CT-based dosimetry for (131)I therapy of metastatic differentiated thyroid cancer. J Nucl Med. 2017;58(7):1146–54.
150. Giovanella L, Duntas LH. Management of endocrine disease: the role of rhTSH in the management of differentiated thyroid cancer: pros and cons. Eur J Endocrinol. 2019;181(4):R133–R45.
151. U.S. Nuclear Regulatory Commission. Regulatory guide 8.39. Revision 1, April 2020. https://www.nrc.gov/docs/ML1923/ML19232A081.pdf.
152. Release of patients administered radioactive material. U.S. Nuclear Regulatory Commission. Regulatory Guide 8.39, Revision 1. April 2020.
153. Vrachimis A, Riemann B, Mader U, Reiners C, Verburg FA. Endogenous TSH levels at the time of (131)I ablation do not influence ablation success, recurrence-free survival or differentiated thyroid cancer-related mortality. Eur J Nucl Med Mol Imaging. 2016;43(2):224–31.
154. Potzi C, Moameni A, Karanikas G, Preitfellner J, Becherer A, Pirich C, et al. Comparison of iodine uptake in tumour and nontumour tissue under thyroid hormone deprivation

and with recombinant human thyrotropin in thyroid cancer patients. Clin Endocrinol. 2006;65(4):519–23.
155. Freudenberg LS, Jentzen W, Petrich T, Fromke C, Marlowe RJ, Heusner T, et al. Lesion dose in differentiated thyroid carcinoma metastases after rhTSH or thyroid hormone withdrawal: 124I PET/CT dosimetric comparisons. Eur J Nucl Med Mol Imaging. 2010;37(12):2267–76.
156. THYROGEN® (thyrotropin alfa) for injection, for intramuscular use. Highlights of prescribing Informtion. Initial U.S. Approval: 1998. Revised 03/2020.
157. Lamartina L, Durante C, Filetti S, Cooper DS. Low-risk differentiated thyroid cancer and radioiodine remnant ablation: a systematic review of the literature. J Clin Endocrinol Metab. 2015;100(5):1748–61.
158. Solans R, Bosch JA, Galofre P, Porta F, Rosello J, Selva-O'Callagan A, et al. Salivary and lacrimal gland dysfunction (sicca syndrome) after radioiodine therapy. J Nucl Med. 2001;42(5):738–43.
159. Alexander C, Bader JB, Schaefer A, Finke C, Kirsch CM. Intermediate and long-term side effects of high-dose radioiodine therapy for thyroid carcinoma. J Nucl Med. 1998;39(9):1551–4.
160. Grewal RK, Larson SM, Pentlow CE, Pentlow KS, Gonen M, Qualey R, et al. Salivary gland side effects commonly develop several weeks after initial radioactive iodine ablation. J Nucl Med. 2009;50(10):1605–10.
161. Almeida JP, Sanabria AE, Lima EN, Kowalski LP. Late side effects of radioactive iodine on salivary gland function in patients with thyroid cancer. Head Neck. 2011;33(5):686–90.
162. An YS, Yoon JK, Lee SJ, Song HS, Yoon SH, Jo KS. Symptomatic late-onset sialadenitis after radioiodine therapy in thyroid cancer. Ann Nucl Med. 2013;27(4):386–91.
163. Schlumberger M, Catargi B, Borget I, Deandreis D, Zerdoud S, Bridji B, et al. Strategies of radioiodine ablation in patients with low-risk thyroid cancer. N Engl J Med. 2012;366(18):1663–73.
164. Lee SM, Lee JW, Kim SY, Han SW, Bae WK. Prediction of risk for symptomatic sialadenitis by post-therapeutic dual (131)I scintigraphy in patients with differentiated thyroid cancer. Ann Nucl Med. 2013;27(8):700–9.
165. Wu JQ, Feng HJ, Ouyang W, Sun YG, Chen P, Wang J, et al. Systematic evaluation of salivary gland damage following I-131 therapy in differentiated thyroid cancer patients by quantitative scintigraphy and clinical follow-up. Nucl Med Commun. 2015;36(8):819–26.
166. Maruoka Y, Baba S, Isoda T, Kitamura Y, Abe K, Sasaki M, et al. A functional scoring system based on salivary gland scintigraphy for evaluating salivary gland dysfunction secondary to (131)I therapy in patients with differentiated thyroid Carcinoma. J Clin Diagn Res. 2017;11(8):TC23–TC8.
167. Allweiss P, Braunstein GD, Katz A, Waxman A. Sialadenitis following I-131 therapy for thyroid carcinoma: concise communication. J Nucl Med. 1984;25(7):755–8.
168. Nakada K, Ishibashi T, Takei T, Hirata K, Shinohara K, Katoh S, et al. Does lemon candy decrease salivary gland damage after radioiodine therapy for thyroid cancer? J Nucl Med. 2005;46(2):261–6.
169. Christou A, Papastavrou E, Merkouris A, Frangos S, Tamana P, Charalambous A. Clinical studies of nonpharmacological methods to minimize salivary gland damage after Radioiodine therapy of differentiated thyroid Carcinoma: systematic review. Evid Based Complement Alternat Med. 2016;2016:6795076.
170. Dottorini ME, Lomuscio G, Mazzucchelli L, Vignati A, Colombo L. Assessment of female fertility and carcinogenesis after iodine-131 therapy for differentiated thyroid carcinoma. J Nucl Med. 1995;36(1):21–7.
171. Yaish I, Azem F, Gutfeld O, Silman Z, Serebro M, Sharon O, et al. A single radioactive iodine treatment has a deleterious effect on ovarian Reserve in Women with thyroid cancer: results of a prospective pilot study. Thyroid. 2018;28(4):522–7.
172. van Velsen EFS, Visser WE, van den Berg SAA, Kam BLR, van Ginhoven TM, Massolt ET, et al. Longitudinal analysis of the effect of Radioiodine therapy on ovarian Reserve in Females with differentiated thyroid cancer. Thyroid. 2020;30(4):580–7.

173. Wu JX, Young S, Ro K, Li N, Leung AM, Chiu HK, et al. Reproductive outcomes and nononcologic complications after radioactive iodine ablation for well-differentiated thyroid cancer. Thyroid. 2015;25(1):133–8.
174. Russo D, Scipioni A, Durante C, Ferretti E, Gandini L, Maggisano V, et al. Expression and localization of the sodium/iodide symporter (NIS) in testicular cells. Endocrine. 2011;40(1):35–40.
175. Poppe K, Bisschop P, Fugazzola L, Minziori G, Unuane D, Weghofer A. 2021 European thyroid association guideline on thyroid disorders prior to and during assisted reproduction. Eur Thyroid J. 2021;9(6):281–95.
176. Canale D, Ceccarelli C, Caglieresi C, Moscatelli A, Gavioli S, Santini P, et al. Effects of radioiodine treatment for differentiated thyroid cancer on testis function. Clin Endocrinol. 2015;82(2):295–9.
177. Dong P, Wang L, Huang R, Li L. Bone marrow suppression in pediatric patients with differentiated thyroid cancer following empirical radioiodine therapy. Medicine (Baltimore). 2020;99(31):e21398.
178. Robeson WR, Ellwood JE, Margulies P, Margouleff D. Outcome and toxicity associated with maximum safe dose radioiodine treatment of metastatic thyroid cancer. Clin Nucl Med. 2002;27(8):556–66.
179. Tuttle RM, Leboeuf R, Robbins RJ, Qualey R, Pentlow K, Larson SM, et al. Empiric radioactive iodine dosing regimens frequently exceed maximum tolerated activity levels in elderly patients with thyroid cancer. J Nucl Med. 2006;47(10):1587–91.
180. Duskin-Bitan H, Leibner A, Amitai O, Diker-Cohen T, Hirsch D, Benbassat C, et al. Bone-marrow suppression in elderly patients following empiric Radioiodine therapy: real-life data. Thyroid. 2019;29(5):683–91.
181. Prinsen HT, Klein Hesselink EN, Brouwers AH, Plukker JT, Sluiter WJ, van der Horst-Schrivers AN, et al. Bone marrow function after (131)I therapy in patients with differentiated thyroid Carcinoma. J Clin Endocrinol Metab. 2015;100(10):3911–7.
182. Padovani RP, Tuttle RM, Grewal R, Larson SM, Boucai L. Complete blood counts are frequently abnormal 1 year after dosimetry-guided radioactive iodine therapy for metastatic thyroid cancer. Endocr Pract. 2014;20(3):213–20.
183. Bikas A, Schneider M, Desale S, Atkins F, Mete M, Burman KD, et al. Effects of dosimetrically guided I-131 therapy on hematopoiesis in patients with differentiated thyroid cancer. J Clin Endocrinol Metab. 2016;101(4):1762–9.
184. Molinaro E, Leboeuf R, Shue B, Martorella AJ, Fleisher M, Larson S, et al. Mild decreases in white blood cell and platelet counts are present one year after radioactive iodine remnant ablation. Thyroid. 2009;19(10):1035–41.
185. Petrich T, Widjaja A, Musholt TJ, Hofmann M, Brunkhorst T, Ehrenheim C, et al. Outcome after radioiodine therapy in 107 patients with differentiated thyroid carcinoma and initial bone metastases: side-effects and influence of age. Eur J Nucl Med. 2001;28(2):203–8.
186. Hebestreit H, Biko J, Drozd V, Demidchik Y, Burkhardt A, Trusen A, et al. Pulmonary fibrosis in youth treated with radioiodine for juvenile thyroid cancer and lung metastases after chernobyl. Eur J Nucl Med Mol Imaging. 2011;38(9):1683–90.
187. Albano D, Bertagna F, Panarotto MB, Giubbini R. Early and late adverse effects of radioiodine for pediatric differentiated thyroid cancer. Pediatr Blood Cancer. 2017;64(11):e26595.
188. Souza MC, Momesso DP, Vaisman F, Vieira Neto L, Martins RA, Corbo R, et al. Is radioactive iodine-131 treatment related to the occurrence of non-synchronous second primary malignancy in patients with differentiated thyroid cancer? Arch Endocrinol Metab. 2016;60(1):9–15.
189. Bhattacharyya N, Chien W. Risk of second primary malignancy after radioactive iodine treatment for differentiated thyroid carcinoma. Ann Otol Rhinol Laryngol. 2006;115(8):607–10.
190. Hall P, Holm LE, Lundell G, Bjelkengren G, Larsson LG, Lindberg S, et al. Cancer risks in thyroid cancer patients. Br J Cancer. 1991;64(1):159–63.
191. Verkooijen RB, Smit JW, Romijn JA, Stokkel MP. The incidence of second primary tumors in thyroid cancer patients is increased, but not related to treatment of thyroid cancer. Eur J Endocrinol. 2006;155(6):801–6.

192. Kim S, Bang JI, Boo D, Kim B, Choi IY, Ko S, et al. Second primary malignancy risk in thyroid cancer and matched patients with and without radioiodine therapy analysis from the observational health data sciences and informatics. Eur J Nucl Med Mol Imaging. 2022;49(10):3547–56.
193. Lang BH, Wong IO, Wong KP, Cowling BJ, Wan KY. Risk of second primary malignancy in differentiated thyroid carcinoma treated with radioactive iodine therapy. Surgery. 2012;151(6):844–50.
194. Teng CJ, Hu YW, Chen SC, Yeh CM, Chiang HL, Chen TJ, et al. Use of radioactive iodine for thyroid cancer and risk of second primary malignancy: a Nationwide population-based study. J Natl Cancer Inst. 2016;108(2):djv314.
195. Silva-Vieira M, Carrilho Vaz S, Esteves S, Ferreira TC, Limbert E, Salgado L, et al. Second primary cancer in patients with differentiated thyroid cancer: does Radioiodine play a role? Thyroid. 2017;27(8):1068–76.
196. Khang AR, Cho SW, Choi HS, Ahn HY, Yoo WS, Kim KW, et al. The risk of second primary malignancy is increased in differentiated thyroid cancer patients with a cumulative (131)I dose over 37 GBq. Clin Endocrinol. 2015;83(1):117–23.
197. Rubino C, de Vathaire F, Dottorini ME, Hall P, Schvartz C, Couette JE, et al. Second primary malignancies in thyroid cancer patients. Br J Cancer. 2003;89(9):1638–44.
198. Sawka AM, Thabane L, Parlea L, Ibrahim-Zada I, Tsang RW, Brierley JD, et al. Second primary malignancy risk after radioactive iodine treatment for thyroid cancer: a systematic review and meta-analysis. Thyroid. 2009;19(5):451–7.
199. Pasqual E, Schonfeld S, Morton LM, Villoing D, Lee C, Berrington de Gonzalez A, et al. Association between radioactive iodine treatment for pediatric and Young adulthood differentiated thyroid cancer and risk of second primary malignancies. J Clin Oncol. 2022;40(13):1439–49.
200. Iyer NG, Morris LG, Tuttle RM, Shaha AR, Ganly I. Rising incidence of second cancers in patients with low-risk (T1N0) thyroid cancer who receive radioactive iodine therapy. Cancer. 2011;117(19):4439–46.
201. Molenaar RJ, Sidana S, Radivoyevitch T, Advani AS, Gerds AT, Carraway HE, et al. Risk of hematologic malignancies after Radioiodine treatment of well-differentiated thyroid cancer. J Clin Oncol. 2018;36(18):1831–9.
202. Little MP, Wakeford R, Borrego D, French B, Zablotska LB, Adams MJ, et al. Leukaemia and myeloid malignancy among people exposed to low doses (<100 mSv) of ionizing radiation during childhood: a pooled analysis of nine historical cohort studies. Lancet Haematol. 2018;5(8):e346–e58.
203. Zhao X, Chen M, Qi X, Zhu H, Yang G, Guo Y, et al. Association of radioiodine for differentiated thyroid cancer and second breast cancer in female adolescent and Young adult. Front Endocrinol (Lausanne). 2021;12:805194.
204. Nappi C, Klain M, Cantoni V, Green R, Piscopo L, Volpe F, et al. Risk of primary breast cancer in patients with differentiated thyroid cancer undergoing radioactive iodine therapy: a systematic review and meta-analysis. Eur J Nucl Med Mol Imaging. 2022;49(5):1630–9.
205. Reinecke MJ, Ahlers G, Burchert A, Eilsberger F, Flux GD, Marlowe RJ, et al. Second primary malignancies induced by radioactive iodine treatment of differentiated thyroid carcinoma—a critical review and evaluation of the existing evidence. Eur J Nucl Med Mol Imaging. 2022;49(9):3247–56.
206. Fallahi B, Adabi K, Majidi M, Fard-Esfahani A, Heshmat R, Larijani B, et al. Incidence of second primary malignancies during a long-term surveillance of patients with differentiated thyroid carcinoma in relation to radioiodine treatment. Clin Nucl Med. 2011;36(4):277–82.
207. Tran TV, Rubino C, Allodji R, Andruccioli M, Bardet S, Diallo I, et al. Breast cancer risk among thyroid cancer survivors and the role of I-131 treatment. Br J Cancer. 2022;127(12):2118–24.
208. Gonzalez Carvalho JM, Gorlich D, Schober O, Wenning C, Riemann B, Verburg FA, et al. Evaluation of (131)I scintigraphy and stimulated thyroglobulin levels in the follow up of

patients with DTC: a retrospective analysis of 1420 patients. Eur J Nucl Med Mol Imaging. 2017;44(5):744–56.
209. Schlumberger M, Brose M, Elisei R, Leboulleux S, Luster M, Pitoia F, et al. Definition and management of radioactive iodine-refractory differentiated thyroid cancer. Lancet Diabetes Endocrinol. 2014;2(5):356–8.
210. Simoes-Pereira J, Mourinho N, Ferreira TC, Limbert E, Cavaco BM, Leite V. Avidity and outcomes of Radioiodine therapy for distant metastasis of distinct types of differentiated thyroid cancer. J Clin Endocrinol Metab. 2021;106(10):e3911–e22.
211. Kim HJ, Lee JI, Kim NK, Min YK, Kim SW, Chung JH. Prognostic implications of radioiodine avidity and serum thyroglobulin in differentiated thyroid carcinoma with distant metastasis. World J Surg. 2013;37(12):2845–52.
212. Lang BH, Wong KP, Cheung CY, Wan KY, Lo CY. Evaluating the prognostic factors associated with cancer-specific survival of differentiated thyroid carcinoma presenting with distant metastasis. Ann Surg Oncol. 2013;20(4):1329–35.
213. Kammori M, Fukumori T, Sugishita Y, Hoshi M, Shimizu K, Yamada T. Radioactive iodine (RAI) therapy for distantly metastatic differentiated thyroid cancer (DTC) in juvenile versus adult patients. Endocr J. 2015;62(12):1067–75.
214. Hirsch D, Levy S, Tsvetov G, Gorshtein A, Slutzky-Shraga I, Akirov A, et al. Long-term outcomes and prognostic factors in patients with differentiated thyroid cancer and distant metastases. Endocr Pract. 2017;23(10):1193–200.
215. Kreissl MC, Janssen MJR, Nagarajah J. Current treatment strategies in metastasized differentiated thyroid cancer. J Nucl Med. 2019;60(1):9–15.
216. Nixon IJ, Ganly I, Patel SG, Palmer FL, Di Lorenzo MM, Grewal RK, et al. The results of selective use of radioactive iodine on survival and on recurrence in the management of papillary thyroid cancer, based on Memorial Sloan-Kettering Cancer Center risk group stratification. Thyroid. 2013;23(6):683–94.
217. Pacini F, Cetani F, Miccoli P, Mancusi F, Ceccarelli C, Lippi F, et al. Outcome of 309 patients with metastatic differentiated thyroid carcinoma treated with radioiodine. World J Surg. 1994;18(4):600–4.
218. Sabra MM, Dominguez JM, Grewal RK, Larson SM, Ghossein RA, Tuttle RM, et al. Clinical outcomes and molecular profile of differentiated thyroid cancers with radioiodine-avid distant metastases. J Clin Endocrinol Metab. 2013;98(5):E829–36.
219. Liu J, Liu R, Shen X, Zhu G, Li B, Xing M. The genetic duet of BRAF V600E and TERT promoter mutations robustly predicts loss of Radioiodine avidity in recurrent papillary thyroid cancer. J Nucl Med. 2020;61(2):177–82.
220. Cancer Genome Atlas Research N. Integrated genomic characterization of papillary thyroid carcinoma. Cell. 2014;159(3):676–90.
221. Durante C, Puxeddu E, Ferretti E, Morisi R, Moretti S, Bruno R, et al. BRAF mutations in papillary thyroid carcinomas inhibit genes involved in iodine metabolism. J Clin Endocrinol Metab. 2007;92(7):2840–3.
222. Anekpuritanang T, Uataya M, Claimon A, Laokulrath N, Pongsapich W, Pithuksurachai P. The association between Radioiodine refractory in papillary thyroid Carcinoma, sodium/iodide symporter expression, and BRAF (V600E) mutation. Onco Targets Ther. 2021;14:3959–69.
223. Tirro E, Martorana F, Romano C, Vitale SR, Motta G, Di Gregorio S, et al. Molecular alterations in thyroid cancer: from bench to clinical practice. Genes (Basel). 2019;10(9):709.
224. Lamartina L, Anizan N, Dupuy C, Leboulleux S, Schlumberger M. Redifferentiation-facilitated radioiodine therapy in thyroid cancer. Endocr Relat Cancer. 2021;28(10):T179–T91.
225. Ho AL, Grewal RK, Leboeuf R, Sherman EJ, Pfister DG, Deandreis D, et al. Selumetinib-enhanced radioiodine uptake in advanced thyroid cancer. N Engl J Med. 2013;368(7):623–32.
226. Rothenberg SM, Daniels GH, Wirth LJ. Redifferentiation of iodine-refractory BRAF V600E-mutant metastatic papillary thyroid cancer with Dabrafenib-response. Clin Cancer Res. 2015;21(24):5640–1.

227. Huillard O, Tenenbaum F, Clerc J, Goldwasser F, Groussin L. Restoring Radioiodine uptake in BRAF V600E-mutated papillary thyroid cancer. J Endocr Soc. 2017;1(4):285–7.
228. Dunn LA, Sherman EJ, Baxi SS, Tchekmedyian V, Grewal RK, Larson SM, et al. Vemurafenib Redifferentiation of BRAF mutant, RAI-refractory thyroid cancers. J Clin Endocrinol Metab. 2019;104(5):1417–28.

# Part II
# Thyroid Ablation

# Chapter 7
# Guidelines for Thyroid Ablation

**Wen-Chieh Chen and Wei-Che Lin**

## Definition of Guideline and Consensus

A clinical guideline consists of recent medical research with high-quality evidence and references from leading experts in the specific field of healthcare, with summarized statements or recommendations on the practice. Each recommendation is often graded according to the strength of evidence available, for example, as *high, moderate,* or *low* [1]. Different strengths of agreement/recommendation by the attending experts are presented (e.g., dividing into the levels of *strong, weak* recommendation, and *not recommended*). The guideline often includes tables that compare diagnostic examinations and treatments and flow charts or checklists for the clinician to follow. Guidelines are mainly written for doctors, but also for nurses, and other healthcare professionals. By defining the important questions in clinical practice, a guideline identifies contents regarding prevention and diagnosis, and categorizes possible treatment options and outcomes. It also weighs the benefits, harms, and cost-effectiveness of each diagnostic procedure and treatment. It helps

W.-C. Chen
Department of Internal Medicine, Division of Endocrinology and Metabolism, Kaohsiung Chang Gung Memorial Hospital, Kaohsiung, Taiwan
e-mail: chingjing@cgmh.org.tw

W.-C. Lin (✉)
Department of Diagnostic Radiology, Kaohsiung Chang Gung Memorial Hospital, Chang Gung University College of Medicine, Kaohsiung, Taiwan

Thyroid Head and Neck Ablation Center, Kaohsiung Chang Gung Memorial Hospital, Kaohsiung, Taiwan

College of Medicine, National Sun Yat-Sen University, Kaohsiung, Taiwan
e-mail: alex@cgmh.org.tw



A. W. Park et al. (eds.), *Thyroid Radiofrequency Ablation*,
https://doi.org/10.1007/978-3-031-65288-2_7

the practitioner decide on appropriate management and helps to ensure that patients receive appropriate treatment and care [2].

Consensuses comprise evidence- and community-based statements on particular medical knowledge and are reached by a representative group of experts. Although it also provides a recommendation with a different grade, a consensus is less likely to provide specific algorithms. Each country or region must develop a consensus that fits its local healthcare system.

## Origin of Thyroid RFA Guidelines

Minimally invasive treatments (MITs), including ultrasound (US)-guided radiofrequency ablation (RFA), are widely applied to thyroid lesions. There is a growing body of data that can be used to formulate guidelines and consensuses for the management of thyroid nodules and differentiated thyroid cancer (DTC). As a modern technology, the American Thyroid Association's 2015 guidelines for the management of thyroid nodules and DTC discussed the use of RFA, for locally recurrent thyroid cancer, with a description of the outcomes mentioned in existing literature at the time. Since the role of RFA was still being explored, it was regarded as most helpful in high-risk surgical patients or patients refusing additional surgery, rather than as a standard alternative to surgical resection [3]. More and more guidelines dedicated to RFA were published in the following years. The guidelines written in English and mainly presented by national representative societies or associations in the last decade are presented in this chapter.

A thorough understanding of currently available guidelines is fundamental for interventionalists to build an RFA program. Data regarding indications, pre- and post-procedural evaluations, treatment techniques, the need to obtain informed consent, and efficacy are most mentioned. Differences in the methodology of guideline formation and RFA indications between guidelines are worth paying attention to.

## Summary of Guidelines

### *KsThR 2017 Guideline*

Presented by the Task Force Committee of the Korean Society of Thyroid Radiology (KSThR), the KSThR guidelines for thyroid RFA were first developed in 2012 [4] using the modified Delphi method [5] and subsequently revised in 2017 [6]. Guideline recommendations are graded as strong, weak, or not recommended according to the level of evidence regarding net benefit, as determined by the Delphi Score. When there is a lack of evidence or limited evidence, an insufficient grading is applied. However, despite high Delphi scores, the strength of a recommendation can be downgraded according to committee consensus [7].

The KSThR 2017 guideline is question-oriented, and it evaluates the use of RFA for both benign nodules and recurrent thyroid cancer. For thyroid nodules, the guideline initially established the requirement of at least two US-guided fine-needle aspiration (FNA) or core needle biopsy (CNB) to confirm benignity before RFA. It also stated that a single benign diagnosis on FNA or CNB is sufficient when the US features of a nodule are highly specific for benignity (*strong recommendation*) or in the case of an autonomously functioning thyroid nodule (AFTNs; *weak recommendation*). Regarding recurrent thyroid cancers, both the 2012 and 2017 guidelines suggest RFA for patients at high surgical risk or for those who refuse surgery. Physicians should evaluate RFA for curative or palliative purposes for patients with cancer. Pre- and post-procedural checklists and checklists for informed consent are also provided within the guideline. For patients taking anticoagulants or antiplatelet drugs before RFA, low levels of evidence were presented, based mainly on previous studies related to gastrointestinal procedures.

The guideline includes a section that describes the appropriate techniques for RFA, which include the trans-isthmic approach and the moving-shot technique. Specific techniques, including peri-nodal lidocaine injection and hydrodissection, are recommended for RFA of recurrent thyroid cancers. The KSThR 2017 guideline also compares the efficiency of ethanol ablation (EA) to that of RFA for the treatment of cystic nodules. It includes a summary of the recommendations, and it further declares RFA as an effective first-line treatment for solid and predominantly solid nodules; EA is recommended as a first-line treatment method for cystic nodules. Situations requiring additional treatment after a single RFA session were also discussed, such as marginal regrowth and remaining cosmetic or symptomatic problems. Debuted as an earlier large guideline, the KSThR 2017 guideline provides a comprehensive evaluation of RFA and has been cited worldwide.

## *Italy MITT Group 2019 Consensus*

In February 2018, the Italian minimally invasive treatments of the thyroid (MITT) group was founded in Milan, Italy, to create cooperation between Italian and international physicians. A Delphi-based consensus regarding MITs for benign thyroid nodules was published in 2019. In addition to the strength of the recommendation, this guideline listed the number of participants that agreed, disagreed, or abstained from each statement. The main content was not much different from previous guidelines, but it concluded with a comprehensive discussion. The management of predominantly cystic nodules and solid nodules were discussed separately. The MITT group recommended a double cytological analysis to confirm benignity before ablation, unless the nodule US appearance is at low risk of malignancy (EU-TIRADS 3) and in AFTN, where a single cytological sample can be achieved before ablation. Thus, the guideline pointed out the necessity of controlled studies to better clarify this issue. Regarding US follow-up after thermal ablation, the MITT group strongly agreed that modalities such as color Doppler or contrast-enhanced US can better differentiate the ablated area. Regarding the RFA of AFTNs, the group agreed on the preferential use of thermal ablation in young patients or patients with subclinical hyperthyroidism and incomplete suppression of normal thyroid tissue to spare thyroid function [8].

In 2022, the MITT group published recommendations for information to patients and referring physicians, with reference to new research within the previous 2 years. In addition to answers to frequently asked questions, the pros and cons of MITs as compared with surgery and radioactive iodine (RAI) treatment (the latter refers to AFTN), were discussed [9].

## Germany 2020 Consensus

In 2020, a consensus was established in Germany regarding the nonsurgical and non-RAI techniques available to treat benign nodules [10]. The Thyroid Section of the German Society for Endocrinology, the Thyroid Working Committee of the German Society for Nuclear Medicine, and the German Association of Endocrine Surgeons came together to develop recommendations that would help both physicians and patients with their decision-making. In addition to RFA, the published report also listed principles, indications, and complications of other techniques, including EA, microwave, laser, and high-intensity focused ultrasound (HIFU) ablation. It proposed that all candidate patients be examined as accurately as those who undergo surgery, such that calcitonin screening and laryngoscopy are mandatory (*strong recommendation*).

The Germany 2020 consensus is more restrictive than other guidelines regarding patient selection, and it clearly defines patient groups in which nonsurgical and non-RAI techniques are not recommended, such as nodules demonstrating Thyroid Imaging Reporting and Data System (TIRADS) and European TIRADS (EU-TIRADS) category 5. Patients with suspicious cervical lymph nodes, follicular neoplasm, high-risk or proven malignancy, and suspicious molecular markers (such as the BRAFV600E mutation) are also not suitable for these procedures (*strong recommendation*).

## ETA 2020 Guideline

The European Thyroid Association (ETA) clinical practice guideline was published in 2020, focusing primarily on benign thyroid nodules, with some mention of EA and other thermal ablations. It divided the recommendation level into strong and weak, and the quality of the evidence grading is given as follows: *very-low, low, moderate,* and *high*. In addition to the presentation of modalities and techniques, the guideline also provided cost estimates of thermal ablation treatments in Europe. For patient eligibility, it stated that thermal ablation should never be performed on nodules with high-risk ultrasound (US features) (EU-TIRADS category 5). Since medullary thyroid cancer may not display suspicious US features or unambiguous cytological findings, determining calcitonin levels was recommended in the evaluation before RFA. The follow-up strategy was similar to previous guidelines. Prolonged regular biochemical follow-up was suggested for AFTN. The guideline also listed the leading predictive factors for recurrence, and it noted the importance of a repeat cytological assessment before retreatment, since nodule regrowth could be a potential sign of overlooked malignancy.

Additional comparisons of outcomes among the different techniques for benign nonfunctioning nodules were made. Based on direct comparison studies, laser ablation (LA) and RFA were recommended as first-line treatment modalities (*strong recommendation*). In the contrast, the ETA guideline suggests that HIFU should be considered only for selected patients who are not suitable for RFA and LA, considering its lower efficacy, higher cost, and limited supporting evidence [11].

## *ACTA 2021 Guideline*

In 2021, the Asian Conference on Tumor Ablation (ACTA) Task Force published recommendations for RFA of benign thyroid nodules. The committee comprised experts from various participating countries and used the modified Delphi method to provide an evidence-based consensus. It was question-oriented and provides discussion and consensus according to a comprehensive analysis of the current literature through August 2019. For example, no definitive cutoff value was available for the size of a benign thyroid nodule suitable for RFA.

It discussed several US stratification systems including the American College of Radiology (ACR) Thyroid Imaging Reporting and Data System (TIRADS), European TIRADS (EU-TIRADS), American Association of Clinical Endocrinologists/American College of Endocrinology and Associazione Medici Endocrinologi (AACE/ACE-AME) medical guideline, and KSThR TIRADS (K-TIRADS). This was the first transnational thyroid RFA consensus, based on an analysis of the similarities and differences among five different countries [12]. In June of the same year, the ACTA guideline was published again in the official journal of the Chinese Taipei Society of Ultrasound in Medicine [13].

## *ETA/CRISE 2021 Guideline*

Many of the earlier guidelines focused on benign nodules. In 2021, the European Thyroid Association (ETA) and Cardiovascular and Interventional Radiological Society of Europe (CIRSE) established guidelines for MITs of malignant thyroid lesions, including both papillary thyroid microcarcinoma (PTMC) and locally recurrent thyroid cancer. The recommendation was ranked as strong and weak. The evidence grading progressed from *very-low, low, moderate,* to *high-quality*. In addition to active surveillance for PTMC, US-guided MITs can achieve good efficacy, prevent the anxiety caused by awareness of harboring a tumor, and were proposed as alternative options to surgery for selected incidental PTMCs. EA and HIFU were not recommended for the treatment of PTMC in the ETA/CIRSE 2021 guideline.

A multidisciplinary team was assembled to assess the individual characteristics of patients with current thyroid malignancy who are eligible for MITs. The guideline presented the criteria for the selection of oncologic patients for MITs. In patients who are a high surgical risk or who refuse surgery, MITs should be considered as a palliative procedure to rapidly decrease tumor burden and improve local symptoms. MIT may be considered in the following conditions: PTMC, unresectable thyroid cancer, neck lymph-node recurrent DTC, and distant metastases. Patients with extensive aggressive disease, central neck involvement, painful metastases, or liver (<3 cm) or lung (<2 cm) metastases can be considered for thermal ablation as a palliative option. The potential of combining thermal ablation with bone consolidation and external beam radiation therapy to treat painful bone metastases was discussed [14]. These recommendations are similar to the 2015 American Thyroid Association (ATA) guidelines, mentioning that unifocal metastatic and recurrent disease can be considered for percutaneous ablation in high-risk patients or those refusing surgery [3].

## *French 2022 Consensus*

The SFE-AFCE-SFMN 2022 consensus on thyroid thermal ablation was established jointly by the French Society of Endocrinology (SFE), the French Association of Endocrine Surgery (AFCE), and the French Society of Nuclear Medicine (SFMN). The consensus suggested absolute contraindications of thermal ablation for nodules as follows: EU-TIRADS 5 nodules >10 mm in size, cytologically indeterminate or malignant (Bethesda class III–VI), toxic multinodular goiters, Graves' disease, and multinodular goiters without a dominant nodule. The contraindications are more stringent and specific than other guidelines. The French consensus discussed a recent issue: thermal ablation for the treatment of hyperthyroidism. Thermal ablation for hyperthyroidism was suggested mainly for autonomous, preferably single nodules in a patient with a thyroid stimulating hormone (TSH) level less than 0.3 μIU/mL. Young patients with a desire for pregnancy, or with persistent uptake in the remaining thyroid parenchyma after RAI, could be considered for thermal ablation. If used as the first- line management, the volume of the nodule should be less than 5–10 mL. A combination of thermal ablation with RAI and ethanol injection was also discussed.

On the other hand, MITs for thyroid cancer was mentioned. Active surveillance is now commonly proposed as an alternative to surgery in selected cases, but it is not always well accepted. Thermal ablation is applied successfully in this indication, whereas FNA is not recommended for EU-TIRADS 5 nodules measuring less than

10 mm, The SFE-AFCE-SFMN 2022 consensus suggests cytological evidence (Bethesda class VI) is essential before considering thermal ablation of a suspected microcarcinoma [15].

## 2022 International Multidisciplinary Consensus

An international multidisciplinary consensus statement directed by the American Head and Neck Society and enrolled multiple societies from USA, Europe, and Asia was published in 2022. A literature search identified eight sentinel articles with the clinical application of thyroid ablation technologies to guide the search, followed by a comprehensive librarian-directed search. A modified Delphi method was applied, and a two-rounded anonymous electronic survey was distributed to the full panel. The scoring section was different from other guidelines; the results were then analyzed using a numerical scale ranging from 1 (strongly disagree) to 9 (strongly agree). Statements were defined as achieving consensus if there was a mean score of 7.0 or greater and 0–2 outlier responses, or a mean greater than or equal to 7.0 and three outliers with no outlier value lower than 5 (neutral). Non-consensus was the default if these criteria were not met.

The management of indeterminate nodules with RFA is not recommended. For recurrent malignancies, if as a curative strategy, the number of lesions must be limited (≤3 foci), confined to the neck, and with a maximum tumor diameter <1.5–2 cm. For the palliative purpose, larger tumors can be targeted with RFA if a reduction in symptoms and an improvement in the quality of life are feasible. More specifically, voice and laryngeal assessment and anticoagulant management strategies are provided in this consensus statement. Patient positioning and the operational setup for the RFA procedure are illustrated. A comparison of efficacy and complexity of ablative techniques (EA and thermal ablations) for solid, predominantly cystic, functional nodules, and PTMC is provided. The international consensus aims to reduce variation in practice and promote responsible global dissemination of the techniques [16].

## Taiwan 2022 Consensus

During late 2022, experts from the Taiwan Academy of Tumor Ablation (TATA), the Endocrine Society of Taiwan, the Taiwan Society of Interventional Radiology (TSIR), and the Taiwan Association of Endocrine Surgeons gathered to develop the first consensus regarding thyroid RFA in Taiwan. The modified Delphi method was applied, with two-round, anonymous, online voting among committee members. A nine-point scale was applied, using the median voting value to decide the level of recommendation. Statements with a high or moderate level of evidence and a median score of 7 or greater were defined as *strong recommendations*. Statements with high or moderate evidence but a median score of 4–6, or those with low evidence levels but more consensus (score ≥ 7) were defined as *weak recommendations*. The Taiwan 2022consensus discusses indications, techniques, efficacy, and complications of benign and malignant thyroid lesions. Most recommendations of indications in the consensus echoed previous guidelines and also referred to the consensus of local experts. A single, benign diagnosis on FNA or CNB is considered insufficient for the confirmation of benignity in AFTN before RFA. In patients with primary thyroid cancer above T1bN0M0, RFA is not recommended due to the current lack of high-quality evidence and discrepant expert opinions [17].

## Conclusion

Several articles with an appraisal or general discussion of the guidelines for thyroid RFA are presented [18–20]. Thyroid RFA is an operator-dependent procedure, and the paths to procedural competence vary according to specific training experiences and clinical practice. Consensus differences within the categories of indications, techniques, and follow-up strategies have been identified. Among so many guidelines, physicians should choose the most appropriate one, based on the individual characteristics of the patient, and follow the medical routine in the region where they practice.

Scientific progress may change the view on the methods of guideline formation. It is worth noting that the content of the guidelines can change, and is usually revised periodically over time with the release of new evidence. New evidence regarding the specificity and sensitivity of diagnostic methods, or the efficacy of management at a longer follow-up period, and the emergence of new therapeutic targets (such as the exploration of locally advanced thyroid cancer) all prompt physicians to follow the latest guidelines. Finally, a guideline must not be legally binding or regarded as the only method. The clinical application needs to be determined by individual conditions, the physician's practice, and willingness of the patient.

## References

1. Gopalakrishna G, et al. Guidelines for guideline developers: a systematic review of grading systems for medical tests. Implement Sci. 2013;8:78.
2. Panteli D, et al. Clinical practice guidelines as a quality strategy. National Institutes of Health, Health Policy Series, 2019. No. 53. https://www.ncbi.nlm.nih.gov/books/NBK549283/.
3. Haugen BR, et al. 2015 American thyroid association management guidelines for adult patients with thyroid nodules and differentiated thyroid cancer: the American thyroid association guidelines task force on thyroid nodules and differentiated thyroid cancer. Thyroid. 2016;26(1):1–133. https://doi.org/10.1089/thy.2015.0020.
4. Na DG, et al. Radiofrequency ablation of benign thyroid nodules and recurrent thyroid cancers: consensus statement and recommendations. Korean J Radiol. 2012;13(2):117–25.

5. Steurer J. The Delphi method: an efficient procedure to generate knowledge. Skeletal Radiol. 2011;40(8):959–61.
6. Kim JH, et al. 2017 thyroid radiofrequency ablation guideline: Korean society of thyroid radiology. Korean J Radiol. 2018;19(4):632–55.
7. Kim JH, et al. Summary of the 2017 thyroid radiofrequency ablation guideline and comparison with the 2012 guideline. Ultrasonography (Seoul, Korea). 2019;38(2):125–34.
8. Papini E, et al. Minimally-invasive treatments for benign thyroid nodules: a Delphi-based consensus statement from the Italian minimally-invasive treatments of the thyroid (MITT) group. Int J Hyperth. 2019;36(1):376–82.
9. Mauri G, et al. Minimally-invasive treatments for benign thyroid nodules: recommendations for information to patients and referring physicians by the Italian minimally-invasive treatments of the thyroid group. Endocrine. 2022;76(1):1–8.
10. Feldkamp J, et al. Non-surgical and non-radioiodine techniques for ablation of benign thyroid nodules: consensus statement and recommendation. Exp Clin Endocrinol Diabetes. 2020;128(10):687–92.
11. Papini E, et al. 2020 European thyroid association clinical practice guideline for the use of image-guided ablation in benign thyroid nodules. Eur Thyroid J. 2020;9(4):172–85.
12. Ha EJ, et al. Radiofrequency ablation of benign thyroid nodules: recommendations from the Asian Conference on Tumor Ablation Task Force. Ultrasonography (Seoul, Korea). 2021;40(1):75–82.
13. Ha EJ, et al. Radiofrequency ablation of benign thyroid nodules: recommendations from the Asian conference on tumor ablation task force—secondary publication. J Med Ultrasound. 2021;29(2):77–83.
14. Mauri G, et al. European thyroid association and cardiovascular and interventional radiological society of Europe 2021 clinical practice guideline for the use of minimally invasive treatments in malignant thyroid lesions. Eur Thyroid J. 2021;10(3):185–97.
15. Ben Hamou A, et al. SFE-AFCE-SFMN 2022 consensus on the management of thyroid nodules: thermal ablation. Ann Endocrinol. 2022;83(6):423–30.
16. Orloff LA, et al. Radiofrequency ablation and related ultrasound-guided ablation technologies for treatment of benign and malignant thyroid disease: an international multidisciplinary consensus statement of the American head and neck society endocrine surgery section with the Asia pacific society of thyroid surgery, associazione medici endocrinologi, British association of endocrine and thyroid surgeons, European thyroid association, Italian society of endocrine surgery units, Korean society of thyroid radiology, Latin American thyroid society, and thyroid nodules therapies association. Head Neck. 2022;44(3):633–60.
17. Lin W-C, et al. Taiwan expert consensus and recommendations for thyroid radiofrequency ablation. Ultrasonography (Seoul, Korea). 2023;42(3):357–75. https://doi.org/10.14366/usg.22126.
18. Suresh NV, et al. Quality appraisal of clinical practice guidelines for the use of radiofrequency ablation in the treatment of thyroid nodules and cancer. Am J Otolaryngol. 2022;43(4):103508.
19. Huber TC. Review of the Korean society of interventional radiology and European thyroid association guidelines regarding the role of radiofrequency ablation for benign and malignant thyroid tumors. Tech Vasc Interv Radiol. 2022;25(2):100817.
20. Lee M, et al. Clinical practice guidelines for radiofrequency ablation of benign thyroid nodules: a systematic review. Ultrasonography (Seoul, Korea). 2021;40(2):256–64.

# Chapter 8
# Image-Guided Thyroid Ablation: Standard Terminology and Reporting Criteria

**Giovanni Mauri**

Image-guided tumor ablation is a commonly performed procedure, used to treat many malignant diseases, such as liver disease (both primary and metastatic) and kidney, lung, or bone lesions. Therefore, in 2003 a document titled "Image-Guided Tumor Ablation: Proposal for Standardization of Terms and Reporting Criteria" [1] was published by the International Working Group on Image-Guided Tumor Ablation, aiming to standardize terminology and data collection to enable a more reliable comparison among the different studies arising on image-guided ablation. In more recent years, the application of image-guided ablations has expanded to include benign conditions, such as benign thyroid nodules [2–7]. However, further inhomogeneity in how data were presented and reported among different studies arose on this matter; Thyroid ablation became highly popular, not only among radiologists but also among other specialists involved in thyroid care, including endocrinologists and surgeons. For this purpose, in 2019, a proposal for the standardization of terminology and reporting criteria on image-guided ablations of benign thyroid nodules based on the previously published document of 2003 was presented by the Italian Working Group on Minimally Invasive Treatments of the Thyroid [8]. In the present chapter, the specific issues related to benign thyroid nodule ablation are discussed, while for the general concepts regarding ablation of cancerous lesions please refer to the 2014 update of the original document [9].

G. Mauri (✉)
Unit of Diagnostic and Interventional Radiology, IRCCS Ospedale Galeazzi - Sant'Ambrogio, Milan, Italy


A. W. Park et al. (eds.), *Thyroid Radiofrequency Ablation*,
https://doi.org/10.1007/978-3-031-65288-2_8

## General Definitions: Review

In the current literature, thyroid ablation therapies have been defined with a series of different terms. According to the 2014 guidelines [9], the term "image-guided ablation" is proposed to identify this kind of procedure. Other terms such as "minimally invasive" or "percutaneous" should be avoided, as they can also identify other types of treatments (e.g., surgical treatments) and could be misleading. When referring to a single intervention, the use of the term "procedure" is recommended. Instead, "course of treatment" should be used to define a series of ablations performed at different time points as a part of a predetermined treatment plan. Devices for image-guided thermal ablation should be generally defined as "applicators" and if an internal cooling is used, the term "internally cooled applicator" should be used.

## Specific Items Related to Image-Guided Ablation of Benign Thyroid Nodules

### *Indications*

Indication(s) for treatment should be reported (e.g., compression symptoms, cosmetic reasons, abnormal thyroid function, others) in all studies [10].

### *Nodule Description*

Currently, no standardized classification of thyroid nodules according to the percentage of solid component has been adopted and nodule classification might vary among different studies. Therefore, a detailed description of the internal structure of each treated nodule should be stated each time. The adoption of the following classification is suggested:

- Solid (<10% of fluid component).
- Predominantly solid (11–50% of fluid component).
- Predominantly cystic (51–90% of fluid component).
- Cystic (>90% of fluid component).

If the cystic portion is aspirated prior to the procedure, it should be stated as such. As a "spongiform" appearance of nodules has been reported to be correlated with benign nodules, it is proposed that "spongiform nodules" be reported differently from other nodules. Spongiform nodules are defined as those nodules containing multiple small cysts <5 mm interspersed within solid tissue for nearly all the volume [10–12].

## *Nodule Size*

Nodule volume should be expressed in milliliters (mL) using the ellipsoid volume formula:

$$\text{Lenght} \times \text{Width} \times \text{Depth} \times 0.524$$

with measures expressed in centimeters. Moreover, nodules should also be classified according to their size. Several different cutoffs have been proposed [3, 5, 10]. To increase uniformity, nodules should be identified as small (<10 mL), medium (11–30 mL), or large (>30 mL) as appropriate.

## *Blood Tests*

Common blood tests performed prior to each procedure should always include thyrotropin (TSH) and free thyroxine (fT4). Free triiodothyronine (fT3) should also be performed in case of TSH and fT4 abnormalities. If fT4 and fT3 are not available in a specific setting, total T4 and total T3 can be performed [10].

## *Finality of Treatment*

To correctly define the "technical success" for each procedure, the treatment goal should be defined by the authors a priori, for example, to achieve a nodular volume ablation of 50% at a specific time point, etc. A 50% volumetric reduction at 1 year is proposed as a reasonable threshold for defining technical success. For autonomously functioning thyroid nodules, the technical purpose of treatment should be to achieve the largest possible extent of nodule ablation to destroy the largest amount of autonomously functioning thyroid tissue, with a proposed threshold of at least 80% nodule volume destruction to define technical success. In association with such a threshold, it should be stressed that the ultimate treatment goal in this case is to achieve a satisfactory normalization of thyroid function.

## *Type of Ablation*

Image-guided thyroid ablation procedures can be performed with several techniques, adopting either thermal energy or chemical agents such as ethanol instillation.

## Energy-Based Ablation

Different types of energy can be used to perform thyroid image-guided thermal ablation [7]. Currently, the most commonly used techniques include radiofrequency ablation (RFA) and laser ablation. Fewer studies have included the adoption of microwave ablation (MWA) or high-intensity focused ultrasound (HIFU-US). The use of definitions other than those provided above is discouraged, as they might be misleading. When referring to all these ablation methods, energy should be reported as "applied." All other definitions (e.g., "irradiation" or "deliverance" and their derivatives) should be avoided, as they can be misleading.

- RFA: RFA applicators should be referred to as "electrodes." Monopolar electrodes are commonly used for this procedure. However, in cases where bipolar electrodes or other modifications are used, this should be noted as such. A description of the applicator should include length, active component, and size expressed preferably by their gauge. Due to the different types of applicators among vendors (e.g., straight tip, umbrella-shape, Christmas tree-shape, other), the exact design of the applicator should be always specified [13].
- Laser ablation: Laser type and precise light wavelength should be specified. Laser ablation applicators should be referred to as "fibers." The number of simultaneous fiber insertions, the type of fibers (e.g., flexible or glass-dome), tip design, and fiber length and diameter should be included in the applicators' description.
- MWA: MWA applicators should be referred to as "antennas." The length of the antennas, active component, and diameter expressed by gauge size should be included in the applicator's description.
- HIFU: The type of guidance for HIFU (e.g., ultrasound (US) or magnetic resonance) and the features of HIFU generator transducer (e.g., frequency, diameter, single, or multiple elements) should be specified.

## Chemical Ablation

This term refers to the use of a chemical agent for the treatment of cystic or predominantly cystic nodules. These procedures should be identified by the name of the chemical agent used followed by the word "ablation," such as ethanol ablation, which is the most common procedure. All other definitions should be avoided. It should always be stated whether the treatment is completed immediately as one procedure or whether it is split into different phases (e.g., nodule aspiration and ablation performed in two different sessions). If treatment is divided into more than one session a priori, then completion of all steps of the procedure will constitute technical success. If different from cyst/nodule shrinkage, any other intended effect should be reported [9, 14, 15].

## Procedure Details

Whenever used, the type, amount, and technique of local anesthesia and/or conscious sedation should be clearly documented. The intra-procedural use of other drugs (e.g., intravenous steroids, nonsteroidal anti-inflammatory drugs [NSAIDs], or painkillers) should be disclosed with justification of their adjuvant use. The adoption of ancillary procedures such as hydrodissection should be declared and thoroughly explained. The technical approach to the nodule should be specified. When the approach to the nodule is through the thyroid isthmus, keeping some normal thyroid tissue in between the nodule and the thyroid capsule puncture site, the adoption of the term "trans-isthmic" is suggested [16]. When the nodule allows a direct puncture approach to achieve a shorter path or insertion along the major axis, the term "direct nodule puncture" is suggested [17]. In case multiple ablations are planned, with multiple expected movements of the applicator into the thyroid nodule to be treated, the term "moving-shot" technique should be used [16, 17]. If treatment planning involves the insertion of the applicator(s) in the deepest part of the nodule, with an eventual subsequent ablation of the more superficial part of the nodule by a simple retraction of the applicator(s), the term "pull-back" technique should be adopted [15]. When a single insertion and ablation is expected, the term "fixed-applicator" technique is suggested [16]. Regarding energy-based ablations, energy application parameters should be provided (i.e., power, duration of application, energy applied per volume, and/or total amount of applied energy). In case of chemical-based ablations, it is recommended to report the concentration and amount of the used chemical agent (e.g., 95% ethanol) and the type and size of needle. The method of delivery should also be stated (e.g., "aspiration of fluid component immediately followed by chemical injection" or "aspiration followed by saline washing and subsequent chemical injection") and also whether ethanol is either re-aspirated after injection or left inside the cavity.

## Results

### *Technical Success*

This term indicates whether the nodule was treated according to the initial planned protocol. With this term, nodules that were treated according to a predefined protocol can be differentiated from those where protocol could not be completed due to a specific reason (which should be stated).

### *Technique Efficacy*

Distinction between technical success and technique efficacy is essential. By the latter term, the ability of the treatment to achieve a predetermined clinical result is indicated and should be assessed using specific clinical or instrumental parameters.

In the setting of ablation of benign nodules, technique efficacy should be defined as a volumetric reduction ≥50% of the initial nodule volume, that is:

$$\frac{\text{Final nodule volume} - \text{Initial volume}}{\text{Initial nodule volume}} \times 100$$

Moreover, the technique efficacy should be always related to specific follow-up time points. Generally, a minimum follow-up of 1 year is considered optimal. Ideally, long-term follow-up should be reported, with a proposed time interval of 1 year after the first year. Primary efficacy rate is defined as the percentage of nodules successfully treated following the initial procedure or at the end of the planned course of treatment. Secondary efficacy rate should include nodules that have undergone successful retreatment after continued nodule regrowth. Nodule regrowth should be defined as nodule volume increase of ≥50% compared to the minimum volume measured at a given follow-up time point [2, 18, 19]. Although some authors have proposed considering the regrowth of nodule periphery as a marker of recurrence, this parameter is not of easy evaluation and difficult to standardize with conventional US techniques [19–21]. For autonomously functioning nodules, a volumetric reduction of at least 80% of the initial nodule volume is proposed as the preferred target for technique efficacy. However, the ultimate goal of treatment for these nodules is to achieve satisfactory normalization of thyroid function [22–25]. In general, nodule volume is evaluated with US as the method of choice, while contrast-enhanced US may provide a more precise evaluation of the ablated area immediately after the procedure.

## *Clinical Success*

By this term, as thyroid ablation is aimed to treat a benign condition (mainly resulting in compression symptoms or cosmetic concerns), a form of novel concept is introduced. The notion of clinical success should be defined as the ability of treatment to resolve the condition itself. Therefore, it is recommended to classify clinical success as:

- Complete (i.e., complete resolution of presenting symptoms).
- Partial (i.e., symptom improvement but still present).
- Absent (i.e., no symptom improvement).

Furthermore, a validated visual analog scale (grade 0–10) may be used to have a semi-quantitative assessment of treatment [10]. Cosmetic assessment should be ideally performed on the basis of a four-point scale [10]:

- 1 = no palpable mass
- 2 = palpable mass without cosmetic problems

- 3 = cosmetic problems on swallowing only
- 4 = visible mass.

For autonomously functioning thyroid nodules, clinical success is defined as the normalization of serum thyroid hormones and TSH followed by the suspension of oral therapy.

## *Procedure-Related Adverse Events*

Regarding adverse events, their assessment is proposed through a combination of the Society of Interventional Radiology (SIR) standardized grading system [26] and the Image-Guided Tumor Ablation: Standardization of Terminology and Reporting Criteria-A 10-Year Update [9]. Adverse events should be reported on a *per session* and *per patient* basis, and their severity should be reported. They should be classified as major complications, minor complications, and side effects. An unexpected event leading to substantial morbidity and disability, which also increases the level of care, should be regarded as a "major complication." All other unexpected adverse events should be regarded as minor. Side effects are defined as those adverse events that are potentially anticipated during or after a procedure and do not result in long-term clinical sequelae. Therefore, peri- or post-procedural discomfort and/or pain that is or is not treated with local ice and/or oral NSAIDs and/or pain-killers and that does not increase the expected level of care should be considered as a side effect and not as a minor complication. Our proposed grading scale for adverse events associated with thyroid thermal ablations is reported in Table 8.1. Events should be also differentiated as immediate (0–24 h), peri-procedural (1–30 days), and delayed (>30 days) [9].

**Table 8.1** Proposed modified classification system for adverse events by outcome in thyroid nodule ablation

| Type | Grade | Description | Occurrence |
|---|---|---|---|
| Side effects | A0 | Undesired events that are somewhat expected during or after a procedure | Unexpected |
| Minor complications | A | No therapy, no consequence | Expected |
| | B | Nominal therapy, no consequence; includes overnight admission for observation only | |
| Major complications | C | Require therapy, minor hospitalization (<48 h) | |
| | D | Require major therapy, unplanned increase in level of care, prolonged hospitalization (>48 h) | |
| | E | Permanent adverse sequelae | |
| | F | Death | |

Note: This table is reported in Mauri et al. [8] as a modification of Table 8.2 reported in the SIR Classification System for Complications by Outcome [26] in combination with what was described in the Image-Guided Tumor Ablation: Standardization of Terminology and Reporting Criteria-A 10-Year Update report concerning side effects [9]

## Follow-Up

As the treatment effect on benign thyroid nodules can only be appreciated over time, results should be reported at standard time points to make results comparable among different studies. Treatment results should be reported at early (between 1 and 3 months), intermediate (6 months), and 1 year follow-up. Afterwards, reporting annual follow-up data for long-term studies is suggested. At each follow-up, the same variables of baseline should be reported. Regarding blood tests, at least, the TSH test should be performed at every reported follow-up. Common topics and reporting criteria for image-guided ablations of benign thyroid nodules are reported in Table 8.2.

**Table 8.2** Common topics and reporting criteria for image-guided ablations of benign thyroid nodules

| Topic | Reporting criteria |
|---|---|
| 1. Indications | Compression symptoms palliation/aesthetic concerns/normalization of thyroid function |
| 2. Patient information | Demographics<br>Relevant comorbidities<br>Inclusion/exclusion criteria<br>Additional previous/ongoing treatments for the same condition; blood tests (fT3, fT4, TSH) |
| 3. Nodule features | Solid, predominantly solid, predominantly cystic, cystic, spongiform<br>Volume in milliliters: Small (<10 mL), medium (11–30 mL), and large (>30 mL) |
| 4. Type of ablation | |
| Energy-based ablation | Device name/model/manufacturer |
| Radiofrequency | Monopolar, bipolar, multipolar<br>Length, active exposure, size (in gauge)<br>Electrode design (straight tip, others) |
| Laser | Type of laser<br>Light wavelength<br>Fiber design and size (in gauge) |
| Microwave | Length, active component, size (in gauge) |
| HIFU | Type of guidance, features of the HIFU generator transducer |
| Chemical ablation | Concentration/amount of chemical agent<br>Type/size of needle (in gauge)<br>Method of delivery<br>Single/multiple phases |
| 5. Procedure details | |
| Anesthesia | Local anesthesia and/or conscious sedation |
| Adjuvant drugs | If any, provide full details |
| Ancillary procedures | Hydrodissection, other |
| Technique | Direct puncture/trans-isthmic<br>Moving shot/pull-back/fixed applicator |

(continued)

**Table 5** (continued)

| Topic | Reporting criteria |
|---|---|
| 6. Energy parameters | Power, duration of application, and total amount of applied energy |
| 7. Results | Technique efficacy<br>Primary efficacy rate<br>Secondary or assisted efficacy rate<br>Nodule regrowth |
| Clinical success | Complete/partial/absent |
| Adverse events | Major complications/minor complications/side effects; immediate (0–24 h)/peri-procedural (1–30 days)/delayed (>30 days) |
| 8. Follow-up | Early (1–3 months)/intermediate (6 months)/1 year/annual follow-up |

Note: *fT3* free triiodothyronine, *fT4* free thyroxine, *TSH* thyrotropin, *HIFU* high-intensity focused ultrasound
The table is reported from Mauri et al. [8]

## Result Stratification

Treatment results might be affected by the amount of solid tissue in the nodule. Therefore, a stratification according to nodule internal structure (i.e., solid, predominantly solid, mixed solid and cystic, predominantly cystic, cystic, spongiform) should be always performed when results are presented.

## Conclusion

The present chapter on "Image-Guided Thyroid Ablation: Proposal for Standardization of Terminology and Reporting Criteria" intends to provide guidance for standardizing benign thyroid nodule ablation procedures. Its adoption is encouraged to facilitate communication and understanding within the field and stimulate further discussion and confrontation on the topic over the coming years.

## References

1. Goldberg SN, Charboneau JW, Dodd GD, Dupuy DE, Gervais DA, Gillams AR, Kane RA, Lee FT, Livraghi T, McGahan JP, et al. Image-guided tumor ablation: proposal for standardization of terms and reporting criteria. Radiology. 2003;228:335–45. https://doi.org/10.1148/radiol.2282021787.
2. Lim HK, Lee JH, Ha EJ, Sung JY, Kim JK, Baek JH. Radiofrequency ablation of benign non-functioning thyroid nodules: 4-year follow-up results for 111 patients. Eur Radiol. 2013;23:1044–9. https://doi.org/10.1007/s00330-012-2671-3.
3. Cesareo R, Naciu AM, Iozzino M, Pasqualini V, Simeoni C, Casini A, Campagna G, Manfrini S, Tabacco G, Palermo A. Nodule size as predictive factor of efficacy of radiofrequency abla-

tion in treating autonomously functioning thyroid nodules. Int J Hyperth. 2018;34:617–23. https://doi.org/10.1080/02656736.2018.1430868.
4. Pacella CM, Mauri G, Cesareo R, Paqualini V, Cianni R, De Feo P, Gambelunghe G, Raggiunti B, Tina D, Deandrea M, et al. A comparison of laser with radiofrequency ablation for the treatment of benign thyroid nodules: a propensity score matching analysis. Int J Hyperth. 2017;33:911–9. https://doi.org/10.1080/02656736.2017.1332395.
5. Pacella CM, Mauri G, Achille G, Barbaro D, Bizzarri G, De Feo P, Di Stasio E, Esposito R, Gambelunghe G, Misischi I, et al. Outcomes and risk factors for complications of laser ablation for thyroid nodules: a multicenter study on 1531 patients. J Clin Endocrinol Metab. 2015;100:3903–10. https://doi.org/10.1210/jc.2015-1964.
6. Mauri G, Cova L, Monaco CG, Sconfienza LM, Corbetta S, Benedini S, Ambrogi F, Milani V, Baroli A, Ierace T, et al. Benign thyroid nodules treatment using percutaneous laser ablation (PLA) and radiofrequency ablation (RFA). Int J Hyperth. 2017;33:295–9. https://doi.org/10.1080/02656736.2016.1244707.
7. Mainini AP, Monaco C, Pescatori LC, De Angelis C, Sardanelli F, Sconfienza LM, Mauri G. Image-guided thermal ablation of benign thyroid nodules. J Ultrasound. 2017;20:11–22. https://doi.org/10.1007/s40477-016-0221-6.
8. Mauri G, Pacella CM, Papini E, Solbiati L, Goldberg SN, Ahmed M, Sconfienza LM. Image-guided thyroid ablation: proposal for standardization of terminology and reporting criteria. Thyroid. 2019;29:611–8. https://doi.org/10.1089/thy.2018.0604.
9. Ahmed M, Solbiati L, Brace CL, Breen DJ, Callstrom MR, Charboneau JW, Chen M-H, Choi BI, de Baère T, Dodd GD, et al. Image-guided tumor ablation: standardization of terminology and reporting criteria—a 10-year update. J Vasc Interv Radiol. 2014;25:1691–1705.e4. https://doi.org/10.1016/j.jvir.2014.08.027.
10. Kim J, Baek JH, Lim HK, Ahn HS, Baek SM, Choi YJ, Choi YJ, Chung SR, Ha EJ, Hahn SY, et al. 2017 thyroid radiofrequency ablation guideline: Korean society of thyroid radiology. Korean J Radiol. 2018;19:632. https://doi.org/10.3348/kjr.2018.19.4.632.
11. Durante C, Grani G, Lamartina L, Filetti S, Mandel SJ, Cooper DS. The diagnosis and Management of Thyroid Nodules. JAMA. 2018;319:914. https://doi.org/10.1001/jama.2018.0898.
12. Andrioli M, Carzaniga C, Persani L. Standardized ultrasound report for thyroid nodules: the Endocrinologist's viewpoint. Eur Thyroid J. 2013;2:37–48. https://doi.org/10.1159/000347144.
13. Pescatori LC, Torcia P, Nicosia L, Mauri G, Rossi UG, Cariati M. Which needle in the treatment of thyroid nodules? Gland Surg. 2018;7:111–6. https://doi.org/10.21037/gs.2018.01.03.
14. Park HS, Yim Y, Baek JH, Choi YJ, Shong YK, Lee JH. Ethanol ablation as a treatment strategy for benign cystic thyroid nodules: a comparison of the ethanol retention and aspiration techniques. Ultrasonography. 2019;38:166–71. https://doi.org/10.14366/usg.18033.
15. Papini E, Gugliemi R, Pacella CM. Laser, radiofrequency, and ethanol ablation for the management of thyroid nodules. Curr Opin Endocrinol Diabetes Obes. 2016;23:400–6. https://doi.org/10.1097/MED.0000000000000282.
16. Ha EJ, Baek JH, Lee JH. Moving-shot versus fixed electrode techniques for radiofrequency ablation: comparison in an ex-vivo bovine liver tissue model. Korean J Radiol. 2014;15:836. https://doi.org/10.3348/kjr.2014.15.6.836.
17. Cervelli R, Mazzeo S, De Napoli L, Boccuzzi A, Pontillo-Contillo B, Materazzi G, Miccoli P, Cioni R, Caramella D. Radiofrequency ablation in the treatment of benign thyroid nodules: an efficient and safe alternative to surgery. J Vasc Interv Radiol. 2017;28:1400–8. https://doi.org/10.1016/j.jvir.2017.07.009.
18. Haugen BR, Alexander EK, Bible KC, Doherty GM, Mandel SJ, Nikiforov YE, Pacini F, Randolph GW, Sawka AM, Schlumberger M, et al. 2015 American thyroid association management guidelines for adult patients with thyroid nodules and differentiated thyroid cancer: the American thyroid association guidelines task force on thyroid nodules and differentiated thyroid cancer. Thyroid. 2016;26:1–133. https://doi.org/10.1089/thy.2015.0020.

19. Sim JS, Baek JH, Lee J, Cho W, Jung S. Il radiofrequency ablation of benign thyroid nodules: depicting early sign of regrowth by calculating vital volume. Int J Hyperth. 2017;33:905–10. https://doi.org/10.1080/02656736.2017.1309083.
20. Suh CH, Baek JH, Ha EJ, Choi YJ, Lee JH, Kim JK, Chung KW, Kim TY, Kim WB, Shong YK. Ethanol ablation of predominantly cystic thyroid nodules: evaluation of recurrence rate and factors related to recurrence. Clin Radiol. 2015;70:42–7. https://doi.org/10.1016/j.crad.2014.09.008.
21. Wang B, Han ZY, Yu J, Cheng Z, Liu F, Yu XL, Chen C, Liu J, Liang P. Factors related to recurrence of the benign non-functioning thyroid nodules after percutaneous microwave ablation. Int J Hyperth. 2017;33:459–64. https://doi.org/10.1080/02656736.2016.1274058.
22. Pacella CM, Mauri G. Is there a role for minimally invasive thermal ablations in the treatment of autonomously functioning thyroid nodules? Int J Hyperth. 2018;34:636–8. https://doi.org/10.1080/02656736.2018.1462537.
23. Gambelunghe G, Stefanetti E, Colella R, Monacelli M, Avenia N, De Feo P. A single session of laser ablation for toxic thyroid nodules: three-year follow-up results. Int J Hyperth. 2018;34:631–5. https://doi.org/10.1080/02656736.2018.1437931.
24. Amabile G, Rotondi M, Pirali B, Dionisio R, Agozzino L, Lanza M, Buonanno L, Di Filippo B, Fonte R, Chiovato L. Interstitial laser photocoagulation for benign thyroid nodules: time to treat large nodules. Lasers Surg Med. 2011;43:797–803. https://doi.org/10.1002/lsm.21114.
25. Bernardi S, Stacul F, Michelli A, Giudici F, Zuolo G, de Manzini N, Dobrinja C, Zanconati F, Fabris B. 12-month efficacy of a single radiofrequency ablation on autonomously functioning thyroid nodules. Endocrine. 2017;57:402–8. https://doi.org/10.1007/s12020-016-1174-4.
26. Cardella JF, Kundu S, Miller DL, Millward SF, Sacks D. Society of interventional radiology clinical practice guidelines. J Vasc Interv Radiol. 2009;20:S189–91. https://doi.org/10.1016/j.jvir.2009.04.035.

# Chapter 9
# Ultrasound Imaging of Thyroid and Perithyroidal Anatomy

**Min Kyoung Lee**

## Introduction

There are various critical structures, including nervous, vascular structures, trachea, and esophagus, within the thyroidal and perithyroidal spaces. The understanding of anatomic locations and variations in critical structures is important to perform thyroid procedures. Muscular structure can be a landmark for assessing the location of critical structures. In this section, we review the anatomical locations and variations in critical structures within the thyroidal and perithyroidal spaces, as well as the relationship between these critical structures and muscular structures.

### *Nervous System*

Nervous structures are the most commonly injured critical structure during a procedure. Careful evaluation of nervous structures can prevent serious complications during a procedure. The nerve shows a round-shaped lesion with hypoechogenicity on US [1, 2]. Understanding the location and variations in nerves may be helpful to differentiate between the metastatic lymph node and neurogenic tumor and to prevent nerve injuries.

M. K. Lee (✉)
Department of Radiology, Yeouido St. Mary's Hospital, Catholic University of Korea School of Medicine, Seoul, South Korea



A. W. Park et al. (eds.), *Thyroid Radiofrequency Ablation*,
https://doi.org/10.1007/978-3-031-65288-2_9

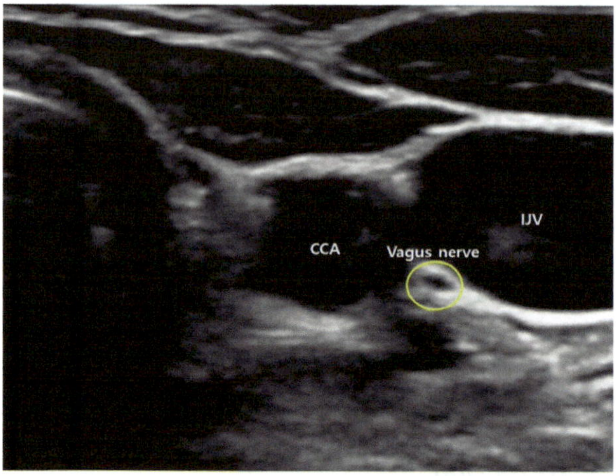


**Fig. 9.1** Common type of vagus nerve location on US. The vagus nerve (yellow round) is commonly located between the CCA and IJV. *CCA* common carotid artery, *IJV* internal jugular vein

## Vagus Nerve

The vagus nerve is the longest cranial nerve. It is typically located within the carotid space and is usually in posterolateral aspect to the common carotid artery (CCA) and posteromedial aspect to the internal jugular vein (IJV) (Fig. 9.1) [3].

There are various variations in the vagus nerve course according to the relation between the CCA and vagus nerve [3]. Anterior variation is relatively common variation with 21.1% prevalence in a previous report [4], but other variations, as medial and posterior variations, have a relatively lower prevalence.

The symptoms of vagus nerve injury are arrhythmia, dysphagia, dyspnea, nausea, and hiccups, and the injury to the vagus nerve may also induce the dysfunction of the inferior recurrent laryngeal nerve (e.g., cough, dysphonia) [2]. A large thyroid mass may change the location of the vagus nerve. Therefore, the physician must carefully evaluate the correlation between the vagus nerve and CCA.

## Superior and Inferior Laryngeal Nerves

The recurrent laryngeal nerve (RLN) is a branch of the vagus nerve and innervates the intrinsic muscles of the larynx [5]. Due to its small size, the RLN cannot be easily detected on US. Although the course of both RLNs is not symmetrical, it is usually located in the tracheoesophageal groove at the neck level (Fig. 9.2) [5].

The non-RLN is a common variation of RLN, which arises from the vagus nerve and directly enters the larynx from the vagus nerve instead of making a loop. The right non-RLN has an association with the aberrant right subclavian artery (Fig. 9.3), and the left non-RLN is associated with the situs inversus [6]. If there is the absence of the brachiocephalic trunk on US, it can predict the presence of non-RLN [7].

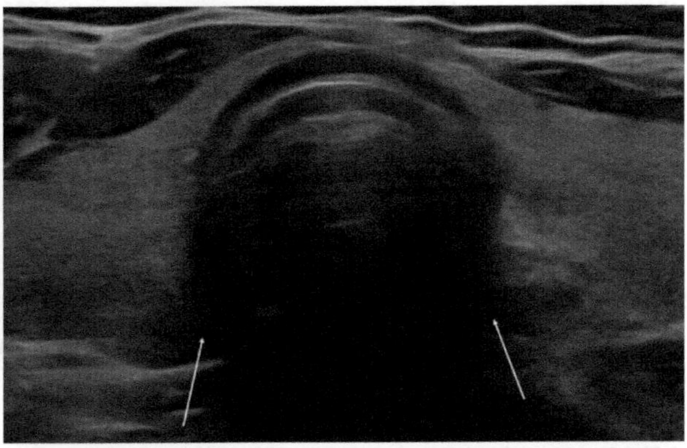

**Fig. 9.2** Relationship of recurrent laryngeal nerves to the thyroid gland. The RLN is usually located in the tracheoesophageal groove (arrows)

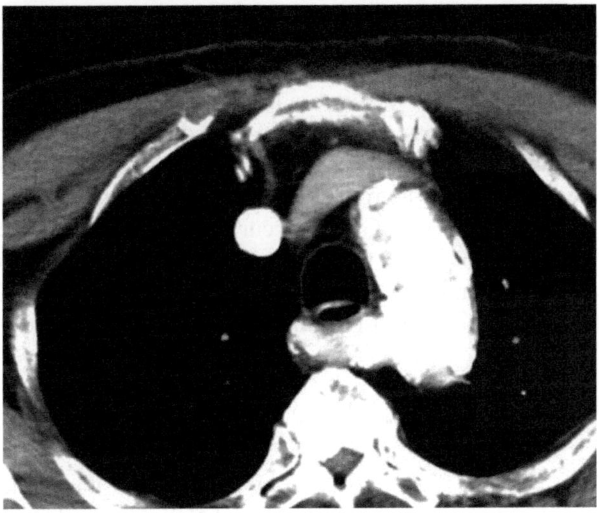

**Fig. 9.3** The aberrant right subclavian artery on post-enhanced neck CT. In patients with a right nonrecurrent laryngeal nerve, the right aberrant subclavian artery arises from the aortic arch

Injury to the RLN causes the symptoms of cough and voice change. Although the identification of the RLN on US is difficult, understanding the course of the RLN may reduce complications during a procedure.

The superior laryngeal nerve (SLN) is another branch of the vagus nerve, and it passes the pharynx and divides into the two branches (internal and external branches). Finally, the SLN enters the vocal cord. Like the RLN, the SLN also is not easily detected on US, but the external branch of the SLN could be located near the superior thyroidal artery (STA) and veins at the superior portion of the thyroid gland [5]. Therefore, if a physician performs the procedure near the superior portion of the thyroid gland, it is necessary to evaluate the patient's symptom (voice change) related with nerve injury.

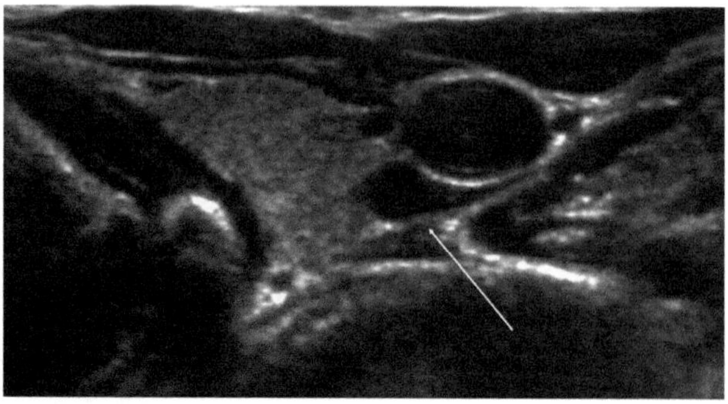

**Fig. 9.4** Transverse US image of the middle cervical sympathetic ganglion. Middle cervical sympathetic ganglion is located inferomedial to the common carotid artery (arrow)

## Middle Cervical Sympathetic Ganglion

The middle cervical sympathetic ganglion (MCSG) is the smallest one among the cervical sympathetic ganglions, and it is located in the anterior portion of the longus coli muscles (C5–7 vertebra level) (Fig. 9.4) [8].

On US images, the MCSG can be detected in 41% of cases [9] and shows a spindle-shaped hypoechoic structure with nerve branches. Because it is usually located near the inferior thyroid artery (ITA), ITA is used as the landmark of the MCSG [9]. The injury of MCSG may occur during a thyroid procedure due to location at the lower portion of the thyroid gland. The Horner syndrome is the typical complication of MCSG injury. Conjunctival injection is the initial finding of MCSG injury, and other symptoms (ptosis, miosis, and an-hidrosis of the face) may be combined.

## Other Nervous Structures

The cervical plexus arises from the plexus of the ventral rami of the upper four cervical spinal nerves, and the brachial plexus arises from the plexus of the ventral rami of the lower four cervical and first thoracic spinal nerves [5]. They are located between the anterior and posterior tubercles and can be easily detected as cordlike hypoechoic structures on US (Fig. 9.5) [10].

The spinal accessory nerve (SAN) is a motor branch of the sternocleidomastoid (SCM) and trapezius muscles. It is located between the posterolateral border of the SCM muscles and anterior border of the trapezius muscle [5]. The SAN may easily be detected within the fat layer between the muscles. Because the SAN is far from the thyroid gland, the injury to SAN is uncommon during a thyroid procedure. However, recurrent thyroid cancer can be located near the SAN. If the SAN is injured during the ablation of recurrent thyroid cancer, patients complain about limitation of abduction of the shoulder and shoulder dropping.

The phrenic nerve arises from the C3–5 spinal nerves, and it passes anteriorly to the anterior scalene muscle and posteriorly to the SCM muscle. The transverse cervical artery is the landmark of the phrenic nerve, due to a crossing course between two structures near the anterior scalene muscle [11].

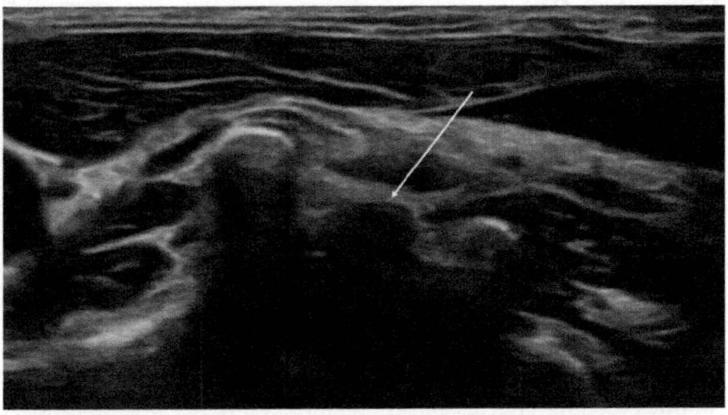

**Fig. 9.5** Transverse US images of the cervical plexus. The cervical plexus (arrow) arises between the anterior and posterior tubercles

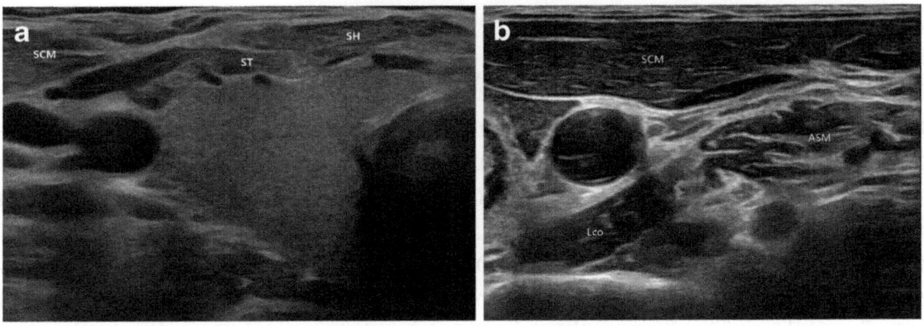


**Fig. 9.6** US images of neck muscles. Transverse US image shows the anterior (**a**) and lateral (**b**) neck muscles. *ASM* anterior scalene muscle, *Lco* longus coli muscle, *SCM* sternocleidomastoid, *SH* sternohyoid, *ST* sternothyroid

## *Muscular Structure*

The neck muscles are an important structure for understanding the location of critical adjacent structures, including nervous and vascular structures.

Anterior neck muscles are composed of the four pairs of strap muscles (thyrohyoid, sternohyoid, omohyoid, and sternothyroid muscles) (Fig. 9.6a) [12]. The strap muscles have a function for swallowing and speech by moving the hyoid bone and larynx. The SCM muscle also consists of the lower part of the anterior neck muscle. Lateral neck muscles area is comprised by large muscles, including SCM, scalene, levator scapulae, and trapezius muscles (Fig. 9.6b). The SCM muscle is used as an anatomical landmark for the identification of neurovascular structures, including CCA, SAN, and cervical or brachial plexus [13, 14]. Posterior neck muscles consist of the longus coli and capitis muscles.

## *Vascular Structure*

The thyroid is supplied by the superior and inferior thyroidal arteries, and has venous drainage through the superior, middle, and inferior thyroid veins [12]. Moreover, there are important vascular structures (CCA and IJV) near the thyroid gland. During a thyroid procedure, vascular injury may occur, and it can induce intrathyroidal, subcapsular, or perithyroidal hematoma. Although the hematoma can be controlled by neck compression, it is important to detect vascular injury early during the procedure. Therefore, the physician must understand the anatomic location of vascular structures near the thyroid gland.

### Superior and Inferior Thyroid Artery

The STA is the first branch of the external carotid artery and supplies the upper and anterior portion of the thyroid gland [5]. The STA is used as the landmark of the external branch of SLN [5]. The inferior thyroid artery (ITA) starts from the thyrocervical trunk and passes anteriorly to the longus coli muscle. It supplies the posterior portion of the thyroid gland. The ITA is used as the landmark of the MCSG due to its close anatomic location to the MCSG [9]. During thyroid biopsy or ablation, STA or ITA may be injured by inserting a needle or an electrode. Therefore, physicians ensure they do not miss the tip of the needle or electrode during procedure, and Doppler US evaluation before the procedure is necessary to reduce vascular injury.

### Common Carotid Artery and Internal Jugular Vein

The CCA and IJV are easily detected during thyroid US evaluation. The CCA runs just on the lateral side of the thyroid gland and the medial side of the IJV. Although CCA injury is not common during the procedure, the thyroid nodule located laterally may cause CCA injury by stylet firing for a core needle biopsy (CNB). Therefore, physicians measure the specimen notch distance from the tip of the CNB needle before firing the stylet [5, 15]. The IJV arises from the jugular foramen of the skull base, and finally forms the brachiocephalic vein by connecting with the subclavian vein [12].

### Superior, Middle, and Inferior Thyroid Veins

The venous drainage of the thyroid consists of three veins (superior, middle, and inferior thyroid veins). The superior and middle thyroid veins drain through the IJV, and the inferior thyroid vein drains through the brachiocephalic veins [12].

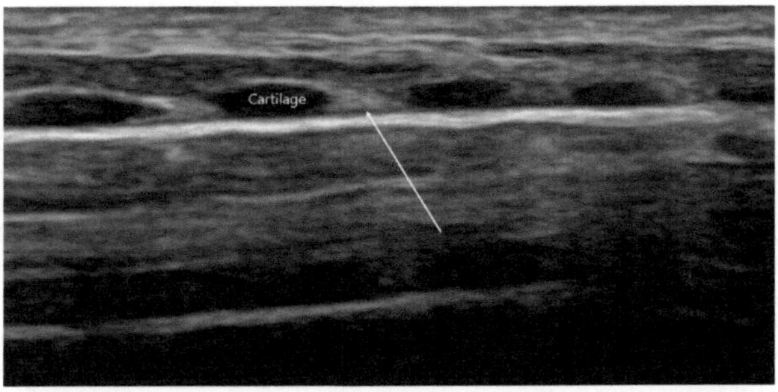


**Fig. 9.7** US anatomy of the trachea. The cartilage ring shows a round-shaped hypoechoic structure, and it is connected by the dense annular ligament (arrow)

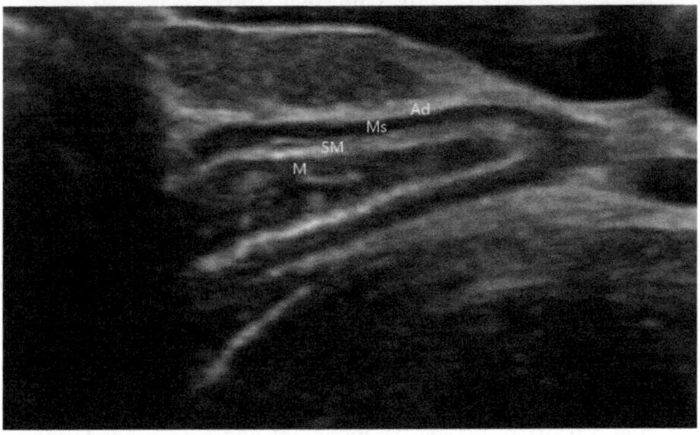


**Fig. 9.8** US anatomy of the esophagus. Four layers, as mucosal (hypoechoic), submucosal (hyperechoic), muscular (hypoechoic), and adventitial (hyperechoic) layers, shown at the posterior aspect of the thyroid gland. *Ad* adventitial layer, *M* mucosal layer, *Ms.* muscular layer, *SM* submucosal layer

## *Esophagus and Trachea*

The trachea is located just posterior to the thyroid gland and consists of 20 incomplete rings of hyaline cartilage at the anterior and lateral walls [16]. The cartilage shows hypoechogenicity on US and connects by annular ligaments with hyperechogenicity (Fig. 9.7).

The posterior wall of the trachea is composed of smooth muscles, but the muscle layer is not well visualized due to shadowing of the air interface. The cervical esophagus is usually located at the left side of the trachea and consists of multiple layers, as mucosa (hypoechoic), submucosa (hyperechoic), muscle (hypoechoic), and adventitia (hyperechoic) [13] (Fig. 9.8). When patients swallow, physician can easily detect the movement of the esophagus.

## References


1. Chiou H-J, Chou Y-H, Chiou S-Y, Liu J-B, Chang C-Y. Peripheral nerve lesions: role of high-resolution US. Radiographics. 2003;23:e15.
2. Giovagnorio F, Martinoli C. Sonography of the cervical vagus nerve: normal appearance and abnormal findings. Am J Roentgenol. 2001;176:745–9.

3. Ha EJ, Baek JH, Lee JH, Kim JK, Shong YK. Clinical significance of vagus nerve variation in radiofrequency ablation of thyroid nodules. Eur Radiol. 2011;21:2151–7.
4. Park J, Jeong S, Lee J-H, Lim G, Chang J. Variations in the course of the cervical vagus nerve on thyroid ultrasonography. Am J Neuroradiol. 2011;32:1178–81.
5. Ha EJ, Baek JH, Lee JH. Ultrasonography-based thyroidal and perithyroidal anatomy and its clinical significance. Korean J Radiol. 2015;16:749–66.
6. Gong R-X, Luo S-H, Gong Y-P, Wei T, Li Z-H, Huang J-B, et al. Prediction of nonrecurrent laryngeal nerve before thyroid surgery—experience with 1825 cases. J Surg Res. 2014;189:75–80.
7. Huang SM, Wu TJ. Neck ultrasound for prediction of right nonrecurrent laryngeal nerve. Head Neck. 2010;32:844–9.
8. Saylam CY, Ozgiray E, Orhan M, Cagli S, Zileli M. Neuroanatomy of cervical sympathetic trunk: a cadaveric study. Clin Anat. 2009;22:324–30.
9. Shin JE, Baek JH, Ha EJ, Choi YJ, Choi WJ, Lee JH. Ultrasound features of middle cervical sympathetic ganglion. Clin J Pain. 2015;31:909–13.
10. Samer NM. Sonoanatomy of the cervical spinal nerve roots implications for brachial plexus block. Reg Anesth Pain Med. 2009;34:616.
11. Canella C, Demondion X, Delebarre A, Moraux A, Cotten H, Cotten A. Anatomical study of phrenic nerve using ultrasound. Eur Radiol. 2010;20:659–65.
12. Standring S. Gray's anatomy e-book: the anatomical basis of clinical practice. Elsevier Health Sciences; 2021.
13. Gervasio A, Mujahed I, Biasio A, Alessi S. Ultrasound anatomy of the neck: the infrahyoid region. J Ultrasound. 2010;13:85–9.
14. Canella C, Demondion X, Abreu E, Marchiori E, Cotten H, Cotten A. Anatomical study of spinal accessory nerve using ultrasonography. Eur J Radiol. 2013;82:56–61.
15. Na DG, Baek JH, Jung SL, Kim J-H, Sung JY, Kim KS, et al. Core needle biopsy of the thyroid: 2016 consensus statement and recommendations from Korean Society of Thyroid Radiology. Korean J Radiol. 2017;18:217–37.
16. Brand-Saberi BE, Schäfer T. Trachea: anatomy and physiology. Thorac Surg Clin. 2014;24:1–5.

# Part III
# Thyroid Radiofrequency Ablation (RFA)

# Chapter 10
# Basic Physics and Equipment for Radiofrequency Ablation

**Brian J. Park and Nincheng (Peter) Li**

## Physics

Radiofrequency (RF) radiation is a type of nonionizing radiation at the lower end of the electromagnetic spectrum, with frequencies from 3 kHz to 300 GHz (Fig. 10.1). For percutaneous ablation, radiofrequency refers to the frequency of electric current oscillation within the body to intentionally produce localized burns. Most medical applications of radiofrequency ablation utilize electric current oscillation in the frequency range of 350–500 kHz. For a typical frequency of 500 kHz, the direction of the current, mediated through agitated tissue cations (e.g., $Na^+$, $K^+$) and anions (e.g., $Cl^-$, $HCO_3^-$), changes one million times per second.

A complete electrical circuit is needed to perform RFA within the body. There are two types of RF circuits based on the electrode: monopolar and bipolar. Monopolar RFA is more established and is the current standard of care in most tumor RF applications. The electric circuit involves the RF power generator, the RF electrode inserted into the target tissue, the patient's body, and the grounding pads attached to the patient's skin (Fig. 10.2). When the circuit is activated, the generated current is passed through the electrode's small conduction surface area, creating high current density near the electrode to produce the desired thermal energy for tissue ablation. Electric current disperses throughout the patient's body until it is collected by the grounding pads, which returns the current back to the generator. The much larger conduction surface area of the grounding pads significantly decreases the current density near the pad, minimizing the risks of unintentional

B. J. Park (✉)
Dotter Department of Interventional Radiology, Oregon Health and Science University, Portland, OR, USA

N (Peter). Li
Department of Radiology, Division of Interventional Radiology, UMass Chan Medical School, Worcester, MA, USA


A. W. Park et al. (eds.), *Thyroid Radiofrequency Ablation*,
https://doi.org/10.1007/978-3-031-65288-2_10

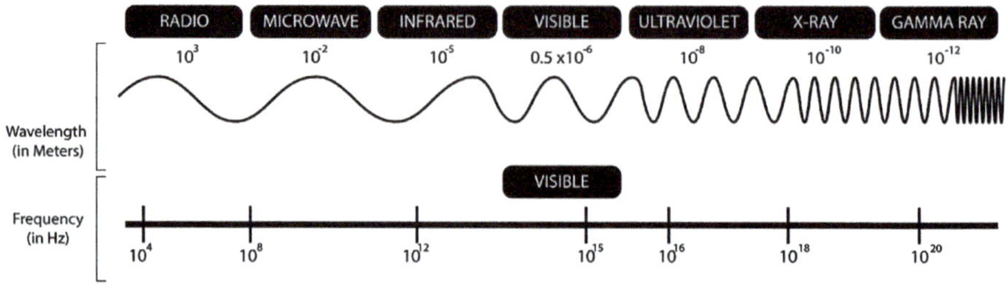


**Fig. 10.1** Radiowaves are on the lower end of the electromagnetic spectrum. [Adapted from Jonathan Urie, distributed under a CC BY-SA 3.0 license]

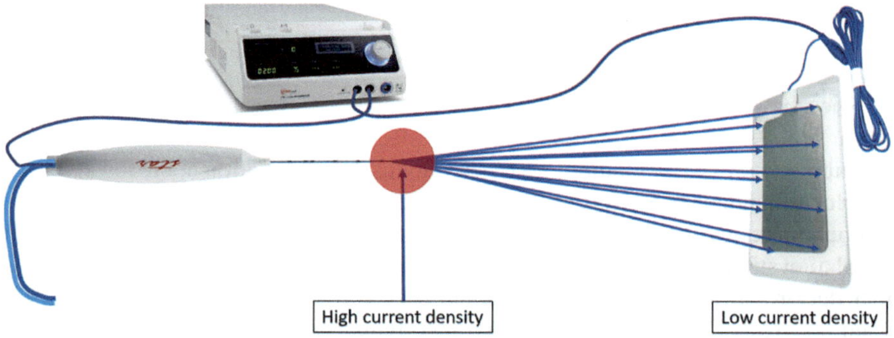


**Fig. 10.2** Monopolar radiofrequency ablation conduction circuit. Current density is highest near the probe, disperses with distance, and is significantly decreased near the grounding pad. (With permission from Park [3])

skin burns. Bipolar RFA is a newer development where both the generation and collection of electric current occurs along the RF electrode. This design eliminates the need for grounding pads. Electric current is localized around the electrode and primarily confined within the target tissue. Minimal to no current passes through distant portions of the body, avoiding global heating of the body, focal burns around embedded metallic materials (e.g., surgical clips), interference with implantable electric medical devices (e.g., cardiac rhythm control devices), and interactions with intrauterine pregnancies [1, 2].

During the RFA process, the target and adjacent tissues experience two types of thermal energy: frictional heat production and conductional heat propagation. Frictional heat is generated as ions in the tissue attempt to follow the changing directions of the alternating current (Fig. 10.3). Frictional heat serves as a direct heating source and is most concentrated in the immediate vicinity of the RF electrode, given the small conduction area and high current density. This heat causes immediate damage to the target tissue within a small radius of few millimeters. Tissues farther away from the electrode are less influenced by changes in the alternating current, with an exponential drop in energy and resultant temperature changes as the distance from the electrode increases [4, 5].

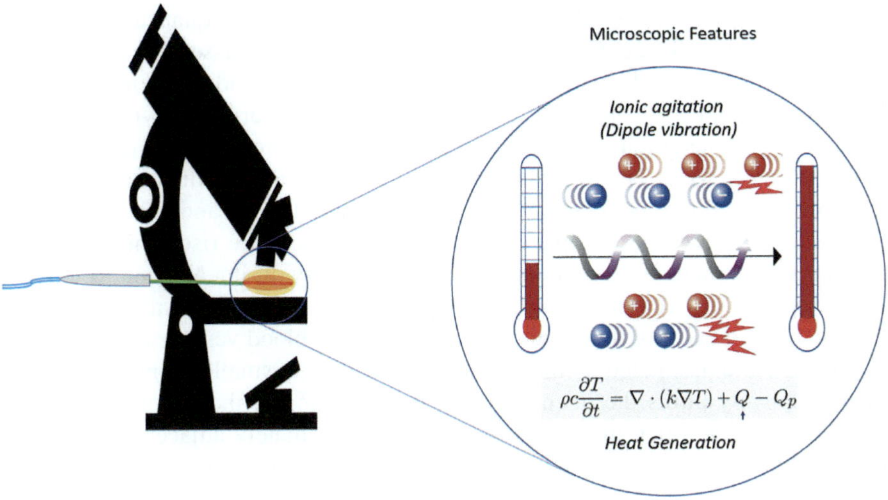


**Fig. 10.3** Rapid change of ion movement direction leads to frictional heat production. (With permission from Park [3])

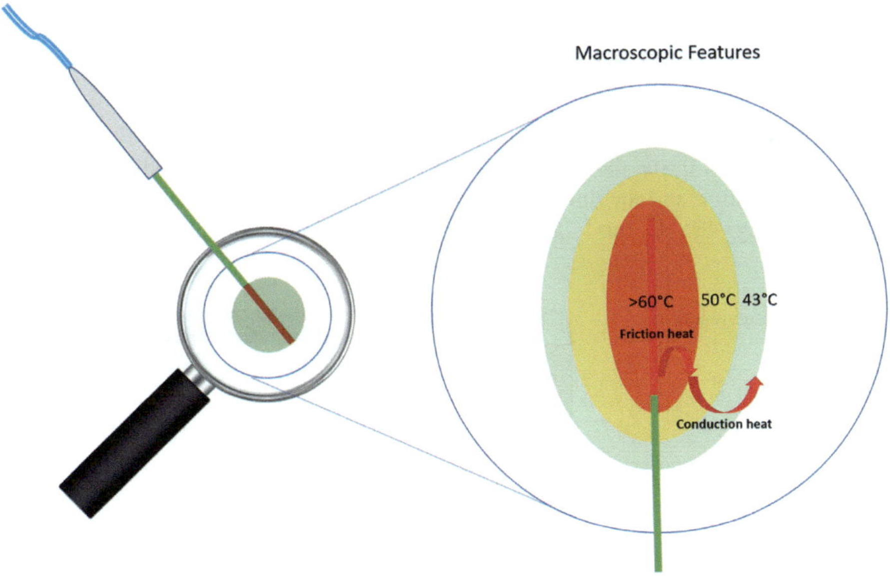


**Fig. 10.4** Frictional heat adjacent to the electrode serves as a direct heating source. Thermal conduction carries the generated heat to tissues farther away. (With permission from Park [3])

In comparison, heat propagation via thermal conduction is slower and indirect (Fig. 10.4). On one hand, this transmission of thermal energy from the RF electrode to adjacent tissues may be desirable to provide additional areas of thermal destruction. On the other hand, the dissipation of heat should be carefully balanced to prevent unintended collateral damage while maintaining an adequate ablation target zone temperature. To control some of these effects, hydrodissection may be performed to create a fluid barrier between the ablation zone and adjacent vital structures (e.g., trachea, esophagus, carotid artery, and recurrent laryngeal nerve). Nonionic solutions, such as dextrose 5% in water, are preferred for hydrodissection in the setting of RFA. The higher thermal conductivity and specific heat capacity of the hydrodissection fluid, compared to those of thyroid gland and adjacent soft tissue, leads to faster heat dissipation and smaller temperature rise. This effectively protects vital structures from unintended thermal injury during ablation [6, 7].

The heat sink effect, in contrast, refers to the inadvertent loss of ablation thermal energy through existing fluid structures, such as large blood vessels and cysts. Heat is absorbed and dissipated by these structures, leading to smaller temperature rises. This effectively limits the intended thermal destruction of the target tissue and is most pronounced when the fluid structures are immediately adjacent to the target tissue. Fluid aspiration, methodical selection of the electrode entry angle to minimize interactions with adjacent fluid structures, artery-first ablation, and marginal venous ablation can mitigate the heat sink effect and optimize ablation outcome [2, 8].

## Tissue Hyperthermia and Necrosis

Localized heat production and conduction around the RF electrode determine the degree of thermal tissue damage (Fig. 10.5). This is influenced by both the achieved tissue temperature and the duration of the temperature exposure. At temperatures of approximately 40 °C, no significant tissue damage takes place. Temperature

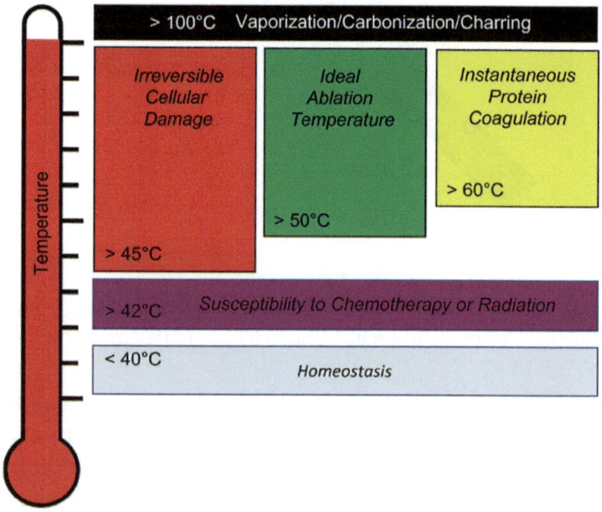


**Fig. 10.5** Tissue reaction to heat. (With permission from Park [3])

elevation to 42–45 °C exerts sublethal thermal damage, resulting in paused metabolism, impaired DNA repair, cytokine and inflammatory marker release, and increased sensitivity to irradiation and chemotherapeutic agents. Continued temperature elevation leads to irreversible cellular damage through a process termed coagulative necrosis. This irreversible destructive process takes place after heat exposure for 60 minutes at temperatures between 46 and 50 °C, 4–6 minutes at temperatures between 50 and 52 °C, and near-immediate at temperatures between 60 and 100 °C.

When temperatures rise above 100 °C, tissues surrounding the electrode undergo dehydration and vaporization with instantaneous tissue death. The release of gases, primarily nitrogen, can result in an audible tissue "popping" sound and tactile feedback as well as the production of microbubbles, or hyperechogenic changes, under real-time ultrasound monitoring. Eventually, the affected tissue becomes carbonized and completely loses its biological status [5, 9–12].

Resistance describes the opposition to current motion in a direct current system and is the source of frictional heat production. The analogous term in an oscillating current system is impedance. Impedance is an important parameter during RFA (Fig. 10.6). Given the presence of physiologic fluid containing large quantities of ions, impedance is typically small at the beginning of an ablation process, facilitating a rapid elevation of tissue temperature. Tissue vaporization and dehydration at temperatures higher than 100 °C deprive the tissue of ion-containing fluid, raising the impedance and gradually limiting further heat production.

During RFA, dehydrated tissue usually starts at the proximal and distal ends of the active tip of the RF electrode and grows toward the middle (Fig. 10.7). This "insulating" layer of dehydrated tissue and gas bubbles also decreases heat conduction. When the electrode is entirely encompassed by nonconducting desiccated tissue, the impedance surges and cuts off the RF conduction circuit. This steep elevation in impedance terminates the ablation process and is referred to as the

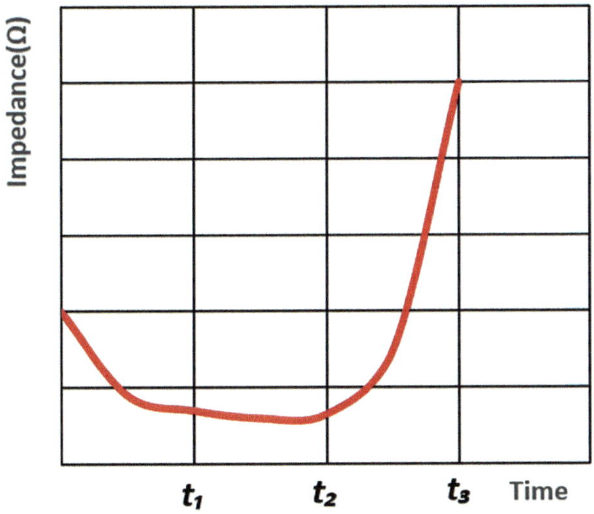


**Fig. 10.6** Impedance between an electrode and grounding pads over time. Rapid rise in impedance is known as the roll-off phenomenon. (With permission from Park [3])

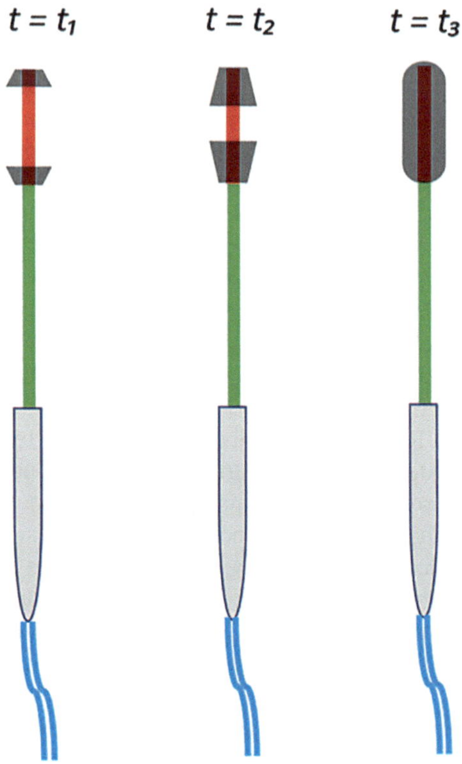


**Fig. 10.7** Growth of dehydrated tissue during RFA over time (*t*). Dehydrated tissue starts at the ends of the active tip of the electrode and grows towards the middle. (With permission from Park [3])

roll-off phenomenon. Continued application of RF power at this stage does not produce additional desired tissue destruction [9, 13–15].

Contrary to RFA in other organs of the body where fast, high-energy, large ablation zones are desired, RFA in the thyroid uses lower energies for smaller, more focal ablation zones. In doing so, unintentional ablation or injury to adjacent tissues and structures are minimized, which is a priority in the neck region with many critical structures including the trachea, esophagus, nerves, and carotid arteries. The moving-shot technique (Fig. 10.8) was developed specifically for thyroid ablation to achieve localized and controlled ablation with minimal collateral damage, focusing on frictional heat immediately adjacent to the electrode as opposed to conductive heat transfer during conventional RFA with fixed electrode technique in larger visceral organs. Briefly, the moving-shot technique involves the RF electrode inserted through the isthmus to the most medial and deepest portion of the target lesion. After adequate ablation at this specific location, the electrode is slowly retracted continuously or in small increments for subsequent ablations along the same electrode-entry angle. The electrode is then reinserted and directed with a slightly more superficial and lateral entry angle into the adjacent, untreated portion of the target lesion, and ablations are performed during pullback along this new entry angle. This process is repeated until the entire nodule is covered. Using this deep-to-superficial and medial-to-lateral approach, the target lesion is compartmentalized into multiple, small, ablation units and comprehensively ablated [16].

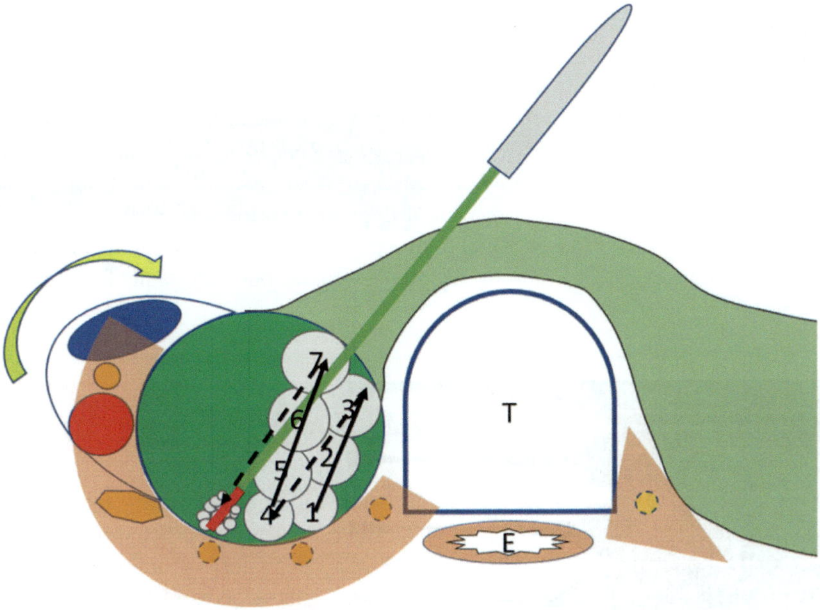


**Fig. 10.8** Moving-shot technique where ablation is performed dynamically with multiple, small, ablation units beginning with the deepest and most medial portion of the nodule to superficial and more lateral portions. *E* esophagus, *T* trachea, 1–7—ablation units; red circle—common carotid artery; blue ellipse—internal jugular vein; yellow circle with solid border—vagus nerve; yellow circles with dotted borders—potential sites of recurrent laryngeal nerve; yellow heptagon—middle cervical sympathetic ganglion. (With permission from Park [3])

## Thyroid RFA Equipment

### *Generator*

A radiofrequency generator (Fig. 10.9) supplies power to the tissue through the RF electrode. Continuous RF mode is specifically designed and used for thyroid ablations. In this mode, RF power is generated and delivered continuously at a set output, typically 5–80 W for thyroid applications. The RF generator also monitors power, impedance, and electrode shaft temperature. These are commonly displayed on the generator panel.

### *Electrodes*

Radiofrequency electrodes come in 18- or 19-gauge needles with an assortment of active tip sizes (5–20 mm) and shaft lengths (7–12 cm). The selection of an appropriate electrode tip size, shaft length, and RF power depends on many

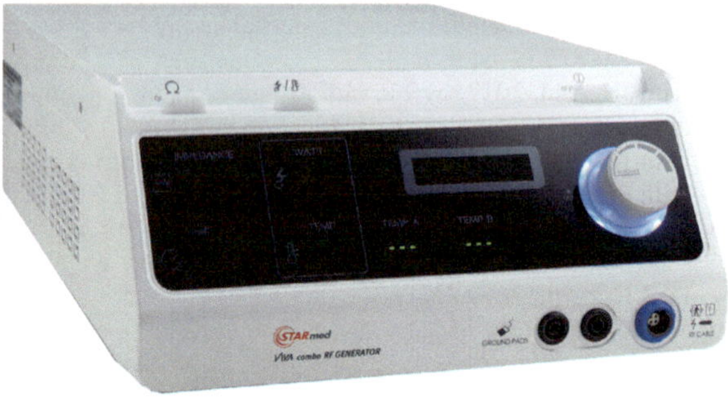


**Fig. 10.9** A 480-kHz radiofrequency generator capable of generating and delivering up to 200 W of power. [Photo Courtesy of STARmed Co., Ltd. Goyang-Si, South Korea]

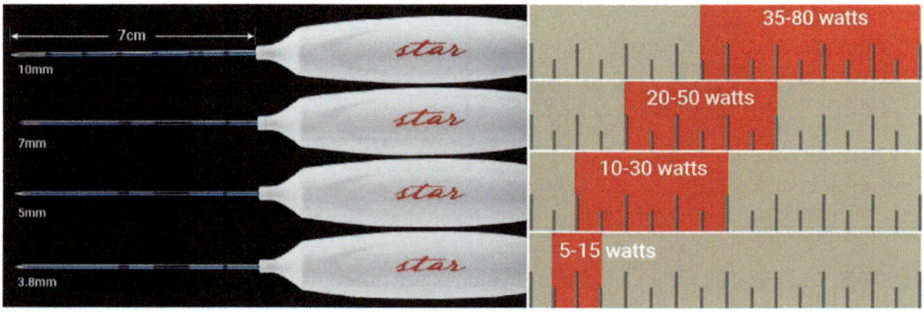


**Fig. 10.10** Various active tip sizes and recommended power settings of a certain brand of RFA electrode. [Photo Courtesy of STARmed Co., Ltd. Goyang-Si, South Korea]

factors, including nodule location, nodule size, nodule composition, proximity to critical structures, and operator preference. Shorter shaft lengths can allow for easier maneuverability as the thyroid gland is located close to the surface of the neck, while longer shaft lengths may be more appropriate for treating deeper lesions. Larger active tip sizes may provide better procedural efficiency. Smaller active tip sizes are preferred for precise control in challenging locations near vital structures.

Electrodes have different recommended RF power settings based on active tip size. In general, electrodes with larger active tip sizes require higher RF power (Fig. 10.10). Within its recommended range specified by the manufacturer, RF power can be adjusted dynamically during the ablation procedure. For example, if a transient hyperechoic zone at the electrode tip does not appear within 5–10 s after application of RF power, RF power may be boosted in 5–10 W increments [2].

Thyroid RFA systems also commonly utilize liquid cooling of the shaft's chamber with chilled water or saline. This reduces heating of the immediately adjacent tissues to allow for greater current deposition without charring or rapid impedance elevation (Fig. 10.11).

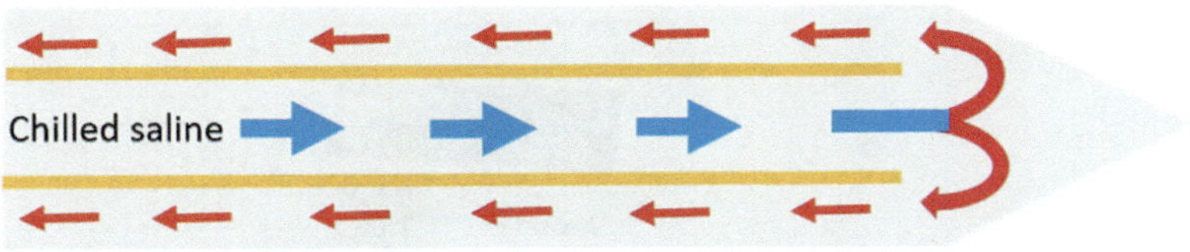


**Fig. 10.11** Internally cooled RF electrode for preventing or minimizing charring. Chilled fluid is pumped through the chamber of the electrode shaft to dissipate heat. (With permission from Park [3])

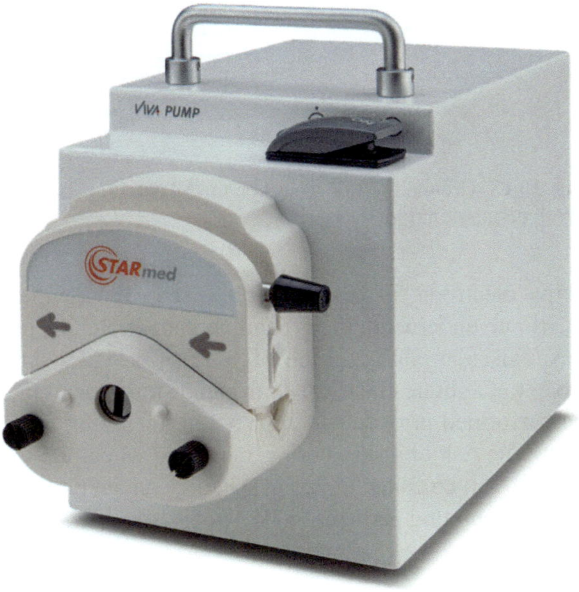


**Fig. 10.12** Peristaltic infusion pump used to reduce electrode tip temperature. [Photo Courtesy of STARmed Co., Ltd. Goyang-Si, South Korea]

## *Pump*

Chilled water or saline (>0 °C) is circulated by a peristaltic pump (Fig. 10.12). The pump continuously reduces the temperature around the electrode tip to prevent or minimize charring. The temperature indicator on the panel of the generator indicates the temperature inside the electrode shaft, not the actual temperature of the ablative tissue.

## *Grounding Pads*

Grounding pads are required to complete a monopolar RF conduction circuit and return the electrical current from the patient back to the generator (Fig. 10.13). Grounding pads are adhered to the patient's skin away from the ablation site. Because the conductive surface area of the grounding pad is much larger than the

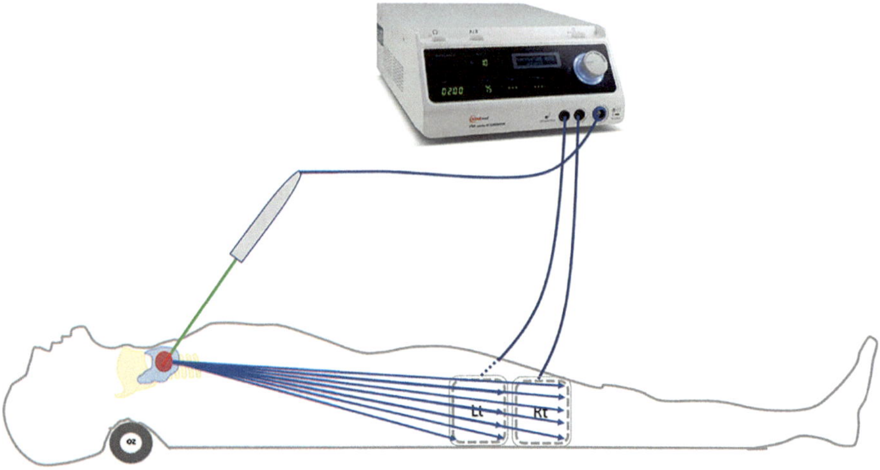


**Fig. 10.13** Grounding pads placed on the bilateral thighs to complete a monopolar RFA circuit. (With permission from Park [3])

active electrode tip, current is dispersed over a wider area, minimizing heating of the tissue underneath the grounding pad. Typically, pads are applied along the convex, muscular portion of the thighs. This provides sufficient distance from the electrode to facilitate electrical equivalence throughout the pad. Site preparation should be performed prior to pad application, including proper shaving and drying of the skin. The risk of a skin burn is increased when pad-to-skin contact is poor because current will be concentrated at specific contact points rather than dispersed over the entire grounding pad area [17].

## References


1. Bruners P, Lipka J, Gunther RW, Schmitz-Rode T, Mahnken AH. Bipolar radiofrequency ablation: is the shape of the coagulation volume different in comparison to monopolar RF-ablation using variable active tip lengths? Minim Invasive Ther Allied Technol. 2008;17(5):267–74.
2. Park HS, Baek JH, Park AW, Chung SR, Choi YJ, Lee JH. Thyroid radiofrequency ablation: updates on innovative devices and techniques. Korean J Radiol. 2017;18(4):615–23.
3. Park AW. Thyroid radiofrequency ablation. 1st ed. Charlottesville: Oz & SE; 2020.
4. Haemmerich D. Biophysics of radiofrequency ablation. Crit Rev Biomed Eng. 2010;38(1):53–63.
5. Hong K, Georgiades C. Radiofrequency ablation: mechanism of action and devices. J Vasc Interv Radiol. 2010;21(8 Suppl):S179–86.
6. Xiaoyin T, Ping L, Dan C, Min D, Jiachang C, Tao W, et al. Risk assessment and hydrodissection technique for radiofrequency ablation of thyroid benign nodules. J Cancer. 2018;9(17):3058–66.
7. IT'IS Database for thermal and electromagnetic parameters of biological tissues [Internet]. 2022.

8. Pillai K, Akhter J, Chua TC, Shehata M, Alzahrani N, Al-Alem I, et al. Heat sink effect on tumor ablation characteristics as observed in monopolar radiofrequency, bipolar radiofrequency, and microwave, using ex vivo calf liver model. Medicine (Baltimore). 2015;94(9):e580.
9. Zhang B, Moser MA, Zhang EM, Luo Y, Liu C, Zhang W. A review of radiofrequency ablation: large target tissue necrosis and mathematical modelling. Phys Med. 2016;32(8):961–71.
10. Goldberg SN. Radiofrequency tumor ablation: principles and techniques. Eur J Ultrasound. 2001;13(2):129–47.
11. Arata MA, Nisenbaum HL, Clark TW, Soulen MC. Percutaneous radiofrequency ablation of liver tumors with the LeVeen probe: is roll-off predictive of response? J Vasc Interv Radiol. 2001;12(4):455–8.
12. Haines DE. Letter by Haines regarding article, "Direct measurement of the lethal isotherm for radiofrequency ablation of myocardial tissue". Circ Arrhythm Electrophysiol. 2011;4(5):e67. author reply e8.
13. Okhai TA, Smith CJ. Principles and application of RF system for hyperthermia therapy. In: Hyperthermia. InTech; 2013. p. 171–84.
14. Castro-López DL, Berjano E, Romero-Mendez R. Radiofrequency ablation combined with conductive fluid-based dopants (saline normal and colloidal gold): computer modeling and ex vivo experiments. Biomed Eng Online. 2021;20(1):4.
15. Trujillo M, Alba J, Berjano E. Relationship between roll-off occurrence and spatial distribution of dehydrated tissue during RF ablation with cooled electrodes. Int J Hyperth. 2012;28(1):62–8.
16. Baek JH, Kim YS, Lee D, Huh JY, Lee JH. Benign predominantly solid thyroid nodules: prospective study of efficacy of sonographically guided radiofrequency ablation versus control condition. AJR Am J Roentgenol. 2010;194(4):1137–42.
17. Goldberg SN, Solbiati L, Halpern EF, Gazelle GS. Variables affecting proper system grounding for radiofrequency ablation in an animal model. J Vasc Interv Radiol. 2000;11(8):1069–75.

# Chapter 11
# Preprocedural Workup for Thyroid RFA

**Ming-Hsun Wu and Wei-Che Lin**

In 2017, the Korean Society of Thyroid Radiology released guidelines for thyroid radiofrequency ablation (RFA). Table 11.1, based on these guidelines, presents the preprocedural checklist for RFA, in accordance with the 2017 KSThR guidelines. The following sections offer comprehensive explanations and discussions on individual components of this checklist.

## Pre-procedure Evaluation for Benign Thyroid Nodules

### *Patient History and Clinical Examination*

A thorough assessment of the patient's complete clinical history is necessary before enrolling them for thyroid RFA, including the presence of other diseases and comorbidities, previous surgeries or radiation therapies, drug history, and drug allergies. Symptoms and physical examination should be included within the patient history. Clinical symptom scores are usually measured on a scale of 0–10, with 0 indicating that the patient is not bothered by symptoms and 10 indicating that the symptoms are persistent and significant to the patient.

M.-H. Wu
Department of Surgery, National Taiwan University Hospital, Taipei, Taiwan

W.-C. Lin (✉)
Department of Diagnostic Radiology, Kaohsiung Chang Gung Memorial Hospital, Chang Gung University College of Medicine, Kaohsiung, Taiwan

Thyroid Head and Neck Ablation Center, Kaohsiung Chang Gung Memorial Hospital, Kaohsiung, Taiwan

College of Medicine, National Sun Yat-Sen University, Kaohsiung, Taiwan



A. W. Park et al. (eds.), *Thyroid Radiofrequency Ablation*,
https://doi.org/10.1007/978-3-031-65288-2_11

**Table 11.1** Preprocedural checklist according to the KSThR 2017 guidelines

| Pathologic thyroid nodule | Recurrent thyroid cancer |
|---|---|
| Pathologic diagnosis | Pathologic and/or serologic diagnosis |
| • Benign diagnosis at least two US-guided FNA or CNB<br>• Benign diagnosis at least one US-guided FNA or CNB in AFTN<br>• Benign diagnosis at least one US-guided FNA or CNB in thyroid nodules with highly specific benign US features | • Cancer recurrence at US-guided FNA or CNB<br>• Increased washout Tg level in aspirate or Tg immunostain of CNB specimen<br>• Increased washout calcitonin level in aspirate or calcitonin immunostaining of CNB specimen in patients with medullary cancer |
| US | US |
| • Features of the nodule and surrounding critical structures<br>• Nodule volume | • Features of the nodule and surrounding critical structures<br>• Tumor volume |
| Symptom score | |
| Cosmetic score | |
| Laboratory tests | Laboratory tests |
| • Complete blood count<br>• Blood coagulation battery<br>• Thyroid function test<br>– Serum TSH<br>– Serum T3<br>– Serum fT4 | • Complete blood count<br>• Blood coagulation battery<br>• Thyroid function test<br>– Serum TSH<br>– Serum T3<br>– Serum fT4 |
| Additional imaging study | Additional imaging study |
| • CT or MRI[a]<br>• $^{99m}$Tc pertechnetate or $^{123}$I thyroid scan[b] | • CT or MRI[a] |

*AFTN* autonomously functioning thyroid nodule, *CNB* core needle biopsy, *CT* computed tomography, *FNA* fine-needle aspiration, *fT4* free thyroxine, *MRI* magnetic resonance imaging, *RFA* radiofrequency ablation, *T3* tri-iodothyronine, *Tg* thyroglobulin, *TSH* thyroid stimulating hormone (thyrotropin), and *US* ultrasound

[a]Selectively indicated

[b]Indicated for AFTN

Physical examination should include documentation of cosmetic score as follows: (1) no palpable mass, (2) no cosmetic problem but palpable mass, (3) a cosmetic problem on swallowing only, and (4) a readily detected cosmetic problem [1]. Voice examination should pay particular attention to any baseline hoarseness. If there is concern about vocal cord dysfunction, a confirmatory evaluation may be required. Some guidelines recommend laryngoscopy to ensure vocal cord mobility in all patients before and after RFA [2].

## *Biochemical Analysis*

Laboratory tests usually include a complete blood count, coagulation profiles (bleeding time, prothrombin time, activated partial thromboplastin time), as well as thyroid function tests (thyrotropin, triiodothyronine, and free thyroxine) [3, 4]. Routine testing of benign thyroid nodules for thyroid antibodies, such as anti-thyroglobulin or anti-microsomal antibodies, prior to RFA is controversial [5–7]. However, it can be evaluated selectively, as patients with elevated autoantibody levels may develop post-RFA subclinical hypothyroidism [8].

Patients taking medications associated with a bleeding tendency should be advised to withhold their medications prior to RFA: 7–10 days for aspirin or clopidogrel, 3–5 days for warfarin, and 4–6 h before heparin [9]. Some guidelines mention the preprocedural process for patients with a bleeding tendency in the contraindication section [10].

## *Image Studies*

Ultrasonography (US) is important to characterize nodules and to assess the relationships between critical structures and the thyroid nodule and should be performed before providing the RFA treatment. US should measure three orthogonal diameters, including the largest diameter, and the nodule or tumor volume could be calculated using the Eq. $V = \pi abc/6$, where $V$ is the volume, $a$ is the largest diameter, and $b$ and $c$ are the other two perpendicular diameters [3, 11, 12]. US characteristics should be documented [13, 14], and several groups have developed risk stratification systems to predict whether nodules are malignant or benign based on these features. US features are now used in current guidelines, such as the 2015 American Thyroid Association (ATA) Guideline Task Force [15] and the American College of Radiology Thyroid Imaging Reporting and Data System (ACR TI-RADS) [16] for clinical judgment. If suspicious findings are found, including extrathyroidal extension or indeterminate lymph nodes, additional tests should be performed to rule out potential malignancy. Caution should be exercised when performing RFA for thyroid nodules with suspicious US features, even if fine-needle aspiration (FNA) or core needle biopsy (CNB) results are benign [11, 13, 14].

US features may also help predict the success of RFA. Pre-ablation cyst components and a spongiform pattern are predictors of a better response, whereas large size and higher echogenicity were identified as predictors of a poorer response [17–20].

Cross-sectional imaging using CT or MRI may be helpful in assessing intrathoracic extension in patients with large thyroid nodules [10, 21, 22]. PET-CT or PET-MRI is not routinely recommended prior to ablation.

### *Cytopathologic Assessment*

Fine-needle aspiration (FNA) or core-needle biopsy is recommended by all groups to confirm the benign nature of the lesion. In most cases, thyroid nodules should be confirmed as benign by at least two separate US-guided fine-needle aspiration (FNA) cytology or core needle biopsy (CNB) prior to RFA [14, 23–25]; however, some guidelines accept a single biopsy result that is confirmed to be benign with typical benign appearances on US or in AFTN [5, 6, 26].

It is recommended to repeat US-guided FNA or CNB for thyroid nodules with suspicious US features or rapidly growing thyroid nodules [10, 22, 27, 28]. Thyroid nodules have a very low rate of malignancy after two confirmations of benignity, so at this point, nodules may be considered benign [24, 25].

## Pre-procedure Evaluation for Thyroid Malignancies

If RFA is intended to treat low-risk papillary thyroid microcarcinoma as well as recurrent thyroid cancers, additional evaluation is required before ablation to ensure a successful outcome and to avoid delay in possible surgery.

Low-risk papillary thyroid microcarcinoma should fulfill the criteria including: (1) cytopathology confirmed papillary thyroid carcinoma (PTC) <1 cm in greatest dimension, which was defined by The World Health Organization (WHO) as PTMC [29], (2) absence of aggressiveness including extrathyroidal extension or clinical metastatic lymph nodes at the time of treatment, and (3) ineligibility for surgery or unwilling to undergo active surveillance [30]. The criteria have been extended in some studies; however, large-scale prospective studies are needed to establish the efficacy of RFA and its use for PTC larger than 1 cm [31].

RFA treatment for follicular neoplasm is more controversial than for PTC, since surgical resection is required to exclude the presence of vascular or capsular invasion and to definitively diagnose whether the nodules is a follicular adenoma or a carcinoma. Thus, if cytological evaluation were shown in the Bethesda IV catalog, even though there are studies showing similar VRR [32], these nodules may not be suitable for RFA treatment. In addition, there is still not enough evidence of RFA treatment for medullary thyroid cancer (MTC), even though it has been demonstrated to be an option for early MTC in patients ineligible for surgery [33].

Pre-ablation laboratory tests should also include tumor markers such as thyroglobulin, anti-thyroglobulin, calcitonin, and CEA. Imaging studies should include US, CT, MRI, or PET-CT to define the location and involvement of all structures and assess disease extensions, such as capsule invasion or lymph node metastases. Cytological results can be reviewed a second time to evaluate whether an aggressive variant of PTC is present. Also, a confirmatory evaluation of laryngoscopy to ensure vocal cord mobility is suggested [2].

A detailed preoperative evaluation may improve patient selection, help in better treatment planning, and ultimately determine a better oncological response to treatment and reduce the possible complications.

## References


1. Lin WC, Wang CK, Wang WH, Kuo CY, Chiang PL, Lin AN, et al. Multicenter study of benign thyroid nodules with radiofrequency ablation: results of 762 cases over 4 years in Taiwan. J Pers Med. 2022;12(1):63.
2. Orloff LA, Noel JE, Stack BC Jr, Russell MD, Angelos P, Baek JH, et al. Radiofrequency ablation and related ultrasound-guided ablation technologies for treatment of benign and malignant thyroid disease: an international multidisciplinary consensus statement of the American head and neck society endocrine surgery section with the Asia Pacific Society of Thyroid Surgery, Associazione Medici Endocrinologi, British Association of Endocrine and Thyroid Surgeons, European thyroid association, Italian Society of Endocrine Surgery Units, Korean Society of Thyroid Radiology, Latin American thyroid society, and thyroid nodules therapies association. Head Neck. 2022;44(3):633–60.
3. Baek JH, Kim YS, Lee D, Huh JY, Lee JH. Benign predominantly solid thyroid nodules: prospective study of efficacy of sonographically guided radiofrequency ablation versus control condition. AJR Am J Roentgenol. 2010;194(4):1137–42.
4. Ahn HS, Kim SJ, Park SH, Seo M. Radiofrequency ablation of benign thyroid nodules: evaluation of the treatment efficacy using ultrasonography. Ultrasonography. 2016;35(3):244–52.
5. Baek JH, Kim YS, Sung JY, Choi H, Lee JH. Locoregional control of metastatic well-differentiated thyroid cancer by ultrasound-guided radiofrequency ablation. AJR Am J Roentgenol. 2011;197(2):W331–6.
6. Torres MR, Nobrega Neto SH, Rosas RJ, Martins AL, Ramos AL, da Cruz TR. Thyroglobulin in the washout fluid of lymph-node biopsy: what is its role in the follow-up of differentiated thyroid carcinoma? Thyroid. 2014;24(1):7–18.
7. Rosario PW, Carvalho M, Mourao GF, Calsolari MR. Comparison of antithyroglobulin antibody concentrations before and after ablation with 131I as a predictor of structural disease in differentiated thyroid carcinoma patients with undetectable basal thyroglobulin and negative neck ultrasonography. Thyroid. 2016;26(4):525–31.
8. Baek JH, Lee JH, Sung JY, Bae JI, Kim KT, Sim J, et al. Complications encountered in the treatment of benign thyroid nodules with US-guided radiofrequency ablation: a multicenter study. Radiology. 2012;262(1):335–42.
9. Kwok A, Faigel DO. Management of anticoagulation before and after gastrointestinal endoscopy. Am J Gastroenterol. 2009;104(12):3085–97. quiz 98.
10. Dobnig H, Zechmann W, Hermann M, Lehner M, Heute D, Mirzaei S, et al. Radiofrequency ablation of thyroid nodules: "good clinical practice recommendations" for Austria: an interdisciplinary statement from the following professional associations: Austrian Thyroid Association (OSDG), Austrian Society for Nuclear Medicine and Molecular Imaging (OGNMB), Austrian Society for Endocrinology and Metabolism (OGES), Surgical Endocrinology Working Group (ACE) of the Austrian Surgical Society (OEGCH). Wien Med Wochenschr. 2020;170(1–2):6–14.
11. Jeong WK, Baek JH, Rhim H, Kim YS, Kwak MS, Jeong HJ, et al. Radiofrequency ablation of benign thyroid nodules: safety and imaging follow-up in 236 patients. Eur Radiol. 2008;18(6):1244–50.
12. Sung JY, Kim YS, Choi H, Lee JH, Baek JH. Optimum first-line treatment technique for benign cystic thyroid nodules: ethanol ablation or radiofrequency ablation? AJR Am J Roentgenol. 2011;196(2):W210–4.
13. Kwak JY, Koo H, Youk JH, Kim MJ, Moon HJ, Son EJ, et al. Value of US correlation of a thyroid nodule with initially benign cytologic results. Radiology. 2010;254(1):292–300.
14. Hahn SY, Shin JH, Oh YL. What is the ideal core number for ultrasonography-guided thyroid biopsy of cytologically inconclusive nodules? AJNR Am J Neuroradiol. 2017;38(4):777–81.
15. Haugen BR, Alexander EK, Bible KC, Doherty GM, Mandel SJ, Nikiforov YE, et al. 2015 American Thyroid Association management guidelines for adult patients with thyroid nodules and differentiated thyroid cancer: the American Thyroid Association guidelines task force on thyroid nodules and differentiated thyroid cancer. Thyroid. 2016;26(1):1–133.

16. Tessler FN, Middleton WD, Grant EG, Hoang JK, Berland LL, Teefey SA, et al. ACR thyroid imaging, reporting and data system (TI-RADS): white paper of the ACR TI-RADS Committee. J Am Coll Radiol. 2017;14(5):587–95.
17. Bisceglia A, Rossetto R, Garberoglio S, Franzin A, Cerato A, Maletta F, et al. Predictor analysis in radiofrequency ablation of benign thyroid nodules: a single center experience. Front Endocrinol (Lausanne). 2021;12:638880.
18. Kuo CY, Wu MH, Ko WC, Cheng SP. Computer-analyzed ultrasound predictors of the treatment efficacy of radiofrequency ablation for benign thyroid nodules. World J Surg. 2022;46(1):112–20.
19. Deandrea M, Garino F, Alberto M, Garberoglio R, Rossetto R, Bonelli N, et al. Radiofrequency ablation for benign thyroid nodules according to different ultrasound features: an Italian multicentre prospective study. Eur J Endocrinol. 2019;180(1):79–87.
20. Wu MH, Chen KY, Chen A, Chen CN. Differences in the ultrasonographic appearance of thyroid nodules after radiofrequency ablation. Clin Endocrinol. 2021;95(3):489–97.
21. Na DG, Lee JH, Jung SL, Kim JH, Sung JY, Shin JH, et al. Radiofrequency ablation of benign thyroid nodules and recurrent thyroid cancers: consensus statement and recommendations. Korean J Radiol. 2012;13(2):117–25.
22. Kim JH, Baek JH, Lim HK, Ahn HS, Baek SM, Choi YJ, et al. 2017 Thyroid radiofrequency ablation guideline: Korean Society of Thyroid Radiology. Korean J Radiol. 2018;19(4):632–55.
23. Shin JH, Baek JH, Chung J, Ha EJ, Kim JH, Lee YH, et al. Ultrasonography diagnosis and imaging-based management of thyroid nodules: revised Korean Society of Thyroid Radiology Consensus Statement and Recommendations. Korean J Radiol. 2016;17(3):370–95.
24. Orlandi A, Puscar A, Capriata E, Fideleff H. Repeated fine-needle aspiration of the thyroid in benign nodular thyroid disease: critical evaluation of long-term follow-up. Thyroid. 2005;15(3):274–8.
25. Ha EJ, Baek JH, Che Y, Chou YH, Fukunari N, Kim JH, et al. Radiofrequency ablation of benign thyroid nodules: recommendations from the Asian conference on tumor ablation task force. Ultrasonography. 2021;40(1):75–82.
26. Jeon SJ, Kim E, Park JS, Son KR, Baek JH, Kim YS, et al. Diagnostic benefit of thyroglobulin measurement in fine-needle aspiration for diagnosing metastatic cervical lymph nodes from papillary thyroid cancer: correlations with US features. Korean J Radiol. 2009;10(2):106–11.
27. Papini E, Pacella CM, Solbiati LA, Achille G, Barbaro D, Bernardi S, et al. Minimally-invasive treatments for benign thyroid nodules: a Delphi-based consensus statement from the Italian minimally-invasive treatments of the thyroid (MITT) group. Int J Hyperth. 2019;36(1):376–82.
28. Garberoglio R, Aliberti C, Appetecchia M, Attard M, Boccuzzi G, Boraso F, et al. Radiofrequency ablation for thyroid nodules: which indications? The first Italian opinion statement. J Ultrasound. 2015;18(4):423–30.
29. Noguchi S, Yamashita H, Uchino S, Watanabe S. Papillary microcarcinoma. World J Surg. 2008;32(5):747–53.
30. Jeong SY, Baek JH, Choi YJ, Lee JH. Ethanol and thermal ablation for malignant thyroid tumours. Int J Hyperth. 2017;33(8):938–45.
31. Muhammad H, Tehreem A, Russell JO. Radiofrequency ablation and thyroid cancer: review of the current literature. Am J Otolaryngol. 2022;43(1):103204.
32. Issa PP, Omar M, Issa CP, Buti Y, Hussein M, Aboueisha M, et al. Radiofrequency ablation of indeterminate thyroid nodules: the First North American Comparative Analysis. Int J Mol Sci. 2022;23(19):11493.
33. Tong MY, Li HS, Che Y. Recurrent medullary thyroid carcinoma treated with percutaneous ultrasound-guided radiofrequency ablation: a case report. World J Clin Cases. 2021;9(4):864–70.

# Chapter 12
# Standard RFA Procedure and Advanced Techniques

**Pi-Ling Chiang and Wei-Che Lin**

## Introduction

Radiofrequency ablation (RFA) is one of the thermal ablations for thyroid tumors, which has developed rapidly with wide application in the last two decades. Within the tissue of a patient, RFA uses the heat generated from ionic agitation by high-frequency alternating electric current oscillating between 200 and 1200 kHz, creating thermally induced coagulation necrosis in the tissue or tumor surrounding the electrode [1]. The clinical application of RFA in thyroid nodules was first introduced in 2006 [2]. A modified "moving-shot technique" was proposed in 2008 [3], and then developed as a standard technique of thyroid RFA. Since then, RFA has been widely used in benign thyroid nodules and recurrent thyroid cancers.

P.-L. Chiang
Department of Diagnostic Radiology, Kaohsiung Chang Gung Memorial Hospital, Chang Gung University College of Medicine, Kaohsiung, Taiwan

Thyroid Head and Neck Ablation Center, Kaohsiung Chang Gung Memorial Hospital, Kaohsiung, Taiwan
e-mail: lovage@cgmh.org.tw

W.-C. Lin (✉)
Department of Diagnostic Radiology, Kaohsiung Chang Gung Memorial Hospital, Chang Gung University College of Medicine, Kaohsiung, Taiwan

Thyroid Head and Neck Ablation Center, Kaohsiung Chang Gung Memorial Hospital, Kaohsiung, Taiwan

College of Medicine, National Sun Yat-Sen University, Kaohsiung, Taiwan
e-mail: alex@cgmh.org.tw



A. W. Park et al. (eds.), *Thyroid Radiofrequency Ablation*,
https://doi.org/10.1007/978-3-031-65288-2_12

In the management of thyroid lesions, RFA, a minimally invasive treatment as an alternative to surgery, has shown good efficacy and safety [4, 5]. Based on the anatomy and location of thyroid glands, the perithyroidal structures, such as trachea, esophagus, recurrent laryngeal, and vagus nerves, are critical and vulnerable to thermal injury. To optimize efficacy and minimize complications, it is important to understand the essential and advanced techniques and to manipulate the electrode properly. This chapter presents the currently developed techniques of thyroid RFA.

## Patient Preparation and Choice of RFA Electrodes

### *Preparation and Monitoring*

Before the ablation procedure, the patient is placed in supine position with neck hyperextended to achieve an optimal exposure of the thyroid gland. Grounding pads are attached to both thighs of the patient. The operator stands at the head of the patient, while the ultrasound screen is positioned in a location that is easily visible to the surgeon, allowing for easy operation during the RFA procedure. For maneuverability, probe and image orientation should be the same as the operator orientation, which may not be the same as the orientation of diagnostic ultrasound (US) images. It is suggested to hold the probe with the hand on same side as the lesion being ablated, and to hold the needle with the contralateral hand. Both hands of the operator should be available for holding the needle.

Regular monitoring of vital signs and checking the voice through conversations are recommended for each patient at the beginning, during, and at the end of an RFA procedure. Prophylactic pain relievers can relieve pain from ablation during the procedure. Patients may undergo RFA procedures under analgesia, sedation, or anesthesia; however, deep sedation or anesthesia may delay the detection of complications [6].

### *The Choices of RFA Electrodes*

The size of coagulation necrosis or ablated zone is dependent on overall energy deposition, which is related to the RF power and duration, and RF electrode's active tip length and gauge. Due to higher nodule-to-parenchyma volume ratios and relatively fewer safety margins of thyroid nodules compared to liver tumors, modified, short (7 cm), and thin (18–19 gauge) electrodes with active tips of various lengths (e.g., 0.5, 0.7, 1.0, or 1.5 cm) can be used [7, 8]. The nodule size, contour, and the relative position of the thyroid capsule and perithyroidal critical structures should be all taken into consideration when choosing RFA electrodes.

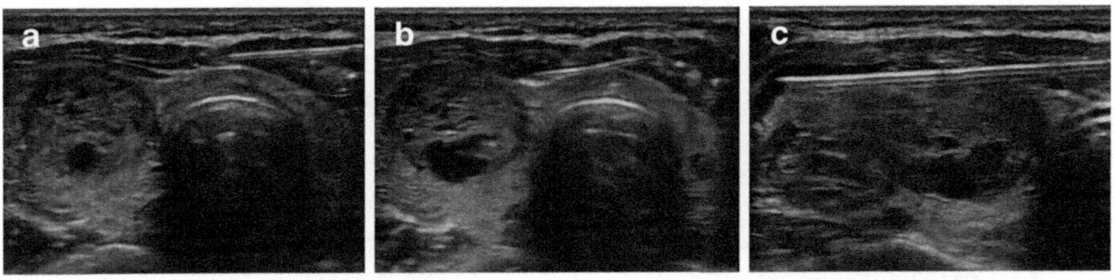


**Fig. 12.1** US-guided local anesthesia is injected into the subcutaneous layer and anterior cervical muscles (**a**), via trans-isthmus approach (**b**), into the perithyroidal space along the thyroid capsule (**c**)

# Standard RFA Techniques

## *Local Anesthesia*

After skin sterilization, local anesthesia with 2% lidocaine is injected at the RFA needle–puncture site, via a trans-isthmus approach, into the perithyroidal space along the thyroid capsule, and also into the subcutaneous tissue and anterior cervical muscles (Fig. 12.1). At this stage, it is important to avoid needle puncture or injury to the thyroid vessels at the capsule to prevent perithyroidal hematoma. Local anesthetic injection into perineural space, such as tracheoesophageal groove and carotid space, can mask thermal injury to the nerve during ablation due to transient nerve palsy caused by local anesthetic injection.

## *RFA Procedures*

The RFA of thyroid nodules is performed using free-hand, percutaneous, trans-isthmic approach, with the "moving-shot" technique (Fig. 12.2) [3, 8], which contrasts with the fixed electrode technique used in the RFA of liver tumors. Under US guidance along the transverse or oblique view of the thyroid glands, an electrode is inserted via the isthmus into the targeted nodule. A trans-isthmic approach through sufficient thyroid parenchyma prevents leakage of ablated fluid or rupture of the ablated thyroid nodule. It also provides more tolerance for changes in the electrode position caused by micro-motion such as swallowing or talking.

During an ablation procedure, a target thyroid nodule is conceptually separated into multiple small units, and ablated unit-by-unit by moving the electrode. The ablated units fill with transient echogenic bubbles, which then turns into a hypoechoic change after the bubbles dissipate in the following minutes. To prevent visual disturbance obscured by ablated bubbles, the ablation electrode tip should be inserted into the deepest unit and then moved back to the superficial and nearest units in a single slice. A thyroid nodule is totally ablated by moving the electrode unit-by-unit

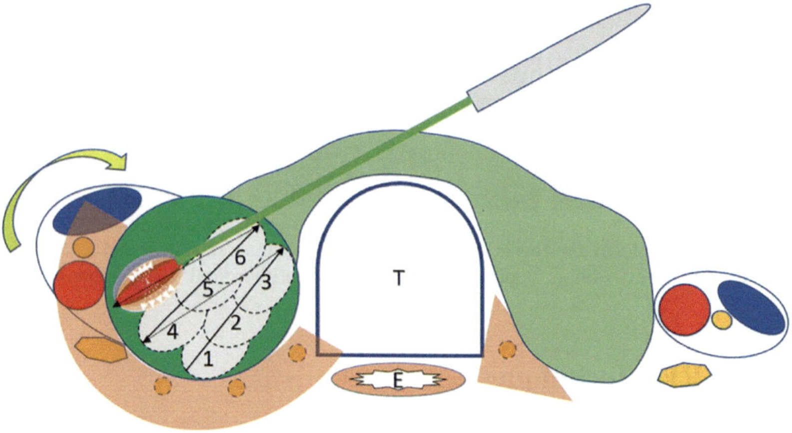


**Fig. 12.2** Moving-shot technique. Ablation is performed dynamically with multiple small ablation units beginning with the deepest and most medial portion of the nodule to superficial and more lateral portions. *E* esophagus, *T* trachea; 1–7—ablation units; red circles—common carotid artery; blue ellipses—internal jugular vein; yellow circles with solid borders—vagus nerve; yellow circles with dotted borders—recurrent laryngeal nerve; and yellow heptagon—middle cervical sympathetic ganglion. (With permission from Park [9])

and then slice-by-slice via single or oligo-punction sites under US guidance along the transverse or oblique view (moving-shot technique) (Fig. 12.2).

The RF power is chosen depending on the size of the active tip and the internal characteristics of the nodules and usually starts at 30 W. With adequate power, a transient echogenic area starts at the electrode tip within 5–10 s and then spreads to the whole ablation zone. If there is no change in echogenicity after more than 10 s of ablation, an increment in RF power of 5–10 W is recommended. If a patient experiences severe pain during ablation, a decrement of RF power or pause of ablation may be considered.

## Advanced RFA Techniques

Hydrodissection is a safe and effective technique to improve ablation completion and reduce damage to surrounding tissues [10–12]. To ensure the safety of ablation, pre-ablation hydrodissection is suggested for thyroid nodules near cervical critical structures (trachea, esophagus, recurrent laryngeal nerve, carotid sheath, etc.). Under sonographic guidance, sterile cold dextrose 5% in water (D5W) is injected using a sterile syringe into the perithyroidal space to separate the thyroid nodules from surrounding tissues. Continuous infusion of cold D5W is also suggested to maintain a thermal buffer during RFA. With adequate hydrodissection, the thyroid nodules can be separated from the perithyroidal critical structures, and the boundary of the thyroid can be well identified, which may provide advantages to minimizing residual viable marginal tissue. There is no need for aspiration of the hydrodissection fluid after the RFA procedure.

## *Medial Hydrodissection*

The tracheoesophageal groove (called as danger triangle) is an important landmark for thyroid ablation, which includes the recurrent laryngeal nerve (RLN), trachea, and esophagus. Medial hydrodissection allows to separate thyroid nodules from these critical structures, especially the RLN. The hydrodissection needle is inserted via a trans-isthmus approach into the danger triangle (Fig. 12.3). Local anesthesia should not be injected into this space to avoid transient palsy of RLN, which may cause transient hoarseness and mask the thermal injury to RLN during ablation procedure.

## *Lateral Hydrodissection*

The carotid sheath is located on the lateral side of the thyroid, contenting common carotid artery (CCA), internal jugular vein (IJV), vagus nerve (VN), and sympathetic plexus. The vagus nerve can be visualized on an ultrasound image, which is typically located between the CCA and the IJV, followed by the most common variation of the vagus nerve passing in front of the CCA [13, 14]. However, a bulging thyroid mass may displace laterally, rotate the carotid sheath, and change the VN's location, abutting and lateral to the thyroid [15] (Fig. 12.4). Adequate lateral hydrodissection between the thyroid and carotid sheath is especially important for a large goiter to prevent unwanted thermal injury to the VN (Fig. 12.5).

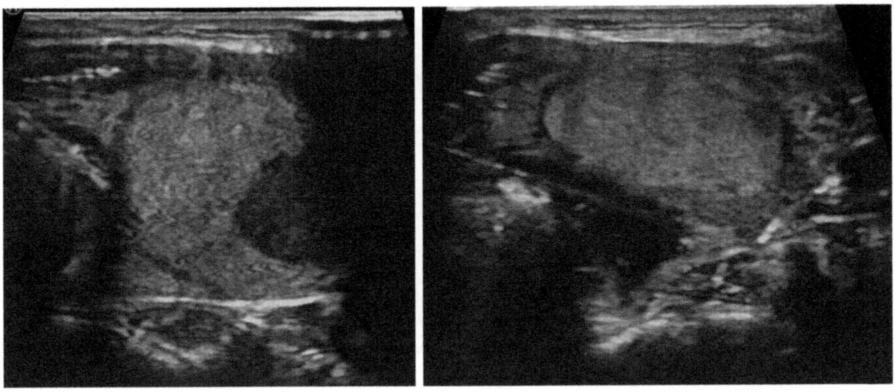

**Fig. 12.3** Medial hydrodissection via trans-isthmus approach to the danger triangle

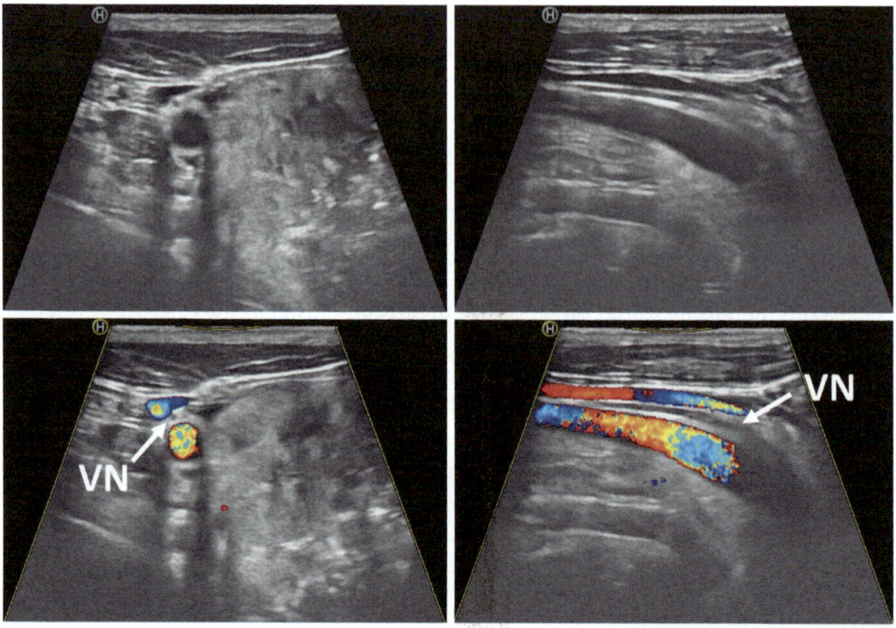


**Fig. 12.4** The VN located between the CCA and the IJV, which is displaced laterally, rotated anteriorly to CCA, and abutting and lateral to the thyroid, due to the bulging thyroid mass

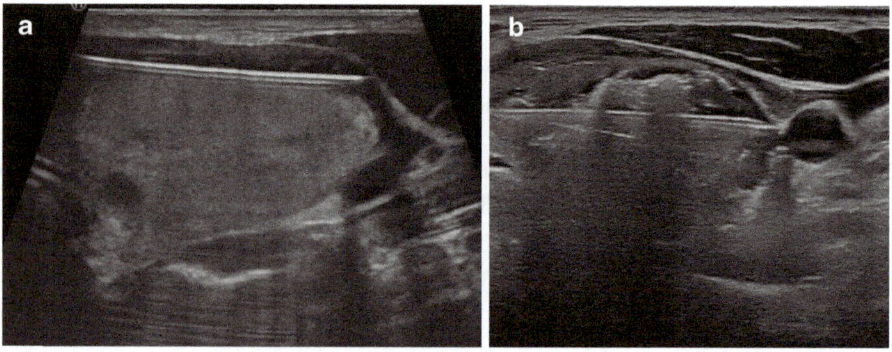


**Fig. 12.5** Lateral hydrodissection can be injected via a needle along the anterior perithyroidal space (**a**) or through trans-thyroidal approach (**b**)

## *Other Hydrodissection*

Dorsal/dorsal-lateral hydrodissection is mainly used to identify the dorsal boundary of thyroid and to separate the middle cervical ganglion (Fig. 12.6). Pretracheal hydrodissection is used to separate isthmic nodules from the trachea to avoid

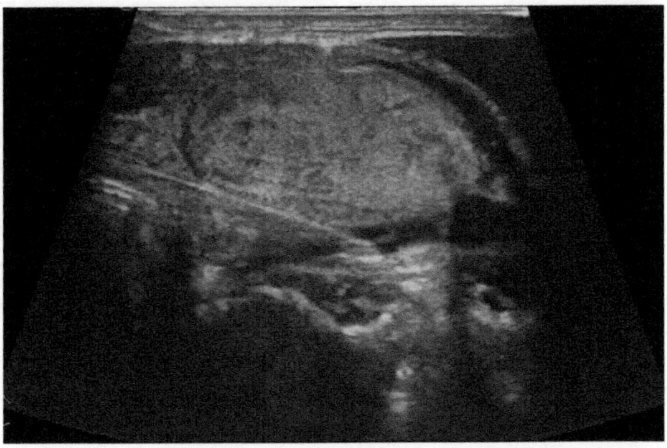

**Fig. 12.6** Dorsal hydrodissection to separate the dorsal boundary of the thyroid and prevertebral space

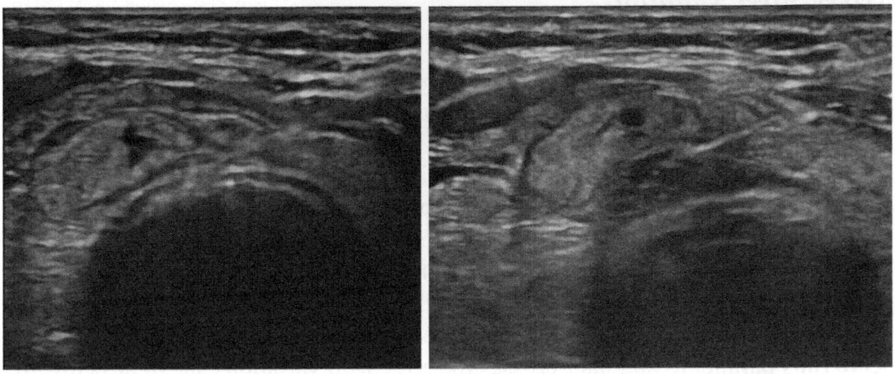

**Fig. 12.7** Pretracheal hydrodissection to elevate the isthmic nodule from the trachea

tracheal thermal injury (Fig. 12.7). Note the paratracheal cold DW5 serves as a temperature stimulus to the trachea and can easily trigger a cough reflex.

## Vascular Ablation

Vascular ablation technique is a useful technique and was first reported by Park et al. [12], including artery-first ablation and marginal venous ablation, which is applied to different nodular characteristics. In another 6-month preliminary result, additional vascular ablation may improve the effectiveness of the RFA, with greater volume reduction rate [16]. Before vascular ablation, administration of adequate local anesthesia and hydrodissection are suggested especially at perithyroidal perivascular site to prevent stronger ablation pain due to capsule injury and higher RF power. A second look of the color Doppler ultrasound may help ensure coagulated vessels before moving the electrode to prevent unwanted vascular bleeding.

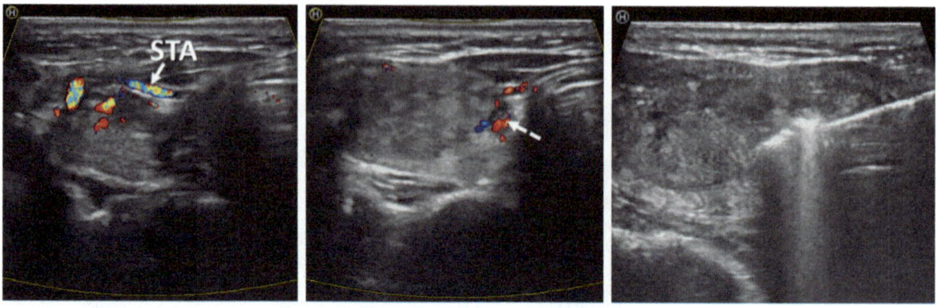


**Fig. 12.8** The superior thyroid artery (solid arrow) enters through the isthmus into the thyroid and supplies feeding arteries (dash arrow) to an upper pole nodule. After administering local anesthesia, artery ablation can be performed if no hoarseness is noted

## *Artery-First Ablation*

For hypervascular thyroid nodules with prominent feeding arteries, the artery-first ablation technique is applicable to decrease arterial flow, reduce the heat-sink effect, and limit intranodular hemorrhage during RFA [12, 17]. In a hypervascular nodule, ablating draining veins but not feeding arteries may result in venous congestion and diffuse edema of the thyroid glands. Doppler ultrasound is useful to distinguish feeding arteries from draining veins. A feeding artery usually enters through the isthmus, which may arise from the superior thyroid artery (STA) supplying upper pole nodules (Fig. 12.8), while the inferior thyroid artery (ITA) supplies lower pole thyroid nodules. It should be noted that the external branch of the superior laryngeal nerve runs parallel to and later crosses the STA with variations above or below the upper pole of the thyroid gland [18]. Ablation of the STA may induce superior laryngeal nerve palsy, causing loss of the high-pitched voice. Sometimes, a wedge-shaped hypoechoic change may be seen in a thyroid nodule after feeding artery ablation owing to arterial infarction.

## *Marginal Venous Ablation*

Marginal venous ablation is useful for most thyroid nodules and can be combined with tissue ablation. It decreases the heat-sink effect during RFA and also provides better outcomes due to the complete ablation of the margin of the target nodule [12, 19]. During initial venous ablation, air bubbles fill in and flow rapidly through the marginal veins of the nodule, and then the bubble flow becomes slow gradually and finally stasis in the marginal veins after a complete ablation. Avoid venous-first ablation in a hypervascular nodule, or congestion and diffuse edema in the thyroid glands may be noted. For thyroid nodules with marginal veins close to the thyroid capsule and critical perithyroidal structures, continuous hydrodissection with cold D5W infusion and monitoring of nerve function are suggested during the ablation.

## Conclusion

In summary, this chapter presents essential and advanced techniques of pre-RFA preparation, local anesthesia, perithyroidal hydrodissection, and nodular and vascular ablation. Knowing and mastering these skills could shorten the learning curve for operators and increase the safety of a patient undergoing thyroid RFA.

## References

1. Rhim H, et al. Essential techniques for successful radio-frequency thermal ablation of malignant hepatic tumors. Radiographics. 2001;21:S17. **21 Spec No**: p. S17–35; discussion S36–9.
2. Kim YS, et al. Radiofrequency ablation of benign cold thyroid nodules: initial clinical experience. Thyroid. 2006;16(4):361–7.
3. Jeong WK, et al. Radiofrequency ablation of benign thyroid nodules: safety and imaging follow-up in 236 patients. Eur Radiol. 2008;18(6):1244–50.
4. Chung SR, et al. Safety of radiofrequency ablation of benign thyroid nodules and recurrent thyroid cancers: a systematic review and meta-analysis. Int J Hyperth. 2017;33(8):920–30.
5. Tong M, et al. Efficacy and safety of radiofrequency, microwave and laser ablation for treating papillary thyroid microcarcinoma: a systematic review and meta-analysis. Int J Hyperth. 2019;36(1):1278–86.
6. Na DG, et al. Radiofrequency ablation of benign thyroid nodules and recurrent thyroid cancers: consensus statement and recommendations. Korean J Radiol. 2012;13(2):117–25.
7. Baek JH, et al. Radiofrequency ablation for the treatment of autonomously functioning thyroid nodules. World J Surg. 2009;33(9):1971–7.
8. Shin JH, et al. Radiofrequency ablation of thyroid nodules: basic principles and clinical application. Int J Endocrinol. 2012;2012:919650.
9. Park AW. Thyroid radiofrequency ablation. OZ & SE; 2020.
10. Xiaoyin T, et al. Risk assessment and hydrodissection technique for radiofrequency ablation of thyroid benign nodules. J Cancer. 2018;9(17):3058–66.
11. Cui D, et al. Efficacy and safety of a combination of hydrodissection and radiofrequency ablation therapy for benign thyroid nodules larger than 2 cm: a retrospective study. J Cancer Res Ther. 2019;15(2):386–93.
12. Park HS, et al. Thyroid radiofrequency ablation: updates on innovative devices and techniques. Korean J Radiol. 2017;18(4):615–23.
13. Park JK, et al. Variations in the course of the cervical vagus nerve on thyroid ultrasonography. AJNR Am J Neuroradiol. 2011;32(7):1178–81.
14. Ha EJ, et al. Clinical significance of vagus nerve variation in radiofrequency ablation of thyroid nodules. Eur Radiol. 2011;21(10):2151–7.
15. Ha EJ, Baek JH, Lee JH. Ultrasonography-based thyroidal and perithyroidal anatomy and its clinical significance. Korean J Radiol. 2015;16(4):749–66.
16. Offi C, et al. The ablation of thyroid nodule's afferent arteries before radiofrequency ablation: preliminary data. Front Endocrinol (Lausanne). 2020;11:565000.
17. Pillai K, et al. Heat sink effect on tumor ablation characteristics as observed in monopolar radiofrequency, bipolar radiofrequency, and microwave, using ex vivo calf liver model. Medicine (Baltimore). 2015;94(9):e580.
18. Dessie MA. Variations of the origin of superior thyroid artery and its relationship with the external branch of superior laryngeal nerve. PLoS One. 2018;13(5):e0197075.
19. Zhao CK, et al. Factors associated with initial incomplete ablation for benign thyroid nodules after radiofrequency ablation: first results of CEUS evaluation. Clin Hemorheol Microcirc. 2017;65(4):393–405.

# Chapter 13
# Postprocedural Care and Follow-Up for Thyroid RFA

**Yoon-Jin Kim**

## Immediate Post-procedural Care

Thyroid radiofrequency ablation (RFA) is an outpatient procedure. After the procedure, patients are transported to the recovery area for post-procedural monitoring (30 min at our institution) prior to discharge. Supportive care for neck soreness and pain is provided with an ice pack. Because patients often receive preprocedural analgesia and intra-procedural subcutaneous anesthesia, additional pain medication prior to discharge is not usually needed but is available. Even for patients who do not receive intravenous sedation, we request they have a ride home in the event of any post-procedural complications or neck soreness that would limit full mobility while driving. Patients are provided with additional ice packs and a written handout for at-home care. They are instructed to limit rigorous activity for 24 h and cautioned that they may have bruising and neck swelling post-procedurally for up to 1 week. We recommend seeking medical attention if a fever occurs or if they experience any of the following symptoms: lightheadedness, difficulty breathing, uncontrolled bleeding, worsening swelling, worsening redness or drainage from the probe insertion site, vomiting, coughing up blood, or any changes in voice. We recommend at home pain control with over-the-counter non-opioid analgesics such as acetaminophen and recommend limiting ibuprofen to minimize the risk of bleeding. Opioids are not routinely prescribed for post-procedural pain management. Patients are asked not to touch or press over the treated area to minimize the risk of rupture.

Y.-J. Kim (✉)
Dotter Department of Interventional Radiology, Oregon Health and Sciences University, Portland, OR, USA



A. W. Park et al. (eds.), *Thyroid Radiofrequency Ablation*,
https://doi.org/10.1007/978-3-031-65288-2_13

## Follow-Up

Follow-up after thyroid RFA should focus on identifying and managing any complications, measuring changes in nodule volume, and tracking the patient's cosmetic and symptom scores. Tables 13.1 and 13.2 outline the follow-up protocols at our institution. Minor specifics do vary from certain society guidelines as the follow-up protocol has evolved over time in response to feedback from patients and limitations of insurance coverage. For example, the Korean Society of Thyroid Radiology (KSThR) recommends performing an ultrasound at every visit [1]. Visits are preferred to be performed in person. However, patients have the option to have a virtual visit to mitigate long-distance travel and facilitate continued follow-up. At each visit, a symptom score and cosmetic score are obtained. If an ultrasound is obtained, the volume of the treated thyroid nodule is calculated to determine the volume reduction ratio by using the formula: [(initial volume – final volume) × 100]/initial volume. The appearance of a treated nodule on the grey scale will be predominantly hypoechoic and may contain echogenic foci. On color Doppler images, a well-treated nodule will have minimal vascularity [2]. Most patients can expect to have a volume reduction ratio (VRR) of 70–90%. Treatment success is defined by improvement in patient's symptoms and technical success by a reduction in nodule size by 50% [2].

Patients with autonomously functioning thyroid nodules (AFTNs) require additional follow-up considerations and are also closely followed by an endocrinologist. Thyroid-stimulating hormone (TSH) values and the patient's hyperthyroid symptoms will guide medication titration after ablation. Unlike benign nonfunctional thyroid nodules, technical success by imaging criteria for an ATFN often requires a larger VRR, often up to 80% [3]. If questions remain about treatment success, a thyroid uptake scan may be helpful [1].

**Table 13.1** Benign nonfunctioning thyroid nodules

| Time post-RFA | Imaging | Labs |
|---|---|---|
| 30 days | None | If indicated[a] |
| 3 months | In-office ultrasound | If indicated[a] |
| 6 months | Formal ultrasound | TSH |
| 12 months | Formal ultrasound | If indicated[a] |
| Yearly—If indicated | Formal ultrasound | In indicated[a] |

[a]Laboratory tests are obtained if there are any symptoms of hyperthyroidism or hypothyroidism.

**Table 13.2** Autonomous functioning thyroid nodules

| Time post-RFA | Imaging | Labs |
|---|---|---|
| 30 days | None | TSH, free T4 |
| 3 months | In-office ultrasound | TSH, free T4 |
| 6 months | Formal ultrasound | TSH, free T4 |
| 12 months | Formal ultrasound | TSH, free T4 |
| Yearly—If indicated | Formal ultrasound | TSH, free T4 |

The decision to retreat a nodule should be guided by the patient's symptoms, a VRR of less than 50%, and/or nodule regrowth. Some physicians advocate treating areas of residual vascularity even with symptom improvement due to the potential for nodule regrowth [1]. For ATFNs, a TSH that does not normalize may guide the decision to retreat despite imaging findings [1]. Nodule regrowth can occur 2–3 years post-ablation, so patients should be followed long term.

## References

1. Kim J, Baek J, Lim H, et al. 2017 Thyroid radiofrequency ablation guideline: Korean Society of Thyroid Radiology. Korean J Radiol. 2018;19(4):632–55.
2. Lim J, Kuo J. Thyroid nodule radiofrequency ablation: complications and clinical follow-up. Tech Vasc Interv Radiol. 2022;25(2):1–7.
3. Sag A, Kazaure H, Kelley C. Role of thyroid RFA in the treatment of autonomously functioning thyroid nodules. Tech Vasc Interv Radiol. 2022;25(2):1–4.

# Chapter 14
# Clinical Efficacy of RFA for Benign Thyroid Nodules

**Jin Yong Sung**

## Introduction

Benign thyroid nodules are prevalent in the adult population and often remain asymptomatic. However, when these nodules become large, they can result in cosmetic concerns and neck pressure symptoms. Additionally, some patients may experience subclinical or overt hyperthyroidism due to the presence of autonomously functioning thyroid nodules (AFTNs) [1, 2]. While surgery is generally well tolerated, it carries the risk of complications such as hypothyroidism, nerve injury, hematoma, and wound infection [3, 4]. As a minimally invasive treatment modality, ultrasound-guided radiofrequency ablation (RFA) has emerged as an alternative to surgery and has rapidly become one of the primary options for managing benign thyroid nodules, demonstrating favorable efficacy and safety [1, 5]. Various national and international societies have developed practical guidelines for thyroid RFA [1, 2, 5–7]. This chapter provides a comprehensive summary of the clinical effects of RFA for benign thyroid nodules, drawing upon relevant literature.

## Metrics for Evaluating the Effects of Thyroid RFA

RFA can be assessed using various metrics. These include the measurement of symptomatic or cosmetic problems using scoring systems. Patients can self-measure symptom scores using a 10-cm visual analog scale (ranging from 0 to 10). Additionally, cosmetic scores can be determined by a physician using the following scale: (1) no palpable mass, (2) no cosmetic problem but palpable mass, (3) a

J. Y. Sung (✉)
Department of Radiology, Thyroid Center, Daerim St. Mary's Hospital, Seoul, South Korea
e-mail: jysrad@drh.co.kr



A. W. Park et al. (eds.), *Thyroid Radiofrequency Ablation*,
https://doi.org/10.1007/978-3-031-65288-2_14

cosmetic problem on swallowing only, and (4) a readily detected cosmetic problem. By comparing pre-RFA scores with follow-up data, the effectiveness of RFA can be evaluated [5, 6].

The size, echogenicity, proportion of solid components, and internal vascularity of each nodule should be carefully evaluated before and after RFA. Three orthogonal diameters, including the largest diameter, should be measured using ultrasound (US), and nodule volume can be calculated using the Eq. $V = \pi abc/6$, where $V$ represents the volume, and $a$, $b$, and $c$ are the perpendicular diameters. The volume reduction ratio (VRR) is calculated as VRR (%) = ([initial volume − final volume] × 100)/initial volume. Therapeutic success is defined as a volume reduction greater than 50% of the initial nodule volume on a follow-up ultrasonography examination. The therapeutic success rate refers to the percentage of successfully treated nodules [5, 8–10].

To predict the recurrence of treated thyroid nodules, three types of nodule volumes can be measured and calculated using US images. These include the total nodule volume (*Vt*), ablated volume (*V*a), and viable volume (*V*v). *Vt* represents the total nodule volume, *V*a represents the ablated nodule volume, which appears as a hypoechoic area without vascularity on US, and *V*v is calculated as $Vv = Vt - Va$, representing the incompletely treated viable nodule volume. The initial ablation ratio (IAR) is the ratio between *V*a and *Vt*, and it is calculated as follows: IAR = $(Va/Vt) \times 100$. The IAR is a semi-quantitative index that measures the amount of ablation induced by RFA and is associated with technique efficacy [11].

Following RFA of AFTN, thyroid function should be monitored by measuring thyroid-stimulating hormone (TSH), triiodothyronine (T3), and thyroxine (T4) at each follow-up [12–15]. Changes in the thyroid nuclear scan can be useful in assessing the efficacy of RFA for AFTN. Thyroid nodules on follow-up nuclear scans are classified into three categories: type 1 (hot nodule), type 2 (nodule uptake similar to extra-nodular thyroid tissue), and type 3 (cold nodule or invisible status) [12, 13]. Based on TSH changes, antithyroid medications can be reduced or stopped after the RFA of AFTN. The therapeutic response of patients depends on the required drug dosage and is classified into three categories: remission (euthyroid state after withdrawal of antithyroid drug), improvement (reducing the medication for euthyroid state), and no response (unchanged medication dose compared to baseline) [15].

## Outcomes of RFA for Benign Nonfunctioning Thyroid Nodule

Multiple randomized controlled trials, including one international study, have demonstrated the effectiveness of RFA for benign nonfunctioning thyroid nodules. These studies have shown that RFA leads to a reduction in nodule volume and alleviation of nodule-related clinical problems. The results obtained from comparisons with similar control groups rule out the possibility of these effects being attributed solely to spontaneous nodule reduction (Fig. 14.1) [16, 17].

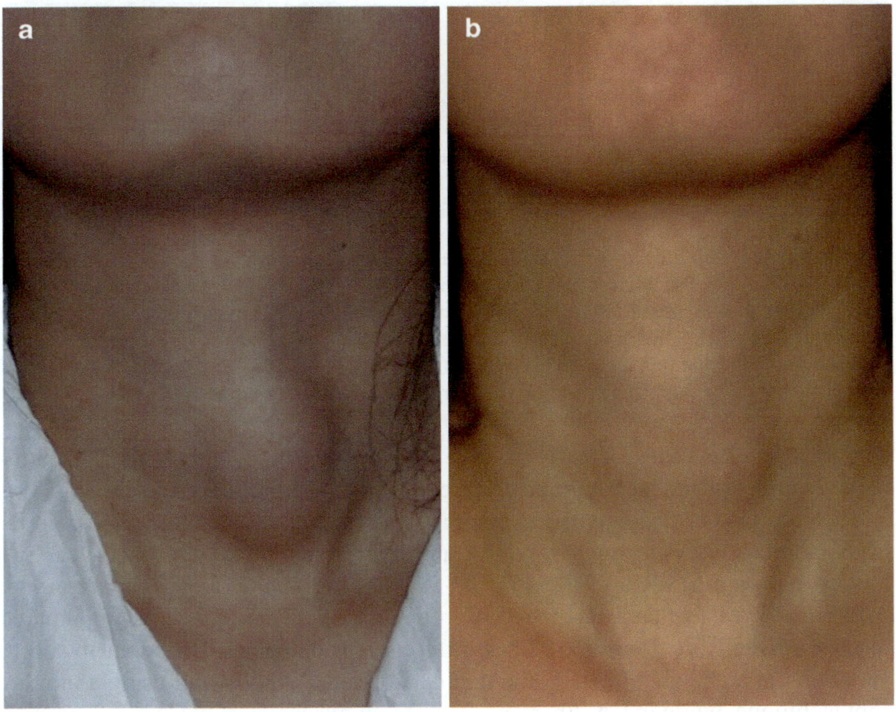


**Fig. 14.1** Improved cosmetic appearance following RFA for a nonfunctioning benign thyroid nodule. (**a**) Initial cosmetic grade 4 due to a nonfunctioning benign thyroid nodule in the left isthmus. (**b**) Cosmetic grade 1 observed at the 2-year post-RFA follow-up

Numerous articles, including retrospective studies, randomized controlled trials, review articles, and systematic reviews with meta-analyses, have consistently demonstrated the favorable efficacy and safety of RFA for benign thyroid nodules [8, 10, 16–34]. The majority of these studies have follow-up periods of less than 2 years, and the VRR at the last follow-up ranges between 50 and 80%. These studies have also shown significant improvement in cosmetic and symptom scores during the follow-up period [3].

A systematic review and meta-analysis focusing on the long-term follow-up results of RFA treatment for benign thyroid nodules, specifically for durations exceeding 3 years, reported the following pooled VRRs: 64.5% at 6 months, 76.9% at 12 months, 80.1% at 24 months, 80.3% at 36 months, and 92.2% at the last follow-up. The study observed a trend of rapid volume reduction in ablated nodules during the first 12 months of follow-up, followed by a plateau phase between 12 and 36 months, and further volume reduction occurring after 36 months, indicating the long-term maintenance of treatment efficacy (Fig. 14.2) [6, 35].

Both surgical resection and RFA have shown efficacy in the treatment of symptomatic thyroid nodules. However, RFA offers several advantages over surgery for

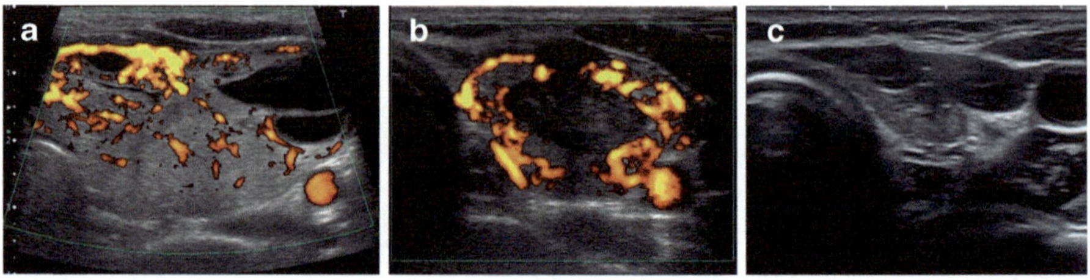


**Fig. 14.2** Long-term efficacy of RFA for nonfunctioning benign thyroid nodule. (**a**) Transverse power Doppler scan of a 28-year-old female with a 38 mL large benign hypervascular left thyroid mass. (**b**) Six months post-RFA follow-up transverse power Doppler scan showing a significant reduction to a 6 mL left thyroid nodule with hypervascular undertreated areas. A second session of RFA was performed at this time. (**c**) Six years after two sessions of RFA, a transverse ultrasound scan demonstrates a completely necrotic left thyroid nodule with a volume of 0.1 mL

benign thyroid nodules. It is associated with fewer complications, better health-related quality of life, and improved preservation of thyroid function [19, 36, 37].

RFA has also been compared to other ablation techniques that are gaining popularity. A meta-analysis comparing RFA and laser ablation (LA) with a 3-year follow-up reported a VRR of 92% in the RFA group and 43% in the LA group. Additionally, 21% of patients in the LA group underwent delayed surgery compared to none in the RFA group [35]. This difference in outcomes can be attributed to variations in technique. In RFA, the nodule is ablated unit by unit using a moving shot technique, while in LA, fibers are focused on the center of the lesion. This may result in incomplete ablation of the nodule margins, which raises concerns about potential regrowth during follow-up. Retrospective and prospective studies comparing RFA with microwave ablation (MWA) for benign thyroid nodules have demonstrated greater VRR in the RFA group compared to the MWA group at 6 months of follow-up [38, 39]. However, it is important to note that the outcomes of these operator-dependent techniques are significantly influenced by the specific skills and training of the performing physicians [1].

## Outcomes of RFA for AFTN

The available data on the effectiveness of RFA for treating hyperthyroidism associated with AFTN is limited, and long-term follow-up data are lacking [6]. The response of AFTNs to RFA is typically lower compared to nonfunctioning cold nodules, as hot nodules exhibit increased vascularity and higher rates of marginal recurrence [12, 13].

A recent systematic review and meta-analysis of RFA for AFTNs reported a TSH normalization rate of 71.2% and VRR of 69.4% at a mean follow-up period of 12.8 months. In terms of treatment sessions, single and multiple sessions of RFA achieved TSH normalization rates of 66.7% and 79.3%, respectively [40, 41]. In a retrospective multicenter study conducted by trained radiologists utilizing the moving-shot technique and modified straight internally cooled electrodes, all patients showed improvement in hyperthyroidism, with a VRR of 81.7%, a normalized TSH rate of 81.8%, and a normalized scan rate of 79.5% at a mean follow-up of 19.9 months (Fig. 14.3) [12].

Patients with smaller nodules (<12 mL) and volume reduction exceeding 80% are more likely to experience symptom resolution and resolution of hyperthyroidism [2, 42]. However, for larger AFTNs (usually >20 mL), RFA is less effective [13, 43–45]. Recently, a combined treatment approach involving LA and radioactive iodine (RAI) therapy has been proposed for large AFTNs. Compared to RAI therapy alone, combination therapy results in faster and greater improvement of local symptoms and biochemical hyperthyroidism, along with reduced RAI activity [44, 45]. Although not yet fully established in the literature, Italian guidelines

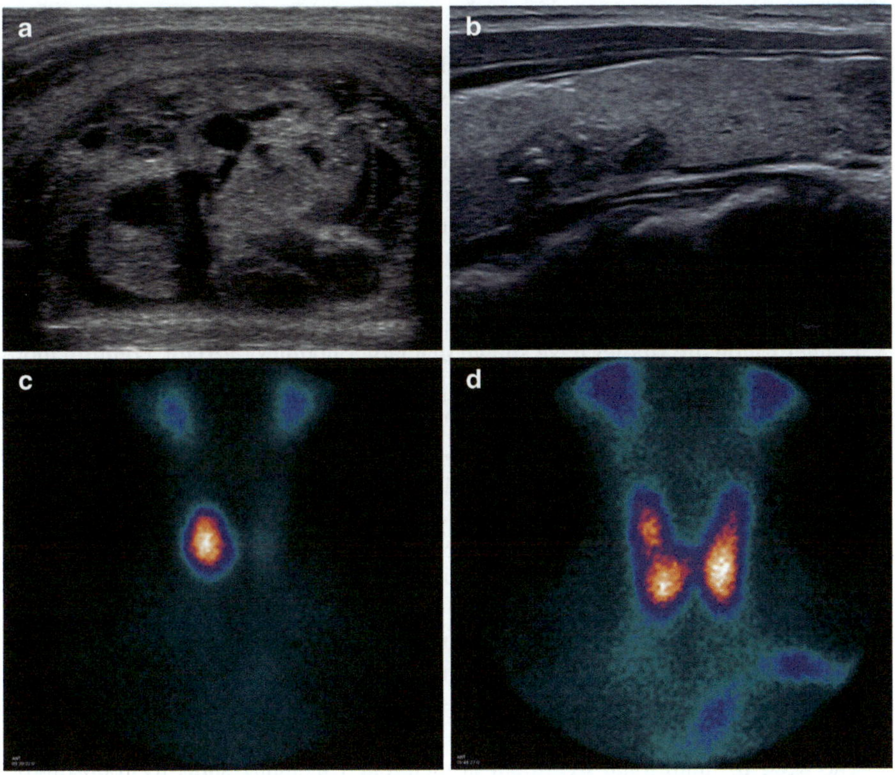


**Fig. 14.3** Long-term efficacy of RFA for autonomously functioning thyroid nodule. (**a**) Transverse ultrasound scan of a 36-year-old female with an 11 mL toxic thyroid nodule in the right thyroid lobe. The initial serum TSH level was 0.04 μIU/mL. (**b**) Ten years after a single session of RFA, a transverse ultrasound scan shows a completely necrotic right thyroid nodule with a volume of 0.3 mL. At that time, the serum TSH level was 1.6 μIU/mL. (**c**) Initial Tc99m-pertechnetate thyroid scan showing a hot nodule in the right thyroid lobe. (**d**) One year after RFA, Tc99m-pertechnetate thyroid scan shows a cold nodule in the right thyroid lobe

recommend the combined use of RFA and RAI treatment for large AFTNs (volume >20 mL) to achieve more rapid improvement of local symptoms [1, 2].

In cases where patients have elevated serum TSH receptor antibodies before RFA, which may indicate a combined status of Graves' disease and AFTNs, post-RFA hormonal changes may be incomplete, despite successful RFA treatment [5]. When compared to surgery, patients undergoing RFA for AFTNs have lower rates of hypothyroidism and procedure-related complications, although a significantly lower proportion achieve normalization of thyroid function [20]. When considering the choice between RAI and RFA, patients are more suitable candidates for RFA if they have solitary AFTNs, are not currently pregnant, but have plans for pregnancy in the relatively near future [46].

## Additional RFA for Benign Thyroid Nodule

The need for additional treatment after RFA may arise based on the size and location of the nodule [5]. If a viable portion with vascularity is detected on gray-scale and color-Doppler ultrasound (US), in addition to persistent symptomatic and cosmetic problems, additional ablation is indicated. This is because the under-ablated portion with vascularity has the potential for regrowth during follow-up [8, 13]. However, color-Doppler US may not be sufficiently sensitive in detecting small vessels and slow blood flow. Some authors have suggested that contrast-enhanced US can serve as an ancillary diagnostic tool for detecting the under-ablated portion after RFA [47, 48].

Longer follow-up studies have shown that larger nodules (>20 mL) require more treatment sessions to achieve a similar VRR compared to smaller nodules [26]. A previous randomized trial and Bayesian network meta-analysis have indicated that two sessions of RFA are more effective, particularly for nodules with a volume greater than 20 mL [49]. These studies suggest that a single treatment session may not maintain the long-term treatment effect, particularly for larger nodules.

In the case of incompletely resolved symptoms or thyroid function, repeat RFA may be necessary for AFTNs. The decision for repeat RFA may be based on the serum TSH level rather than the scan or under-ablated portion observed on US. Repeat RFA can be considered 1–3 months after the initial RFA, as rapid volume reduction of the nodule occurs during this period [12]. Previous studies have reported a mean number of treatment sessions ranging from 1.8 to 2.2 (1–6 sessions) for AFTNs [12, 13].

The need for additional treatment is mentioned in many short-term and long-term follow-up studies, but the proper timing for additional treatment remains unclear. Indications for additional treatment can be summarized as follows: incomplete symptom relief after treatment, VRR less than 50%, and tumor regrowth [8, 25]. In a study by Sim et al. [11], after 7 years of follow-up based on US, the authors divided the ablated nodule area into two parts: (1) the low-echogenic area with RFA and (2) the residual viable area, typically isoechoic and located at the periphery of the ablation zone. While the volume of the ablation zone decreases over time, the volume of the viable area may increase during regrowth. Monitoring the volume of the viable area rather than the entire nodule can be useful in determining the timing of additional ablation [11]. Few studies have explored factors associated with a lower treatment response or regrowth, but several proposals include intrinsic factors such as nodule volume, solidity, and functionality, as well as extrinsic factors like the positional relationship with surrounding tissues [34, 47].

## Conclusion

RFA has emerged as an effective non-surgical treatment option for both benign nonfunctioning thyroid nodules and AFTNs. However, further investigation is needed, particularly in areas such as the timing of additional RFA in cases of regrowth or incomplete ablation, as well as the long-term efficacy of RFA for various applications in thyroid treatment. Continued research and studies will contribute to enhancing our understanding and optimizing the use of RFA in the management of thyroid nodules.

## References

1. Papini E, Monpeyssen H, Frasoldati A, Hegedüs L. European thyroid association clinical practice guideline for the use of image-guided ablation in benign thyroid nodules. Eur Thyroid J. 2020;9(4):172–85.
2. Papini E, Pacella CM, Solbiati LA, et al. Minimally-invasive treatments for benign thyroid nodules: a Delphi-based consensus statement from the Italian minimally-invasive treatments of the thyroid (MITT) group. Int J Hyperth. 2019;36(1):376–82.
3. Muhammad H, Santhanam P, Russell JO, Kuo JH. RFA and benign thyroid nodules: review of the current literature. Laryngosc Investig Otolaryngol. 2021;6(1):155–65.
4. Reeve T, Thompson NW. Complications of thyroid surgery: how to avoid them, how to manage them, and observations on their possible effect on the whole patient. World J Surg. 2000;24(8):971–5.
5. Kim J-H, Baek JH, Lim HK, et al. Thyroid radiofrequency ablation guideline: Korean Society of Thyroid Radiology. Korean J Radiol. 2017;19(4):632–55.
6. Orloff LA, Noel JE, Stack BC Jr, et al. Radiofrequency ablation and related ultrasound-guided ablation technologies for treatment of benign and malignant thyroid disease: an international multidisciplinary consensus statement of the American Head and Neck Society Endocrine Surgery Section with the Asia Pacific Society of Thyroid Surgery, Associazione Medici Endocrinologi, British Association of Endocrine and Thyroid Surgeons, European Thyroid Association, Italian Society of Endocrine Surgery Units, Korean Society of Thyroid Radiology, Latin American Thyroid Society, and Thyroid Nodules Therapies Association. Head Neck. 2022;44(3):633–60.
7. Dobnig H, Zechmann W, Hermann M, et al. Radiofrequency ablation of thyroid nodules: "good clinical practice recommendations" for Austria: an interdisciplinary statement from the following professional associations: Austrian Thyroid Association (ÖSDG), Austrian Society for Nuclear Medicine and Molecular Imaging (OGNMB), Austrian Society for Endocrinology

and Metabolism (ÖGES), Surgical Endocrinology Working Group (ACE) of the Austrian Surgical Society (OEGCH). Wien Med Wochenschr. 2020;170:6–14.
8. Jeong WK, Baek JH, Rhim H, et al. Radiofrequency ablation of benign thyroid nodules: safety and imaging follow-up in 236 patients. Eur Radiol. 2008;18:1244–50.
9. Baek JH, Kim YS, Lee D, Huh JY, Lee JH. Benign predominantly solid thyroid nodules: prospective study of efficacy of sonographically guided radiofrequency ablation versus control condition. AJR Am J Roentgenol. 2010;194:1137–42.
10. Sung JY, Kim YS, Choi H, Lee JH, Baek JH. Optimum first-line treatment technique for benign cystic thyroid nodules: ethanol ablation or radiofrequency ablation? AJR Am J Roentgenol. 2011;196:W210–4.
11. Sim JS, Baek JH, Lee J, Cho W, Jung SI. Radiofrequency ablation of benign thyroid nodules: depicting early sign of regrowth by calculating vital volume. Int J Hyperth. 2017;33:905–10.
12. Sung JY, Baek JH, Jung SL, et al. Radiofrequency ablation for autonomously functioning thyroid nodules: a multicenter study. Thyroid. 2015;25:112–7.
13. Baek JH, Moon WJ, Kim YS, Lee JH, Lee D. Radiofrequency ablation for the treatment of autonomously functioning thyroid nodules. World J Surg. 2009;33:1971–7.
14. Faggiano A, Ramundo V, Assanti AP, et al. Thyroid nodules treated with percutaneous radiofrequency thermal ablation: a comparative study. J Clin Endocrinol Metab. 2012;97:4439–45.
15. Bernardi S, Stacul F, Michelli A, et al. 12-Month efficacy of a single radiofrequency ablation on autonomously functioning thyroid nodules. Endocrine. 2017;57:402–8.
16. Baek JH, Kim YS, Lee D, Huh JY, Lee JH. Benign predominantly solid thyroid nodules: prospective study of efficacy of sonographically guided radiofrequency ablation versus control condition. Am J Roentgenol. 2010;194(4):1137–42.
17. Deandrea M, Sung JY, Limone P, et al. Efficacy and safety of radiofrequency ablation versus observation for nonfunctioning benign thyroid nodules: a randomized controlled international collaborative trial. Thyroid. 2015;25(8):890–6.
18. Kim YS, Rhim H, Tae K, Park DW, Kim ST. Radiofrequency ablation of benign cold thyroid nodules: initial clinical experience. Thyroid. 2006;16:361–7.
19. Bernardi S, Dobrinja C, Fabris B, et al. Radiofrequency ablation compared to surgery for the treatment of benign thyroid nodules. Int J Endocrinol. 2014;2014:934595.
20. Che Y, Jin S, Shi C, et al. Treatment of benign thyroid nodules: comparison of surgery with radiofrequency ablation. AJNR Am J Neuroradiol. 2015;36:1321–5.
21. Ugurlu MU, Uprak K, Akpinar IN, Attaallah W, Yegen C, Gulluoglu BM. Radiofrequency ablation of benign symptomatic thyroid nodules: prospective safety and efficacy study. World J Surg. 2015;39:961–8.
22. Ahn HS, Kim SJ, Park SH, Seo M. Radiofrequency ablation of benign thyroid nodules: evaluation of the treatment efficacy using ultrasonography. Ultrasonography. 2016;35:244–52.
23. Hong MJ, Baek JH, Choi YJ, et al. Radiofrequency ablation is a thyroid function-preserving treatment for patients with bilateral benign thyroid nodules. J Vasc Interv Radiol. 2015;26:55–61.
24. Baek JH, Ha EJ, Choi YJ, Sung JY, Kim JK, Shong YK. Radiofrequency versus ethanol ablation for treating predominantly cystic thyroid nodules: a randomized clinical trial. Korean J Radiol. 2015;16:1332–40.
25. Huh JY, Baek JH, Choi H, Kim JK, Lee JH. Symptomatic benign thyroid nodules: efficacy of additional radiofrequency ablation treatment session—prospective randomized study. Radiology. 2012;263:909–16.
26. Lim HK, Lee JH, Ha EJ, Sung JY, Kim JK, Baek JH. Radiofrequency ablation of benign nonfunctioning thyroid nodules: 4-year follow-up results for 111 patients. Eur Radiol. 2013;23:1044–9.
27. Cesareo R, Pasqualini V, Simeoni C, et al. Prospective study of effectiveness of ultrasound-guided radiofrequency ablation versus control group in patients affected by benign thyroid nodules. J Clin Endocrinol Metab. 2015;100:460–6.
28. Aysan E, Idiz UO, Akbulut H, Elmas L. Single-session radiofrequency ablation on benign thyroid nodules: a prospective single center study: radiofrequency ablation on thyroid. Langenbecks Arch Surg. 2016;401:357–63.

29. Baek JH, Jeong HJ, Kim YS, Kwak MS, Rhim HC, Chang SH. Percutaneous radiofrequency ablation for benign nodules of the thyroid gland. J Korean Radiol Soc. 2005;52:379–84.
30. Li XL, Xu HX, Lu F, et al. Treatment efficacy and safety of ultrasound-guided percutaneous bipolar radiofrequency ablation for benign thyroid nodules. Br J Radiol. 2016;89:20150858.
31. Sung JY, Baek JH, Kim KS, et al. Single-session treatment of benign cystic thyroid nodules with ethanol versus radiofrequency ablation: a prospective randomized study. Radiology. 2013;269:293–300.
32. Kim TH, Kim SM, Jung AL, et al. Efficacy and safety of radiofrequency ablation performed by an endocrinologist for benign thyroid nodules. Int J Thyroidol. 2015;8:183–6.
33. Valcavi R, Tsamatropoulos P. Health-related quality of life after percutaneous radiofrequency ablation of cold, solid, benign thyroid nodules: a 2-year follow-up study in 40 patients. Endocr Pract. 2015;21:887–96.
34. Yue WW, Wang SR, Lu F, et al. Radiofrequency ablation vs. microwave ablation for patients with benign thyroid nodules: a propensity score matching study. Endocrine. 2017;55:485–95.
35. Cho SJ, Baek JH, Chung SR, Choi YJ, Lee JH. Long-term results of thermal ablation of benign thyroid nodules: a systematic review and meta-analysis. Endocrinol Metab. 2020;35:339–50.
36. Che Y, Jin S, Shi C, et al. Treatment of benign thyroid nodules: comparison of surgery with radiofrequency ablation. Am J Neuroradiol. 2015;36(7):1321–5.
37. Yue WW, Li XL, Xu HX, et al. Quality of life and costeffectiveness of radiofrequency ablation versus open surgery for benign thyroid nodules: a retrospective cohort study. Sci Rep. 2016;6:37838. https://doi.org/10.1038/srep37838.
38. Cheng Z, Che Y, Yu S, et al. US-guided percutaneous radiofrequency versus microwave ablation for benign thyroid nodules: a prospective multicenter study. Sci Rep. 2017;7(1):9554.
39. Hu K, Wu J, Dong Y, Yan Z, Lu Z, Liu L. Comparison between ultrasound-guided percutaneous radiofrequency and microwave ablation in benign thyroid nodules. J Cancer Res Ther. 2019;15(7):1535–40.
40. Ha EJ, Baek JH, Che Y, et al. Radiofrequency ablation of benign thyroid nodules: recommendations from the Asian conference on tumor ablation task force. Ultrasonography. 2021;40:75–82.
41. Kim HJ, Cho SJ, Baek JH, Suh CH. Efficacy and safety of thermal ablation for autonomously functioning thyroid nodules: a systematic review and meta-analysis. Eur Radiol. 2020;31:605.
42. Cesareo R, Palermo A, Pasqualini V, et al. Radiofrequency ablation on autonomously functioning thyroid nodules: a critical appraisal and review of the literature. Front Endocrinol (Lausanne). 2020;11:317. https://doi.org/10.3389/fendo.2020.00317.
43. Spiezia S, Garberoglio R, Milone F, et al. Thyroid nodules and related symptoms are stably controlled two years after radiofrequency thermal ablation. Thyroid. 2009;19:219–25.
44. Garberoglio R, Aliberti C, Appetecchia M, Attard M, Boccuzzi G, Boraso F, et al. Radiofrequency ablation for thyroid nodules: which indications? The first Italian opinion statement. J Ultrasound. 2015;18:423–30.
45. Chianelli M, Bizzarri G, Todino V, Misischi I, Bianchini A, Graziano F, et al. Laser ablation and 131-iodine: a 24-month pilot study of combined treatment for large toxic nodular goiter. J Clin Endocrinol Metab. 2014;99:E1283–6.
46. Cervelli R, Mazzeo S, Boni G, et al. Comparison between radioiodine therapy and single-session radiofrequency ablation of autonomously functioning thyroid nodules: a retrospective study. Clin Endocrinol. 2019;90:608–16.
47. Zhao CK, Xu HX, Lu F, Sun LP, He YP, Guo LH, et al. Factors associated with initial incomplete ablation for benign thyroid nodules after radiofrequency ablation: first results of CEUS evaluation. Clin Hemorheol Microcirc. 2017;65:393–405.
48. Tang X, Cui D, Chi J, Wang Z, Wang T, Zhai B, et al. Evaluation of the safety and efficacy of radiofrequency ablation for treating benign thyroid nodules. J Cancer. 2017;8:754–60.
49. Ha EJ, Baek JH, Kim KW, Pyo J, Lee JH, Baek SH, et al. Comparative efficacy of radiofrequency and laser ablation for the treatment of benign thyroid nodules: systematic review including traditional pooling and Bayesian network metaanalysis. J Clin Endocrinol Metab. 2015;100:1903–11.

# Chapter 15
# Complications of Thyroid RFA

**Gary Tse and Michael Douek**

## Introduction

Radiofrequency ablation (RFA) has been performed internationally for over 10 years and has proven to be efficacious in the treatment of symptomatic benign thyroid nodules and toxic nodules. A number of studies have reported on the safety of thyroid RFA, which compares favorably to that of surgical alternatives [1]. Certain procedural modifications, namely, the "transisthmic" approach, use of the "moving shot" technique, and avoidance of the "danger triangle" have helped mitigate complications. Nonetheless, though infrequent, both major and minor complications do occur. A large retrospective series of 1543 thyroid nodules reported a complication rate of 3.3%, with their authors defining 20 as major and 28 as minor complications [2]. Major complications included voice changes, brachial plexus injury, nodule rupture, and permanent hypothyroidism (Table 15.1). Minor complications included hematoma, skin burns, and vomiting. All patients are reported to have recovered spontaneously with only one case of permanent hypothyroidism. As RFA of thyroid nodules has increased in utilization, it is important to review the clinical and imaging findings of thyroid RFA complications and how to avoid and manage them.

G. Tse (✉) · M. Douek
Department of Interventional Radiology, UCLA, Los Angeles, CA, USA
e-mail: gtse@mednet.ucla.edu


A. W. Park et al. (eds.), *Thyroid Radiofrequency Ablation*,
https://doi.org/10.1007/978-3-031-65288-2_15

**Table 15.1** Complications and side effects in 1459 patients who underwent RFA of thyroid nodules[a]

| Complications or side effects | Number of complications | Time of detection (days) | Time to recovery (days) |
|---|---|---|---|
| **Major** | **20 (1.4%)** | **1–180** | **1–90** |
| Voice change | 15 (1.02%) | 1–2 | 1–90 |
| Nodule rupture | 2 (0.14%) | 22–30 | <30 |
| Nodule rupture with abscess formation | 1 (0.07%) | 50 | None |
| Hypothyroidism | 1 (0.07%) | 180 | None |
| Brachial plexus injury | 1 (0.07%) | 1 | 60 |
| **Minor** | **28 (1.92%)** | **1–2** | **1–30** |
| Hematoma | 15 (1.02%) | 1 | <30 |
| Vomiting | 9 (0.62%) | 1–2 | 1–2 |
| Skin burn | 4 (0.27%) | 1 | <7 |
| **Side effects** | **46 (3.15%)** | **1** | **1–2** |
| Pain | 38 (2.6%) | 1 | 1–2 |
| Vasovagal reaction | 5 (0.34%) | 1 | 1 |
| Coughing | 3 (0.21%) | 1 | 1 |

[a]Baek et al. Radiology 2012 [2]

## *Major Complications*

Major complications are defined by the Society of Interventional Radiology (SIR) as those complications that can lead to substantial morbidity and disability, may increase the level of care, result in hospital admission, or lengthen hospital stay [3]. These will be reviewed in this section.

### Voice Change (1%)

Voice change is considered a major complication as it can lead to substantial morbidity and disability. The location of the recurrent laryngeal nerve (RLN) in the tracheoesophageal groove puts it at risk for thermal injury if ablation is performed in this region. Typically, the voice change is noticed during or immediately after the ablation. Knowledge of this "danger triangle"—the area that encompasses the esophagus, trachea, and medial thyroid gland—and avoiding ablation in this region, is paramount in mitigating this complication. On the right side, a "danger zone" concept applies to the area from the tracheoesophageal groove medially to the carotid sheath laterally that encompasses the right RLN and its variable locations in addition to the vagus nerve and the middle sympathetic ganglion (Fig. 15.1).

Using the moving shot technique to spread the thermal energy is important to avoid over-ablating near the danger triangle. Administering local lidocaine only or minimizing sedation so that the patient can verbalize throughout the case is helpful in identifying nerve injury earlier, which can allow for rescue maneuvers.

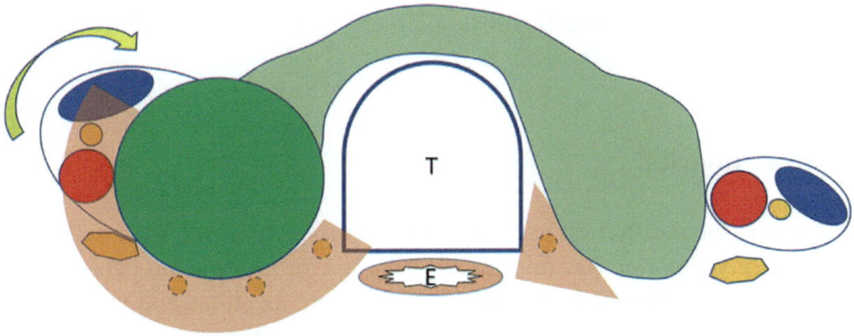


**Fig. 15.1** Danger triangle vs danger zone. *T* trachea, *E* esophagus; red circle—common carotid artery; blue oval—internal jugular vein; yellow solid circle—vagus nerve; yellow dotted circle—recurrent laryngeal nerve; and yellow heptagon—middle sympathetic ganglion. (With permission from Park AW 2020 [4])

**Fig. 15.2** Hydrodissection as a rescue maneuver in voice changes: *T* trachea, *E* esophagus; red circle—common carotid artery; blue oval—internal jugular vein; yellow solid circle—vagus nerve; yellow dotted circle—recurrent laryngeal nerve; and yellow heptagon—middle sympathetic ganglion. (With permission from Park AW 2020 [4])

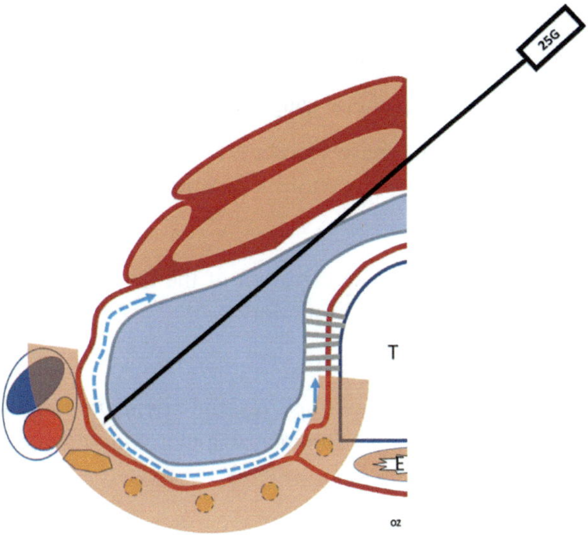


If voice changes are detected during the procedure, a technique known as Dextrose 5% in water (D5W) rescue has been proposed, consisting of the following steps:

- Immediately turn off radiofrequency output.
- Advance a 23–25 G needle to the medial inferior margin of the carotid artery or directly near the tracheoesophageal groove (Fig. 15.2).
- Instill 10–20 cc of cold D5W to hydrodissect the issue around the nerve.

This technique has proven to be an effective method to allow for quick recovery of voice change [5]. A short course of steroids may also be considered if the voice change is persistent. Fortunately, most voice changes spontaneously recover within 3 months.

### Other Nerve Injuries

Understanding the perithyroid neck anatomy is critical to avoid other nerve injuries. These are rarely reported but important to recognize as they can cause significant morbidity and disability. Knowledge of typical nerve locations and variant anatomy is important. These types of injury appear to occur more commonly in RFA of recurrent thyroid cancers and may be due to adjacent desmoplastic reaction and lack of normal surrounding thyroid gland [6]. With a 10 mm active tip electrode, the recommended minimal distance from the nerve structures should be 3 mm, with 6 mm adding a layer of safety [7].

- Brachial plexus
  - Injury could cause sensory and/or motor dysfunction in the upper extremity.
- Cervical sympathetic ganglion
  - Injury can cause Horner's syndrome, a classic triad of ptosis, miosis, and anhidrosis with conjunctival injection as an early sign.
- Phrenic nerve
  - Injury can cause elevation of the hemidiaphragm, which may result in dyspnea and chest discomfort.
- Spinal accessory nerve
  - Injury can cause trapezius and sternocleidomastoid dysfunction resulting in drooping of the shoulder, scapular winging, and/or weakness.

### Nodule Rupture (0.2–0.5%)

Thyroid nodule rupture following RFA is thought to be due to thyroid capsular breakdown and extrusion of the thyroid components, usually into the anterior neck soft tissues. Patients present with abrupt neck bulging and pain. This complication is thought to be caused by delayed hemorrhage secondary to microvascular leakage, as there are often high attenuation products observed on CT with volume expansion and subsequent tear of the capsule at its weakest point (Fig. 15.3). Post-procedural massaging or neck movement has also been suggested as possible etiologies [8]. Abscess formation is also possible. Interestingly, most of the nodule ruptures reported occur weeks to months post-procedure, and therefore follow-up is key.

Conservative management is recommended with observation and gentle compression of the rupture site, as the vast majority of reported cases have resolved spontaneously. However, US-guided needle aspiration may be considered to help

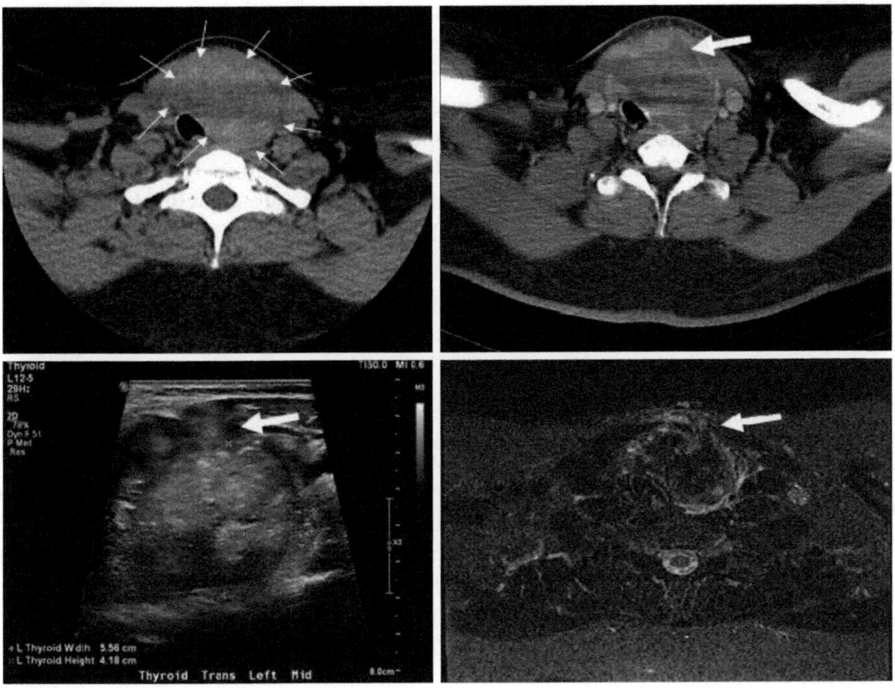


**Fig. 15.3** **Top left**: Pre-ablation CT. 6 cm left inferior thyroid gland nodule before ablation. **Top right**: Post-ablation CT. 2 weeks post left thyroid nodule ablation. The nodule has increased in size and is hypoattenuating with peripheral enhancement. A small focal defect can be seen anteriorly where the rupture has occurred with extrusion of the nodule into the anterior neck soft tissues (arrow). **Bottom left**: Post-ablation US. The left thyroid nodule is heterogenous in echotexture 2 weeks post ablation. Focal extrusion of the nodule is seen anteriorly (arrow). **Bottom right**: Post-ablation MRI. T2 Inversion recovery weighted sequence showing the nodule rupture into the anterior neck soft tissues (arrow)

improve bulky symptoms or if abscess formation is suspected. Antibiotics may be considered in cases of suspected infection. In rare cases of severe compressive symptoms in the confined neck space (deviation of trachea, esophagus, neurovascular structures, for example), surgical incision and drainage or resection may be required.

## Hypothyroidism (0.07%)

Permanent hypothyroidism is exceedingly rare after thyroid RFA. Conversely, this complication is reported to occur in approximately 30–40% of patients after surgical hemithyroidectomy [9, 10]. Avoiding permanent hypothyroidism and the need for lifelong thyroid replacement is one of the key reasons why some patients choose ablation over surgery.

When hypothyroidism does occur after ablation, the etiology is unclear. Baek et al. reported a single case of permanent hypothyroidism in 1459 patients treated with RFA, which occurred 6 months after treatment [2]. Their patient had elevated thyroperoxidase antibodies before and after RFA. Previous reports on ethanol ablation also reported that patients who developed hypothyroidism had increased thyroperoxidase antibodies and/or thyroglobulin antibodies before RFA. Therefore, it may be prudent to discuss the risk of hypothyroidism in patients with already known thyroid antibodies before RFA, although the routine preoperative check for thyroid antibodies is controversial.

Treatment would be levothyroxine replacement.

#### Tracheoesophageal Injury

Thermal injury to the trachea or esophagus is possible given that these structures reside posterior to the thyroid gland. Thermal injury to the trachea may result in intraprocedural cough. Minor thermal injury to the esophagus or trachea may be managed conservatively. However, perforation of either the esophagus or trachea may lead to abscess formation and/or tracheoesophageal fistulae and would require surgical management.

### *Minor Complications*

A minor complication is defined as an adverse event that either does not require therapy or only nominal therapy with no significant consequence. These will be reviewed in this section.

#### Hematoma (1%)

Hematomas may occur in the perithyroidal, intranodular, or subcapsular spaces and are generally self-limited. This hemorrhage is thought to be secondary to mechanical injury to the perithyroidal arteries by the RFA electrode. This usually presents as gradual mass-like enlargement, which may have mixed hyperechoic and hypoechoic components. The hematoma may compress the thyroid parenchyma in cases of intranodular or subcapsular hematomas or adjacent structures in cases of perithyroidal hemorrhage (Fig. 15.4).

Conservative management with manual compression and observation is recommended. Ablation of the culprit vessels may be helpful in certain cases. Fortunately, most hematomas resolve within 1–2 weeks. Diligent preoperative screening is important to identify patients with bleeding diatheses and coagulopathies as well as stopping aspirin and blood thinners. Serious perithyroidal hemorrhage secondary to injury of the systemic arteries and their branches (carotid, subclavian, superior

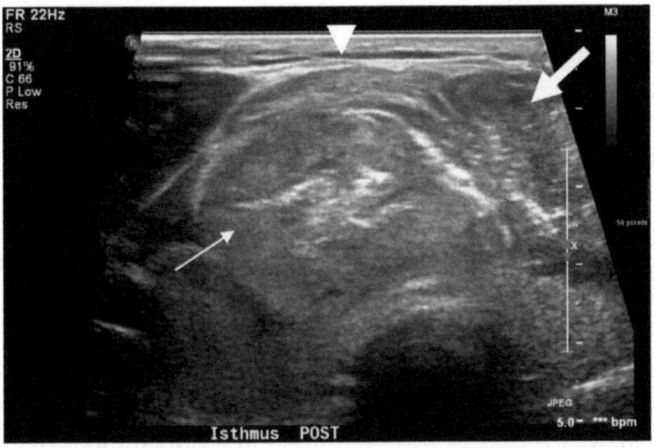


**Fig. 15.4** Postoperative hematoma. Transverse ultrasound post-RFA. Patient presented with immediate pain and swelling after the removal of the probe. The ablated nodule with internal hyperechogenicities can be seen in the right isthmus (thin arrow). There is an adjacent heterogeneously mixed echogenic subcapsular hematoma (thick arrow) just midline to the nodule at the probe insertion site that can be seen having a slight mass effect on the adjacent thin strap muscle (arrowhead). Pressure was held and the swelling stabilized. This hematoma resolved in 3 days

thyroid, and inferior thyroid arteries, for example) may occur if the electrode tip is poorly visualized and where manual compression may not be helpful. In these cases, careful observation of the patient's oxygenation and vitals is important as severe compression of the trachea and other neck structures may occur and result in escalation of care.

## Nausea and Vomiting (0.6%)

Few patients may experience nausea and vomiting either during or after the procedure. The etiology is unknown but may be related to vagus nerve irritation as the nerve runs in the adjacent carotid sheath.

Management would be with IV or oral antiemetics and usually resolves within 1–2 days.

## Skin Burn (0.3%)

Skin burns have been reported primarily at the puncture site and are caused by direct thermal injury from the RFA probe. Patients present within 1–2 days of the procedure with skin color change, mild pain, and discomfort. This is usually a self-limited complication, which resolves within a week.

## *Side Effects*

### Pain

Pain is the most common side effect of thyroid RFA. Almost every patient will experience some degree of discomfort during the ablation procedure, but generally this is well tolerated and can be mitigated by decreasing power or briefly turning off the generator, or alternatively, administering additional perithyroidal lidocaine. Patients may complain of pain in the lower neck, which may or may not radiate to the head, ears, shoulders, chest, back, or teeth, but this is usually self-limited. Postoperative pain is well managed with a few days of analgesics, if necessary.

### Vasovagal Reaction (0.3%)

Patients with a vasovagal reaction may present with sweating or difficulty breathing. Stopping the ablation and elevating the legs can help to mitigate the symptoms.

In conclusion, the overall complication rate among patients who undergo thyroid RFA is low. Major complications are rare and even when they do occur, they appear to mostly resolve with time. Proficient ultrasound visualization of the electrode needle tip and knowledge of the neck anatomy are paramount to minimize these complications, as well as familiarity with rescue techniques. These findings hopefully may help in preventing such complications and present strategies for the proper management of these complications if they do occur.

## References

1. Che Y, Jin S, Shi C, Wang L, Zhang X, Li Y, Baek JH. Treatment of benign thyroid nodules: comparison of surgery with radiofrequency ablation. AJNR Am J Neuroradiol. 2015;36(7):1321–5. https://doi.org/10.3174/ajnr.A4276. Epub 2015 Mar 26. PMID: 25814656; PMCID: PMC7965284.
2. Baek JH, Lee JH, Sung JY, Bae JI, Kim KT, Sim J, Baek SM, Kim YS, Shin JH, Park JS, Kim DW, Kim JH, Kim EK, Jung SL, Na DG, Korean Society of Thyroid Radiology. Complications encountered in the treatment of benign thyroid nodules with US-guided radiofrequency ablation: a multicenter study. Radiology. 2012;262(1):335–42. https://doi.org/10.1148/radiol.11110416. Epub 2011 Oct 13.
3. Khalilzadeh O, Baerlocher MO, Shyn PB, Connolly BL, Devane AM, Morris CS, Cohen AM, Midia M, Thornton RH, Gross K, Caplin DM, Aeron G, Misra S, Patel NH, Walker TG, Martinez-Salazar G, Silberzweig JE, Nikolic B. Proposal of a new adverse event classification by the Society of Interventional Radiology Standards of Practice Committee [Erratum in: J Vasc Interv Radiol. 2018 Jan;29(1):146.]. J Vasc Interv Radiol. 2017;28(10):1432–1437.e3. https://doi.org/10.1016/j.jvir.2017.06.019. Epub 2017 Jul 27.
4. Park AW. Thyroid radiofrequency ablation. 1st ed. Charlottesville: Oz & SE; 2020.
5. Chung SR, Baek JH, Choi YJ, Lee JH. Management strategy for nerve damage during radiofrequency ablation of thyroid nodules. Int J Hyperth. 2019;36(1):204–10. https://doi.org/10.1080/02656736.2018.1554826. Epub 2019 Jan 14.

6. Kim C, Lee JH, Choi YJ, Kim WB, Sung TY, Baek JH. Complications encountered in ultrasonography-guided radiofrequency ablation of benign thyroid nodules and recurrent thyroid cancers. Eur Radiol. 2017;27(8):3128–37. https://doi.org/10.1007/s00330-016-4690-y. Epub 2016 Dec 14.
7. Ha EJ, Baek JH, Lee JH. Moving-shot versus fixed electrode techniques for radiofrequency ablation: comparison in an ex-vivo bovine liver tissue model. Korean J Radiol. 2014;15(6):836–43. https://doi.org/10.3348/kjr.2014.15.6.836. Epub 2014 Nov 7. PMID: 25469097; PMCID: PMC4248641.
8. Shin JH, Jung SL, Baek JH, Kim JH. Rupture of benign thyroid tumors after radio-frequency ablation. AJNR Am J Neuroradiol. 2011;32(11):2165–9. https://doi.org/10.3174/ajnr.A2661. Epub 2011 Sep 15. PMID: 21920870; PMCID: PMC7964385.
9. Wilson M, Patel A, Goldner W, Baker J, Sayed Z, Fingeret AL. Postoperative thyroid hormone supplementation rates following thyroid lobectomy. Am J Surg. 2020;220(5):1169–73. https://doi.org/10.1016/j.amjsurg.2020.06.052. Epub 2020 Jul 1.
10. Guan SH, Wang H, Teng DK. Comparison of ultrasound-guided thermal ablation and conventional thyroidectomy for benign thyroid nodules: a systematic review and meta-analysis. Int J Hyperth. 2020;37(1):442–9. https://doi.org/10.1080/02656736.2020.1758802.

# Chapter 16
# Ultrasonographic Changes Following Thyroid RFA

**Jung Hee Shin**

Thyroid radiofrequency ablation (RFA) has been developed and performed for over a decade. RFA is performed under ultrasound (US) guidance, and US is the imaging tool for follow-up after RFA of thyroid nodules. However, ultrasonographic changes that occur after thyroid RFA have not been well described. The ultrasonographic features of thyroid tissue after RFA will be reviewed and presented in this chapter.

## US Features Before RFA

US imaging is superior to other modalities for characterizing thyroid nodules. Based on US images, thyroid nodules are classified into four types by composition (Table 16.1), as defined by the 2021 Korean Thyroid Imaging Reporting and Data System (K-TIRADS) [1].

RFA is used to treat the solid component of a thyroid nodule. The US features of the solid component are separated into three categories: hypoechoic, isoechoic, and hyperechoic, relative to the normal thyroid tissue. In multinodular goiter, heterogeneous echogenicity can be observed. Necrosis, fibrosis, or calcifications can also show heterogeneity on US.

J. H. Shin (✉)
Samsung Medical Center, Seoul, South Korea


A. W. Park et al. (eds.), *Thyroid Radiofrequency Ablation*,
https://doi.org/10.1007/978-3-031-65288-2_16

**Table 16.1** Classification of thyroid nodules by composition

| Classification | Composition |
|---|---|
| Cystic nodule | No obvious solid component |
| Predominantly cystic nodule | Cystic portion >50% |
| Predominantly solid nodule | Cystic portion ≤50% |
| Solid nodule | No obvious cystic component |

## US Features During RFA

When the tissue temperature increases due to the friction (resistance) heat generated by radiofrequency, vaporization of tissue gases or fluid occurs. During vaporization, a large amount of gas is formed, which appears on US as echogenic microbubbles. During the RFA procedure, heterogenous echogenicity is a common US feature depicting a mixture of ablated and non-ablated zones. At the end of the procedure or during periods of the procedure without further ablation, condensation of the vaporized tissue gases or fluid occurs due to a gradual loss of heat by conduction and a heat sink effect. At this point, the ablated zone can be differentiated from the non-ablated zone (Fig. 16.1). Because the US distinction between the ablated and non-ablated zones is made within a target nodule, three US features can be expected at the end of the procedure, as shown in Fig. 16.2.

After RFA of a hyperechoic target nodule, hypoechoic US change is easily detectable by the contrast in echogenicity (Fig. 16.2a). In an isoechoic target nodule, hypoechoic change could be subtle, but the ablated zone still can be differentiated from the non-ablated zone (Fig. 16.2b). However, in a hypoechoic target nodule, the detection of post-ablation changes could be very subtle or imperceptible (Fig. 16.2c).

## US Features After RFA

US findings of successful ablation are as follows:

- Loss of intra-nodular vascular signal in Doppler US examination
- Decreased nodule volume (i.e., >50% decrease)
- Decreased echogenicity of the ablated nodule (which looks like a malignancy)

Edematous changes by post-ablation inflammatory reaction appear hypoechoic, which can be distinct from the non-ablated zone of the thyroid nodule. At 6 months post-RFA, they are more clearly seen (Fig. 16.3).

After three or more years post-RFA, nodule volume is reduced, and the ablated zones sometimes have calcified echogenic dots (Fig. 16.4). The area of calcification could be enlarged in size or multiplied with the appearance of macrocalcification or rim calcification over time (Fig. 16.4c). Although it was initially a nodule with no calcification at all, the echogenic dots that occur in the 3 years following RFA can

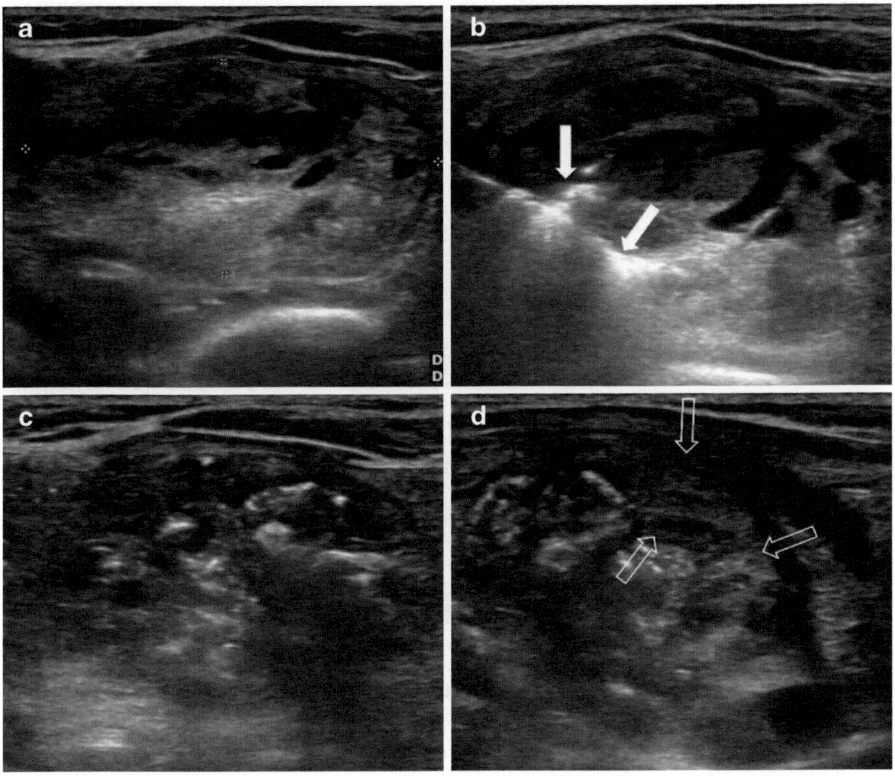


**Fig. 16.1** (**a**) A large thyroid nodule (crosses) in the isthmus. (**b**) Echogenic microbubbles (white solid arrows) from the electrode tip are noted at the start of RFA. (**c**) Heterogeneous echogenicity of the thyroid nodule is seen during RFA. (**d**) Longitudinal image of the thyroid nodule shows a non-ablated zone (white hollow arrows) in the anterior portion of the nodule

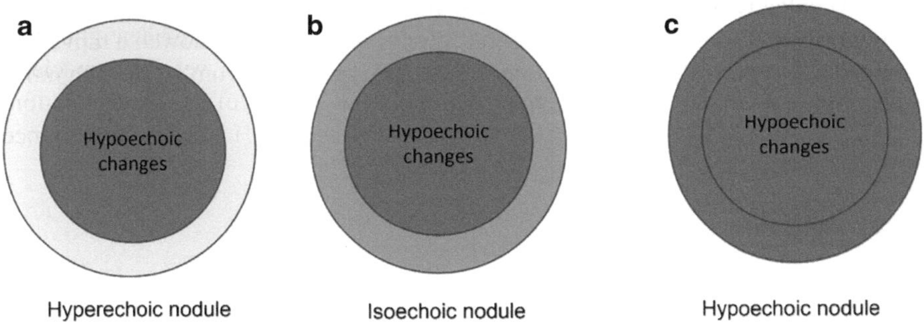


**Fig. 16.2** Depending on the background echogenicity of a target nodule, US changes of the ablated zone in contrast to the non-ablated zone after RFA can be (**a**) distinct, (**b**) subtle, and (**c**) indistinct

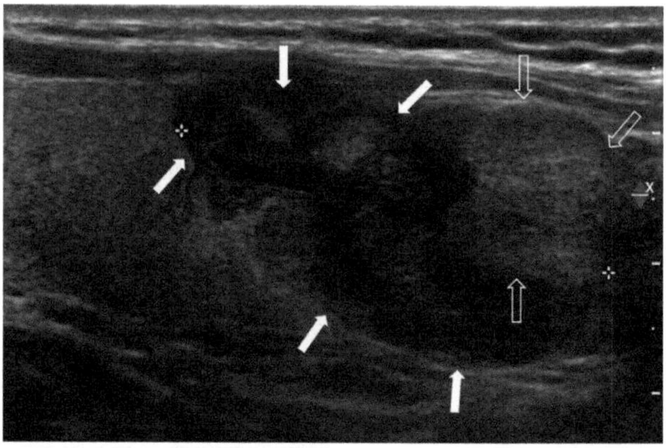

**Fig. 16.3** At 6 months post-RFA, ablated hypoechoic (white solid arrow) and non-ablated isoechoic (white hollow arrow) zones of a thyroid nodule (crosses) are seen

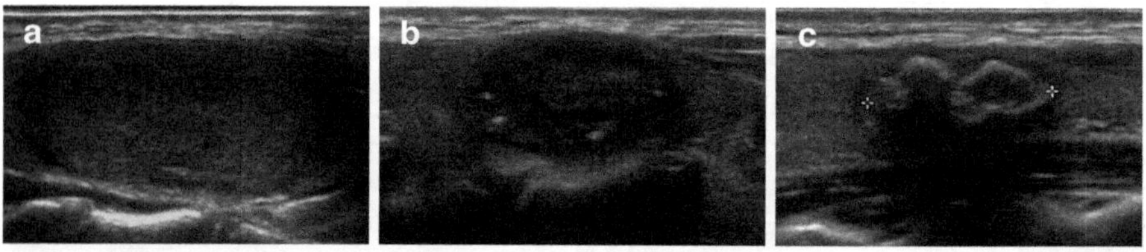


**Fig. 16.4** A thyroid nodule (**a**) before ablation, (**b**) macrocalcifications in the nodule at 1 year post-RFA, and (**c**) a degenerating nodule with rim calcification at 7 years post-RFA

look like malignant microcalcifications. As the nodule degenerates over time, the calcification increases in size and coalesces.

The ablated area decreases with time and shows an irregular margin, nonparallel orientation, and echogenic dots that resemble malignancy (Fig. 16.5). However, it can be distinguished from malignancy if there is no vascularity within the nodule and by considering the history of previous RFA. In some cases, the lesion disappears completely or remains only as a scar-like hypoechoic line.

Reported pooled volume-reduction rates for ablated nodules showed a rapid volume reduction during the first 12 months post-RFA, a plateau from 12 to 36 months, and additional volume reduction after 36 months [1].

## Regrowth After RFA

Regrowth is defined as a greater than 50% increase in nodule volume compared with the smallest volume recorded previously during the postprocedural follow-up evaluation [2]. Regrowth of treated nodules can occur due to insufficient treatment or the malignant potential of the nodule.

Common features of a regrowing nodule after RFA include marginal regrowth as undertreated peripheral lobulation with a contracted ablated core and increased

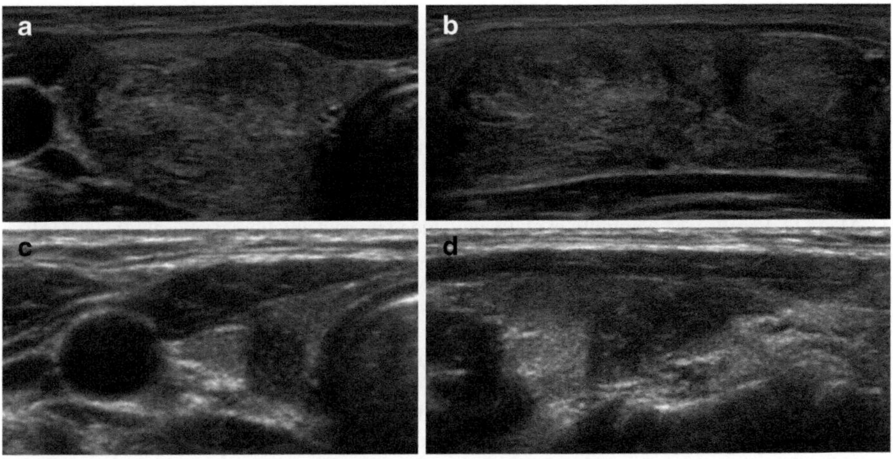


**Fig. 16.5** A large nodule (**a**, **b**) before ablation, and (**c**, **d**) a decreased nodule with an irregular margin, nonparallel orientation, and echogenic dots, which looks like malignancy at 3 years post-RFA

**Fig. 16.6** A nodule that was previously treated with RFA showing marginal regrowth (white solid arrows) and an ablated core (white hollow arrow)

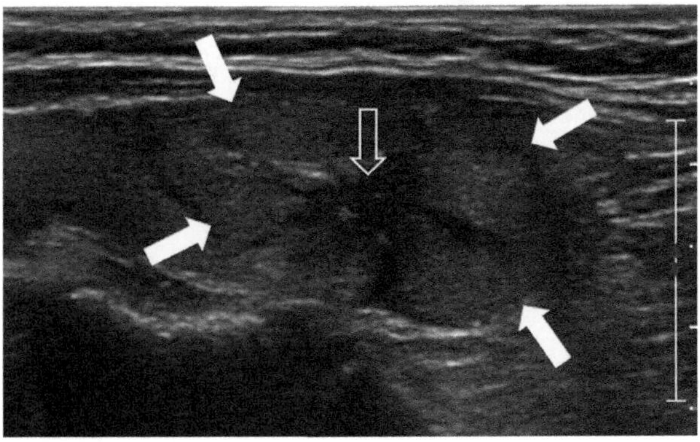

vascularity in a Doppler US scan (Fig. 16.6). If a viable portion with vascularity is found on Doppler US images, additional treatment should be considered to achieve the maximal ablation effect.

Although rare, the malignant potential of an ablated nodule should be considered if its volume reduction is minimal, if the nodule is larger, or if it is newly hypervascular at the post-RFA follow-up evaluation. It should be noted that for nodules ≥3 cm in diameter, the false-negative cytology rate is 11.7% [3, 4]. Because follicular thyroid carcinoma and the follicular variant of papillary thyroid carcinoma are common histologic types that are later diagnosed as cancer in the RFA-treated benign nodule, US-guided core needle biopsy can be helpful to exclude the diagnosis of follicular neoplasm [5–7]. In addition, molecular testing might be considered as a helpful diagnostic marker in large solid nodules.

## References

1. Ha EJ, Chung SR, Na DG. Korean thyroid imaging reporting and data system and imaging-based management of thyroid nodules: Korean Society of Thyroid Radiology Consensus Statement and Recommendations. Korean J Radiol. 2021;22:2094–123.
2. Cho SJ, Baek JH, Chung SR, Choi YJ, Lee JH. Long-term results of thermal ablation of benign thyroid nodules: a systematic review and meta-analysis. Endocrinol Metab. 2020;35:339–50.
3. Mauri G, Pacella CM, Papini E, et al. Image-guided thyroid ablation: proposal for standardization of terminology and reporting criteria. Thyroid. 2019;29:611–8.
4. Rossi ED, Bizzarro T, Fadda G, Pontecorvi A, Bernet V, Nassar A. The cytological diagnosis of a 'benign thyroid lesion': is it a real safe diagnosis for the patient? Cytopathology. 2016;27(3):168–75.
5. Giles WH, Maclellan RA, Gawande AA, Ruan DT, Alexander EK, Moore FD Jr, Cho NL. False negative cytology in large thyroid nodules. Ann Surg Oncol. 2015;22(1):152–7.
6. Park KW, Shin JH, Hahn SY, et al. Ultrasound-guided fine-needle aspiration or core needle biopsy for diagnosing follicular thyroid carcinoma. Clin Endocrinol. 2020;92(5):468–74.
7. Kim MK, Shin JH, Hahn SY, Kim H. Delayed cancer diagnosis in thyroid nodules initially treated as benign with radiofrequency ablation: ultrasound characteristics and predictors for cancer. Korean J Radiol. 2023;24:903–11.

# Chapter 17
# Volume Measurements of Thyroid Nodules Following RFA

**Jung Suk Sim**

## Introduction

Benign thyroid nodules (BTN) treated with thermal ablation (TA) exhibit two distinct areas: an ablated region necrotized by device-generated heat and a viable area primarily located at the periphery [1]. Following TA, nodules experience a temporary increase in volume due to hemorrhage and edema, followed by continuous reduction thereafter [2]. In most cases, volume reduction occurs within approximately 1 year as the ablated tissue is absorbed [3, 4]. It is well known that the volume of TA-treated nodules remains relatively stable for up to 2 or 3 years [5, 6]. Once the ablated tissue is completely absorbed, no further volume reduction can be expected. Subsequently, if regrowth occurs in the non-ablated viable tissue, the nodule volume may increase [2]. Ultrasound imaging allows monitoring of these phenomena by measuring three volumes: Total nodule volume (*Vt*), Ablated volume (*V*a), and Viable volume (*V*v) [2]. Utilizing these measurements, an effective management plan can be developed for the follow-up of TA-treated nodules [2, 7, 8]. This chapter provides definitions of terminology used in monitoring TA-treated nodules using ultrasound and introduces various measurable and calculable indicators along with their utilization.

J. S. Sim (✉)
Department of Radiology, Withsim Clinic, Seongnam-si, Gyeonggi-do, South Korea


A. W. Park et al. (eds.), *Thyroid Radiofrequency Ablation*,
https://doi.org/10.1007/978-3-031-65288-2_17

## Terminology

### Initial Nodule Volume

The initial nodule volume refers to the volume of the nodule prior to TA treatment. Other terms such as baseline nodule volume and index nodule volume convey the same meaning, but this handbook will adopt the term "initial nodule volume" [9].

### Total Nodule Volume (*Vt*)

Total nodule volume (*Vt*) is the volume of a nodule that is commonly measured at follow-up examinations. This volume is the sum of the ablated volume (*V*a) and viable volume (*V*v), as described in the following paragraphs [2].

### Ablated Volume (*V*a)

Ablated volume (*V*a) represents the volume of centrally located ablated tissue within a TA-treated nodule. TA treatment primarily focuses on the central area of the nodule. Depending on the anatomical location of the nodule, the peripheral margin may be intentionally left unablated to a certain thickness to prevent thermal damage to adjacent critical structures, such as nerves, trachea, and esophagus. The volume of the centrally located ablated area can be separately measured using the same methodology employed for nodule volume measurement, and it is defined as *V*a [2].

### Viable Volume (*V*v)

Viable volume (*V*v) is the volume of peripherally located viable tissue that is not ablated during the TA treatment. Unlike *Vt* or *V*a, this volume cannot be directly measured. However, as illustrated in Figs. 17.1 and 17.2, *V*v can be calculated using the formula $V\text{v} = Vt - V\text{a}$ [2].

### Subscripts Indicating the Time of Measurement

To provide useful information using *Vt*, *V*a, and *V*v, it is sometimes necessary to indicate the time when the measurement was obtained. For example, the time stamp before TA treatment can be expressed as "initial," the time stamp 1 month after TA treatment can be expressed as "1 month," and the first follow-up after TA treatment can be expressed as "first f/u," etc. This time stamp is marked with a subscript. For example, $Vt_{1\ \text{month}}$ refers to *Vt* at 1 month after TA, and $V\text{v}_{1\text{st f/u}}$ refers to *V*v at the first follow-up after TA.

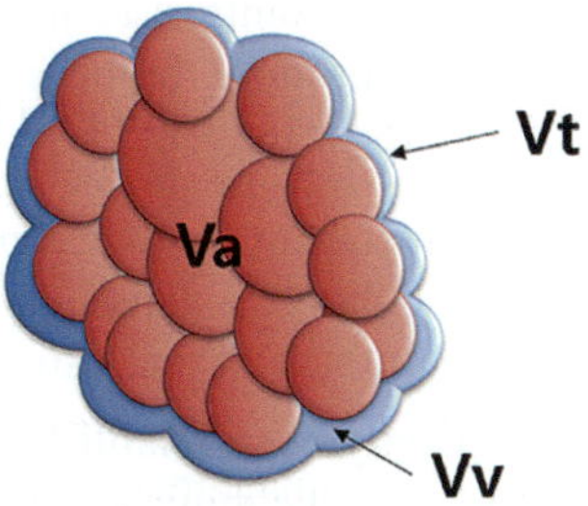


**Fig. 17.1** Diagram of benign thyroid nodules after radiofrequency ablation (RFA) using the moving-shot technique. The small circles at the center represent conceptual units ablated by the moving-shot technique, which combine to form the ablated area (*V*a). To safeguard surrounding critical structures from thermal damage, the periphery of the nodule is intentionally left unablated. The remaining viable nodule tissue constitutes *V*v. Total nodule volume (*Vt*) and *V*a can be calculated by measuring the length in three dimensions. *V*v is obtained by the equation $V\text{v} = Vt - V\text{a}$

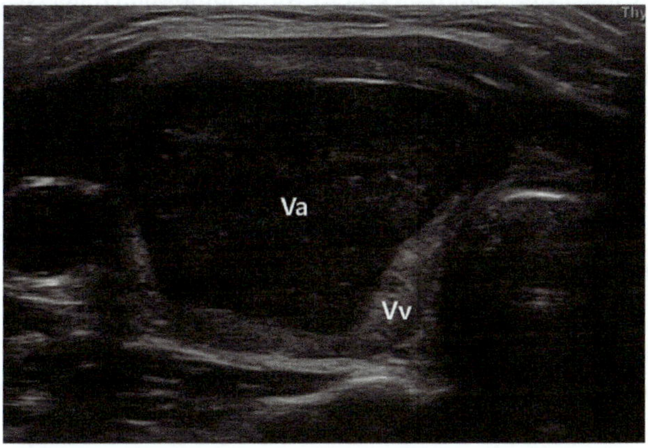


**Fig. 17.2** Ultrasound image of a 35-year-old woman taken 1 month after the treatment of a 27-mL benign thyroid nodule (BTN) with RFA. The centrally located ablated area (*V*a) appears hypoechoic, while the viable nodule tissue left unablated is distributed in the peripheral area (*V*v). The *V*v is predominantly located in the medial aspect, where the recurrent laryngeal nerve runs, as well as near the carotid sheath and in the posterior aspect. The anterior aspect, with relatively few critical structures, shows minimal viable tissue

## Long-Term

The term "long-term" is frequently used in the context of follow-up after TA treatment. However, there is still a lack of consensus regarding the specific duration that qualifies as long-term. Two aspects, time period vs. clinical significance, can be considered. Long-term is generally used when referring to a follow-up period of at least 2 years or longer, typically 3 years or more. Another perspective considers the clinical significance of long-term follow-up, often focusing on the occurrence of regrowth. According to Sim et al. regrowth usually becomes apparent after 3 years

[2]. Taking into account these two viewpoints, it is most reasonable to define long-term as a follow-up period of 3 years or more. In this chapter, the term "long-term" refers to a follow-up period of 3 years or longer.

### Regrowth

The definition of regrowth has recently been established by consensus, referring to a volume increase of 50% or more over the minimum recorded value during follow-up [10, 11].

### Recurrence

The term "recurrence" is sometimes used interchangeably with "regrowth" or in a different context, but a consensus on its definition has not been reached [12, 13]. While it may be used to indicate an increase in nodule volume, the term "recurrence" is often associated with the reoccurrence of symptoms or cosmetic issues [14]. In this chapter and the subsequent chapter, the term "regrowth" has been predominantly utilized. However, in cases where the original paper used the term "recurrence," it has been quoted verbatim.

## *Initial Ablation Ratio (IAR)*

The initial ablation ratio (IAR) is a value that represents the extent of nodule tissue ablation during the RFA procedure, specifically, the percentage of initial ablated volume ($Va_{\text{initial}}$) to the initial total volume ($Vt_{\text{initial}}$). The calculation for IAR is as follows [7]:

$$\text{IAR}(\%) = \frac{Va_{\text{initial}}}{Vt_{\text{initial}}} \times 100(\%).$$

While this formula seems straightforward, it is challenging to directly obtain $Vt$ and $Va$ immediately after RFA. The ultrasound image cannot clearly differentiate between $Vt$ and $Va$ due to factors like hemorrhage and edema. To address this limitation, we propose an indirect method that utilizes images obtained during the first follow-up, typically conducted within 1–6 months after the procedure.

The revised formula for IAR is as follows:

$$\text{IAR}(\%) = \frac{Vt_{\text{initial}} - Vv_{\text{first f/u}}}{Vt_{\text{initial}}} \times 100(\%).$$

The primary difference between this formula and the previous one lies in the numerator. We replaced $Va_{\text{initial}}$ with $Vt_{\text{initial}} - Vv_{\text{first f/u}}$. We cannot directly measure

$Vv_{initial}$. Thus, we substitute it with $Vt_{initial} - Vv_{first\ f/u}$. It is worth noting that $Vv_{initial}$ and $Vv_{first\ f/u}$ are interchangeable because they represent the same value. $Vv_{first\ f/u}$ can be calculated by the equation, $Vt_{first\ f/u} - Va_{first\ f/u}$.

IAR holds clinical significance as it demonstrates a linear correlation with the 1-year volume reduction ratio (VRR). It quantifies the extent of nodule tissue ablation achieved during the RFA procedure. Consequently, higher IAR values correspond to higher expected 1-year VRR, indicating a more successful outcome. In fact, a study reported that an IAR exceeding 70% predicts a 1-year VRR of over 50% [7]. This finding enables early prediction of whether the 1-year VRR will exceed the commonly used threshold of 50%, which serves as an indicator for short-term therapeutic success [11].

Furthermore, IAR can be utilized as an index to evaluate the operator's performance. While the 1-year VRR is a valuable indicator of treatment efficacy, it is important to consider other factors specific to the nodule. Even if the same degree of ablation is achieved in nodules with the same volume, variations in composition, such as the presence of a cystic component or differences in absorption rates within the patient's body, can affect the 1-year VRR [15]. These intrinsic nodule factors are beyond the operator's control. However, since IAR directly reflects the volume ablated immediately after treatment, it provides a more direct measure of the operator's performance. Novice operators can initially aim for a lower target IAR to prevent complications, gradually increasing it (e.g., 70%, 80%, and 90%) as their experience accumulates. In this way, IAR serves as a valuable reference for operators to engage in self-driven quality control and improvement.

## *Vv* Increase: An Early Sign of Regrowth

Regrowth in this context refers to a scenario where the *Vt* increases by 50% or more compared to the minimum recorded *Vt* during the follow-up after TA treatment. On the other hand, *Vv* increase signifies a case where the non-ablated residual *Vv* increases by 50% or more compared to the minimum recorded *Vv* [2].

Interestingly, *Vv* increase precedes the increase in *Vt*, indicating regrowth by 1 year. The authors coined the term "*Vv* increase" as an early sign of regrowth. The rationale behind this sequence is as follows:

During the first year after TA treatment, *Vt* experiences a rapid decrease. This decrease primarily occurs due to the reduction in *Va*. *Va* represents the volume of the tissue treated with TA, and its reduction is a result of the absorption of necrotized tissue. However, after 1 year, *Va* stabilizes at a minimized state as there is no further necrotized tissue to be absorbed.

On the other hand, *Vv* represents the volume of the remaining tissue that was not ablated during TA, and it possesses the potential for growth. Within the first year after TA, while *Va* undergoes rapid reduction, the change in *Vv* is slower compared to *Va*. Consequently, even if there is an increase in *Vv*, it is offset by the reduction in *Va*. Therefore, when measuring *Vt*, the increase in *Vv* tends to be masked.

However, by separately measuring *Vv*, it becomes possible to observe its increase earlier, before the increase in *Vt*. Regrowth (i.e., *Vt* increase) can only be confirmed when the increase in *Vv* surpasses the reduction in *Va*. Hence, *Vv* increase can be detected earlier than regrowth by monitoring *Vt*.

## References


1. Na DG, Lee JH, Jung SL, Kim JH, Sung JY, Shin JH, et al. Radiofrequency ablation of benign thyroid nodules and recurrent thyroid cancers: consensus statement and recommendations. Korean J Radiol. 2012;13(2):117–25.
2. Sim JS, Baek JH, Lee J, Cho W, Jung SI. Radiofrequency ablation of benign thyroid nodules: depicting early sign of regrowth by calculating vital volume. Int J Hyperth. 2017;33(8):905–10.
3. Papini E, Guglielmi R, Bizzarri G, Graziano F, Bianchini A, Brufani C, Pacella S, et al. Treatment of benign cold thyroid nodules: a randomized clinical trial of percutaneous laser ablation versus levothyroxine therapy or follow-up. Thyroid. 2007;17(3):229–35.
4. Jeong WK, Baek JH, Rhim H, Kim YS, Kwak MS, Jeong HJ, et al. Radiofrequency ablation of benign thyroid nodules: safety and imaging follow-up in 236 patients. Eur Radiol. 2008;18(6):1244–50.
5. Papini E, Rago T, Gambelunghe G, Valcavi R, Bizzarri G, Vitti P, et al. Long-term efficacy of ultrasound-guided laser ablation for benign solid thyroid nodules. Results of a 3-year multicenter prospective randomized trial. J Clin Endocrinol Metab. 2014;99(10):3653–9.
6. Ha EJ, Baek JH, Kim KW, Pyo J, Lee JH, Baek SH, et al. Comparative efficacy of radiofrequency and laser ablation for the treatment of benign thyroid nodules: systematic review including traditional pooling and Bayesian network meta-analysis. J Clin Endocrinol Metab. 2015;100(5):1903–11.
7. Sim JS, Baek JH, Cho W. Initial ablation ratio: quantitative value predicting the therapeutic success of thyroid radiofrequency ablation. Thyroid. 2018;28(11):1443–9.
8. Sim JS, Baek JH. Long-term outcomes of thermal ablation for benign thyroid nodules: the issue of regrowth. Int J Endocrinol. 2021;2021:9922509.
9. Ahmed M, Solbiati L, Brace CL, Breen DJ, Callstrom MR, Charboneau JW, et al. Image-guided tumor ablation: standardization of terminology and reporting criteria—a 10-year update. Radiology. 2014;273(1):241–60.
10. Haugen BR, Alexander EK, Bible KC, Doherty GM, Mandel SJ, Nikiforov YE, et al. 2015 American Thyroid Association management guidelines for adult patients with thyroid nodules and differentiated thyroid cancer: the American Thyroid Association guidelines task force on thyroid nodules and differentiated thyroid cancer. Thyroid. 2016;26(1):1–133.
11. Mauri G, Pacella CM, Papini E, Solbiati L, Goldberg SN, Ahmed M, et al. Image-guided thyroid ablation: proposal for standardization of terminology and reporting criteria. Thyroid. 2019;29(5):611–8.
12. Lim HK, Lee JH, Ha EJ, Sung JY, Kim JK, Baek JH. Radiofrequency ablation of benign non-functioning thyroid nodules: 4-year follow-up results for 111 patients. Eur Radiol. 2013;23(4):1044–9.
13. Baek JH. Factors related to the recurrence of benign thyroid nodules after thermal ablation. Int J Hyperth. 2017;33(8):957–8.
14. Ji Hong M, Baek JH, Choi YJ, Lee JH, Lim HK, Shong YK, et al. Radiofrequency ablation is a thyroid function-preserving treatment for patients with bilateral benign thyroid nodules. J Vasc Interv Radiol. 2015;26(1):55–61.
15. Negro R, Greco G, Deandrea M, Rucco M, Trimboli P. Twelve-month volume reduction ratio predicts regrowth and time to regrowth in thyroid nodules submitted to laser ablation: a 5-year follow-up retrospective study. Korean J Radiol. 2020;21(6):764–72.

# Chapter 18
# Long-term Management Following RFA: Controlling Regrowth

**Jung Suk Sim**

## Introduction

The efficacy and safety of thermal ablation (TA) have primarily been evaluated through short-term follow-ups of up to 1 year. These studies have consistently demonstrated a volume reduction ratio (VRR) of 50% or more, regardless of the specific modality employed [1]. TA has proven effective in alleviating pressure-related symptoms and resolving cosmetic concerns associated with benign thyroid nodules [2–4].

However, it has been reported that there may be regrowth from long-term follow-up results of more than 3 years [5]. A single-institution study reported a regrowth rate of 24% following a single session of radiofrequency ablation (RFA) after more than 3 years of follow-up [5]. Subsequent publications have also reported cases of regrowth [6]. Based on current reports, the regrowth rate in long-term follow-ups after a single session of TA is estimated to be approximately 20–30% [7].

In this chapter, we present the concept of marginal regrowth, which is considered the most probable cause of regrowth, and examine factors associated with regrowth. Furthermore, we will propose the goal for TA based on long-term management.

## Marginal Regrowth

The volume reduction observed after TA can be attributed to the absorption of ablated tissue by the patient's body [8]. Generally, absorption of ablated tissue occurs within the first year following treatment. Since TA primarily targets the

J. S. Sim (✉)
Department of Radiology, Withsim Clinic, Seongnam-si, Gyeonggi-do, South Korea



A. W. Park et al. (eds.), *Thyroid Radiofrequency Ablation*,
https://doi.org/10.1007/978-3-031-65288-2_18

central region of the nodule, the absorption of ablated tissue predominantly takes place at the center [5].

Conversely, the peripheral portion of the nodule is intentionally spared from ablation to prevent thermal damage to the surrounding tissues. The volume of viable tissue located at the periphery is relatively smaller compared to the centrally ablated tissue. The volume change of viable tissue during this period is relatively insignificant, as the absorption of ablated tissue primarily occurs within the first year after TA [5].

However, over an extended period, the volume of the peripherally located viable tissue, initially occupying a relatively small volume, may increase. Following the termination of ablated tissue absorption, the volume change of the remaining viable tissue becomes more pronounced. Ultimately, if the regrowth of residual viable tissue exceeds the absorbed volume of ablated tissue, an increase in the total nodule volume is observed, indicating regrowth [5].

The majority of regrowth cases originate from the remaining viable tissue, which is predominantly situated at the margin of the nodule. Therefore, the regrowth of the nodule after TA can be largely attributed to marginal regrowth [9].

## Factors Related to Regrowth

Achieving favorable long-term outcomes in TA relies on effectively controlling regrowth [10]. Therefore, it is crucial to understand the factors that contribute to regrowth in order to maintain favorable long-term results [11]. Regrowth-related factors can be classified into nodule factors and technical factors [7].

### *Nodule Factors*

Nodule factors that influence regrowth include initial nodule volume, vascularity, nodule composition, and anatomical location [7].

#### Initial Nodule Volume

A larger, initial nodule volume is associated with lower short-term and long-term VRR and a higher regrowth rate [12, 13]. A prospective study with a 1-year follow-up after RFA reported a slight inverse correlation between baseline nodule volume and VRR [12]. Retrospective studies that followed patients within 1 year after a single session of RFA indicated greater volume reduction in the small-volume group compared to the large-volume group [13, 14]. Another study investigating predictive factors for clinical outcomes of at least 2 years after a single session of RFA reported that patients with baseline nodule volumes less than 22.4 mL were more likely to achieve a VRR >75% after 12 months [15].

Deandrea et al. [16] reported the 5-year follow-up results after a single session of RFA. The final VRRs for the three groups categorized by initial nodule volume (<10 mL, 10–20 mL, and >20 mL) were 82%, 75%, and 65%, respectively. In another study by Lim et al. [9], who conducted a 4-year follow-up after multiple-session RFA, VRR and treatment sessions were compared between groups with initial nodule volumes <10 mL and >20 mL. The <10 mL group achieved a higher VRR (94.5% vs. 88.5%) with fewer treatment sessions (1.7 vs. 3.8). The authors also found that the initial nodule volume was an independent predictor of the final VRR. In a study with a 3-year follow-up after single-session laser ablation (LA) for autonomous functioning thyroid nodules (AFTNs), it was reported that a larger initial nodule volume was associated with a lower likelihood of discontinuing medication [17].

Considering the aforementioned evidence, large, initial nodule volume is not only related to lower short-term and long-term VRR but can also be considered a significant factor influencing regrowth. However, there is limited data available on the regrowth rate based on initial nodule volume. A study investigating risk factors for recurrence after a single session of microwave ablation (MWA) with a follow-up of more than 12 months reported that initial nodule volume and vascularity were factors associated with regrowth. However, this study had a relatively short follow-up period of 1 year [18].

## Vascularity

High vascularity in the nodule can result in a heat sink effect during TA treatment, leading to reduced therapeutic effectiveness [19]. A study investigating recurrence factors after a follow-up of 12 months or more following a single session of MWA reported that nodule vascularity, along with initial volume and input energy, was associated with recurrence [18].

If vascularity develops in the remaining viable tissue during the follow-up period or if existing vascularity increases, it can predispose the nodule to regrowth [7]. Consequently, widely accepted guidelines recommend routine vascularity assessments during regular follow-up after TA [4]. However, there is currently limited direct research data available on this specific issue.

## Nodule Composition

The composition of thyroid nodules, particularly the presence of cystic components, has been found to influence the short-term VRR after thermal ablation. Studies have shown that nodules with more cystic components tend to have higher short-term VRR. In a prospective study evaluating the correlation between ultrasound findings and VRR at a 1-year follow-up after RFA, Deandrea et al. reported that spongiform nodules had a higher volume reduction compared to nodules with a mixed or solid pattern [12]. Another study found that nodules with a higher proportion of solid components were more prevalent in the "less than 50%" VRR group compared to the "greater than or equal to 50%" VRR group in short-term outcomes [20].

However, there are conflicting reports regarding the impact of nodule composition on long-term VRR and regrowth rate. A study investigating predictive factors for clinical outcomes after a follow-up of at least 2 years after a single session of RFA reported that nodules with macrocystic components were more likely to achieve VRR greater than 75% after 12 months [15]. In a 3-year follow-up study after multiple-session MWA, the cystic component was found to be a prognostic factor for VRR at the 1-, 3-, and 6-month follow-ups but did not significantly affect VRR at the 12-, 24-, and 36-month follow-ups [21]. These findings suggest that nodule composition may influence short-term VRR but have little effect on VRR after 1 year. Another study reported that solid nodules showed a tendency for regrowth at long-term follow-up [22].

#### Anatomical Location

The anatomical location of thyroid nodules can also impact the regrowth rate after TA. If a nodule is located close to critical structures such as the recurrent laryngeal nerve, carotid sheath, and airway, a portion of the nodule close to these structures may be intentionally left unablated to avoid thermal damage [23, 24]. Consequently, the location of the nodule can affect the regrowth rate [25].

However, studies on the impact of anatomical location on regrowth rate are limited, and the results are inconsistent. A study that examined the factors contributing to recurrence after a follow-up of more than 12 months after a single session of MWA reported that nodules located close to critical structures might not receive sufficient thermal energy, which could be a factor contributing to regrowth [18]. On the other hand, another study reported no significant difference in the anatomical location of nodules when studying factors affecting the therapeutic success rate after a follow-up within 1 year after multiple-session RFA [26].

### *Technical Factors*

#### Difference Among Devices

Studies have compared the outcomes of different TA devices, mainly focusing on comparisons between LA and RFA [27, 28]. Randomized trials have shown that RFA achieved higher VRR compared to LA at 6 and 12 months after TA [27, 29]. However, a retrospective study comparing LA and RFA reported similar results at the 1-year follow-up [3].

In a multicenter retrospective study that used propensity score matching to compare LA and RFA, RFA demonstrated higher VRR at 1 year (72% vs. 54%), lower regrowth rate (17% vs. 34%), and lower retreatment rate (14% vs. 32%) at 5 years [6]. A systematic review and meta-analysis comparing long-term follow-up results of LA and RFA for over 2 years reported that RFA had higher VRR at 2 or 3 years compared to LA. This difference was attributed to the greater maneuverability of the RFA electrode, allowing for more intensive treatment of the residual viable portion during multiple-session treatment [28, 30].

However, a study using propensity score matching for 1-year follow-up data after RFA and LA reported higher VRR in LA than in RFA [31]. The authors of this study suggested that the operator's skills could play a crucial role in determining the extent of nodule volume reduction, regardless of the technique used.

MWA and high-intensity focused ultrasound (HIFU) were introduced later than LA and RFA, so there are fewer comparative studies involving these modalities. Regarding HIFU, the 2-year VRR was reported to be approximately 33.3%, 43.3%, and 70.4%, while the 3-year VRR was approximately 31.9%, generally lower than other modalities [2, 32, 33]. In a meta-analysis comparing the 12-month efficacy of MWA and RFA, the VRR at 3 and 6 months was similar, but the 12-month VRR was lower in RFA (86.2% vs. 80.0%) [34]. In a retrospective study by Luo et al. [21] involving 659 benign thyroid nodules treated with multiple-session MWA and followed for 3 years, the VRRs after 1, 2, and 3 years were reported as 87.4%, 90.1%, and 93.2%, respectively. These results indicate a high VRR similar to those reported by Lim et al. [9]. Considering that both Lim et al. and Luo et al. used the moving-shot technique, it suggests that the maneuverability highlighted by Cho et al. [30] and Ha et al. [28] was advantageous in controlling the marginal tissue.

In summary, there are differences in outcomes among various TA devices. RFA has generally shown higher VRR and lower regrowth rates compared to LA, while MWA and HIFU have shown promising results but have fewer comparative studies available. The operator's skills and maneuverability of the devices may also play a role in the extent of nodule volume reduction and overall treatment success.

## Energy Delivery

Multiple studies have suggested that the amount of energy delivered during the TA procedure has an impact on the outcomes. One study investigating VRR 1 year after RFA found that the amount of energy delivered was proportional to VRR [35]. Another study reported that delivering 756 J/mL and 2670 J/mL of energy resulted in a probability of VRR > 50% in 50% and 99% of patients, respectively, at 1 year [36]. In a study with a long-term follow-up of over 5 years after RFA, RFA with a cutoff of 1360 J/mL predicted VRR > 50%, while RFA with a cutoff of 918 J/mL predicted the need for retreatment [6].

### Recently Proposed Methods to Control Marginal Residual Tissue

Recently, several techniques have been introduced to achieve complete or near-complete ablation of residual marginal tissue that can contribute to regrowth [37]. Artery-first ablation is a technique that involves ablating the feeding arteries before ablating the nodule tissue. Marginal venous ablation is a technique used to ablate draining veins distributed in the nodule margin. Hydrodissection is a technique that involves injecting 5% dextrose around the nodule margin to facilitate complete ablation of the marginal nodule tissue while creating a distance between critical structures and the nodule margin. Offi et al. reported that ablation of the feeding artery first resulted in a higher VRR compared to the conventional method (83.0% VRR vs. 70.0% at 6 months) [38].

### Multiple Ablation

Kim et al. divided nodules that met the criteria for additional treatment into two groups: a group that received additional treatment and a group that did not. They found that the final VRRs between the two groups differed significantly, with 84.6% in the additional treatment group and 39.8% in the nontreatment group. The criteria for additional treatment included unresolved or recurrent patient symptoms or cosmetic problems, regrowth or an increase in viable volume (Vv), an initial ablation ratio (IAR) below 70%, and the presence of increased vascularity with or without volume increase [39]. Both recently published guidelines from Korea and Europe have recognized the need for additional ablation in thermal ablation for benign thyroid nodules [4, 40]. Systematic reviews and meta-analyses have also indicated that further volume reduction can be achieved with multiple ablations [28, 30]. Studies with follow-up periods of more than 4 years after multiple-session RFA and more than 3 years after multiple-session MWA have reported VRRs exceeding 90%. However, the optimal timing and number of additional ablations still need to be studied in the future.

## What Is the Goal of Thermal Ablation?

The goal of TA has not been extensively studied yet. However, Sim et al. have argued that since TA is an alternative to surgery, the effect of volume reduction should be long-lasting, similar to surgery, and that the permanent avoidance of surgery should be a new clinical goal of TA [10].

## References

1. Kuo JH, et al. A comprehensive review of interventional ablation techniques for the management of thyroid nodules and metastatic lymph nodes. Surgery. 2022;171(4):920–31.
2. Trimboli P, et al. High-intensity focused ultrasound (HIFU) for benign thyroid nodules: 2-year follow-up results. Endocrine. 2019;65(2):312–7.
3. Mauri G, et al. Benign thyroid nodules treatment using percutaneous laser ablation (PLA) and radiofrequency ablation (RFA). Int J Hyperthermia. 2017;33(3):295–9.
4. Kim JH, et al. 2017 thyroid radiofrequency ablation guideline: Korean Society of Thyroid Radiology. Korean J Radiol. 2018;19(4):632–55.
5. Sim JS, et al. Radiofrequency ablation of benign thyroid nodules: depicting early sign of regrowth by calculating vital volume. Int J Hyperthermia. 2017;33(8):905–10.
6. Bernardi S, et al. Five-year results of radiofrequency and laser ablation of benign thyroid nodules: a multicenter study from the Italian minimally invasive treatments of the thyroid group. Thyroid. 2020;30:1759.
7. Sim JS, Baek JH. Long-term outcomes of thermal ablation for benign thyroid nodules: the issue of regrowth. Int J Endocrinol. 2021;2021:9922509.
8. Nikfarjam M, Christophi C. Interstitial laser thermotherapy for liver tumours. Br J Surg. 2003;90(9):1033–47.
9. Lim HK, et al. Radiofrequency ablation of benign non-functioning thyroid nodules: 4-year follow-up results for 111 patients. Eur Radiol. 2013;23(4):1044–9.
10. Sim JS, Baek JH. Unresolved clinical issues in thermal ablation of benign thyroid nodules: regrowth at longterm follow-up. Korean J Radiol. 2021;22:1436.
11. Baek JH. Factors related to the efficacy of radiofrequency ablation for benign thyroid nodules. Ultrasonography. 2017;36(4):385–6.
12. Deandrea M, et al. Radiofrequency ablation for benign thyroid nodules according to different ultrasound features: an Italian multicentre prospective study. Eur J Endocrinol. 2019;180(1):79–87.
13. Cesareo R, et al. Prospective study of effectiveness of ultrasound-guided radiofrequency ablation versus control group in patients affected by benign thyroid nodules. J Clin Endocrinol Metab. 2015;100(2):460–6.
14. Feroci F, et al. Radiofrequency thermal ablation of benign thyroid nodules: the correlation between ultrasound nodule characteristics and results. Surg Innov. 2020;27(4):342–51.
15. Bisceglia A, et al. Predictor analysis in radiofrequency ablation of benign thyroid nodules: a single center experience. Front Endocrinol (Lausanne). 2021;12:638880.
16. Deandrea M, et al. Long-term efficacy of a single session of RFA for benign thyroid nodules: a longitudinal 5-year observational study. J Clin Endocrinol Metab. 2019;104(9):3751–6.
17. Gambelunghe G, et al. A single session of laser ablation for toxic thyroid nodules: three-year follow-up results. Int J Hyperthermia. 2018;34(5):631–5.
18. Wang B, et al. Factors related to recurrence of the benign non-functioning thyroid nodules after percutaneous microwave ablation. Int J Hyperthermia. 2017;33(4):459–64.
19. Pillai K, et al. Heat sink effect on tumor ablation characteristics as observed in monopolar radiofrequency, bipolar radiofrequency, and microwave, using ex vivo calf liver model. Medicine (Baltimore). 2015;94(9):e580.
20. Negro R, et al. Twelve-month volume reduction ratio predicts regrowth and time to regrowth in thyroid nodules submitted to laser ablation: a 5-year follow-up retrospective study. Korean J Radiol. 2020;21:764.
21. Luo F, et al. Microwave ablation of benign thyroid nodules: 3-year follow-up outcomes. Head Neck. 2021;43:3437.
22. Negro R, Salem TM, Greco G. Laser ablation is more effective for spongiform than solid thyroid nodules. A 4-year retrospective follow-up study. Int J Hyperthermia. 2016;32(7):822–8.
23. Shin JH, et al. Radiofrequency ablation of thyroid nodules: basic principles and clinical application. Int J Endocrinol. 2012;2012:919650.

24. Wang JF, et al. Complications following radiofrequency ablation of benign thyroid nodules: a systematic review. Chin Med J (Engl). 2017;130(11):1361–70.
25. Sim JS, Baek JH. Long-term outcomes following thermal ablation of benign thyroid nodules as an alternative to surgery: the importance of controlling regrowth. Endocrinol Metab (Seoul). 2019;34(2):117–23.
26. Lee GM, et al. Successful radiofrequency ablation strategies for benign thyroid nodules. Endocrine. 2019;64(2):316–21.
27. Cesareo R, et al. Laser ablation versus radiofrequency ablation for benign non-functioning thyroid nodules: six-month results of a randomised, parallel, open-label, trial (LARA trial). Thyroid. 2020;30:847.
28. Ha EJ, et al. Comparative efficacy of radiofrequency and laser ablation for the treatment of benign thyroid nodules: systematic review including traditional pooling and Bayesian network meta-analysis. J Clin Endocrinol Metab. 2015;100(5):1903–11.
29. Cesareo R, et al. Laser ablation versus radiofrequency ablation for thyroid nodules: 12-month results of a randomized trial (LARA II study). J Clin Endocrinol Metab. 2021;106(6):1692–701.
30. Cho SJ, et al. Long-term results of thermal ablation of benign thyroid nodules: a systematic review and meta-analysis. Endocrinol Metab (Seoul). 2020;35(2):339–50.
31. Pacella CM, et al. A comparison of laser with radiofrequency ablation for the treatment of benign thyroid nodules: a propensity score matching analysis. Int J Hyperthermia. 2017;33(8):911–9.
32. Monpeyssen H, et al. High-intensity focused ultrasound (HIFU) therapy for benign thyroid nodules: a 3-year retrospective multicenter follow-up study. Int J Hyperthermia. 2020;37(1):1301–9.
33. Lang BHH, Woo YC, Chiu KW. Two-year efficacy of single-session high-intensity focused ultrasound (HIFU) ablation of benign thyroid nodules. Eur Radiol. 2019;29(1):93–101.
34. Guo DM, et al. Comparison of radiofrequency ablation and microwave ablation for benign thyroid nodules: a systematic review and meta-analysis. Clin Endocrinol (Oxf). 2021;95(1):187–96.
35. Trimboli P, Deandrea M. Treating thyroid nodules by radiofrequency: is the delivered energy correlated with the volume reduction rate? A pilot study. Endocrine. 2020;69(3):682–7.
36. Deandrea M, et al. Determining an energy threshold for optimal volume reduction of benign thyroid nodules treated by radiofrequency ablation. Eur Radiol. 2021;31:5189.
37. Park HS, et al. Thyroid radiofrequency ablation: updates on innovative devices and techniques. Korean J Radiol. 2017;18(4):615–23.
38. Offi C, et al. The ablation of thyroid Nodule's afferent arteries before radiofrequency ablation: preliminary data. Front Endocrinol (Lausanne). 2021;11:565000.
39. Kim HJ, et al. Long-term follow-up of the radiofrequency ablation of benign thyroid nodules: the value of additional treatment. Ultrasonography. 2022;41:661.
40. Papini E, et al. 2020 European Thyroid Association clinical practice guideline for the use of image-guided ablation in benign thyroid nodules. Eur Thyroid J. 2020;9(4):172–85.

# Chapter 19
# RFA for the Treatment of Primary Thyroid Cancer

**Ji-hoon Kim**

## Introduction

Primary thyroid cancers encompass a diverse spectrum of aggressiveness, with the majority displaying indolent behavior. In recent years, the efficacy and safety of radiofrequency ablation (RFA) for treating papillary thyroid microcarcinoma (PTMC) have been extensively reported, following a series of initial case reports. Moreover, investigations into the outcomes of RFA for other types of primary thyroid cancer have also emerged. This chapter aims to present an overview of the outcomes and recent guidelines pertaining to RFA in the management of primary thyroid cancer, in line with the current trends in medical practice. Notably, numerous academic societies have begun endorsing RFA and thermal ablation as viable therapeutic approaches for primary thyroid cancer. The chapter provides a comprehensive summary of the reported outcomes of RFA, while also delving into the emerging guidelines and discussing potential future considerations for the field.

## Radiofrequency Ablation for Papillary Thyroid Microcarcinoma

RFA has been widely recognized as a safe and effective treatment for low-risk PTMC (Fig. 19.1). A number of studies have consistently reported positive outcomes in terms of safety and efficacy.

---

J. Kim (✉)
Department of Radiology, Seoul National University Hospital, Seoul National University College of Medicine, Seoul, South Korea
e-mail: jihnkim@snu.ac.kr


A. W. Park et al. (eds.), *Thyroid Radiofrequency Ablation*, https://doi.org/10.1007/978-3-031-65288-2_19

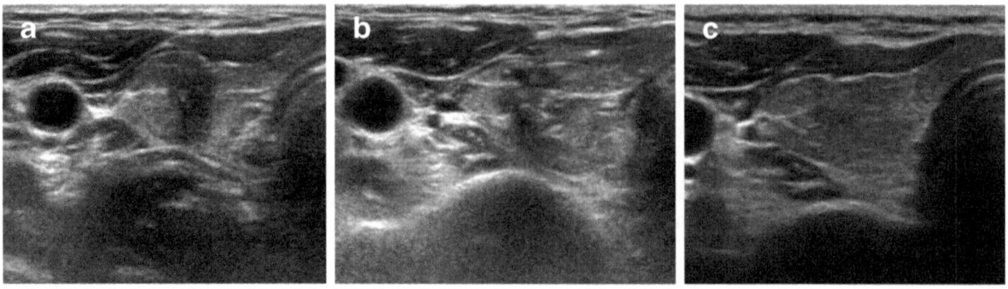


**Fig. 19.1** Outcome of radiofrequency ablation for papillary thyroid microcarcinoma (PTMC) in a 63-year-old woman. Pre-ablation ultrasonography (**a**) reveals a 0.7 × 0.6 × 0.7 cm PTMC in the right thyroid gland. Ultrasonography (**b**) obtained immediately after radiofrequency ablation (RFA) shows a larger ablation zone than the initial PTMC. Ultrasonography (**c**) obtained 3 years later after RFA presents complete disappearance of the PTMC

Zhang et al. conducted the first prospective study on RFA for low-risk PTMC in 2016 [1]. In a mean follow-up period of 7.8 months, complete resolution was achieved in 10 out of 98 PTMC cases (10.2%), while 23 cases (23.5%) showed only needle tracks with no major complications. No residual or recurrent tumors or lymph node metastasis were detected. Follow-up ultrasound-guided RFA at 3 months did not reveal any residual or recurrent tumors.

Long-term follow-up studies have demonstrated encouraging results. Cho et al. reported 100% complete disappearance rates after a 60-month follow-up, with a major complication rate of 1.4% (1/74) after a mean of 1.2 RFA sessions over a mean follow-up of 72 months [2]. Although four newly developed cancers were identified in three patients, there was no local tumor progression, lymph node metastasis, or distant metastasis. Yan et al. presented the mean 42-month follow-up outcome of a large cohort study involving 414 patients [3]. During the study period, a mean volume reduction rate of 98.81 ± 6.41% (range 50–100%) was observed, along with an 88.41% complete disappearance rate, a 3.62% local tumor progression rate, a 0.97% new lymph node metastasis rate, and a 2.42% recurrent PTMC rate. Additional RFA was performed in 13 patients, resulting in complete disappearance of 11 lesions.

Systematic reviews and meta-analyses have further confirmed the safety and efficacy of RFA for PTMC. van Dijk et al. analyzed 1822 PTMC cases from 1770 patients and reported a pooled complete disappearance rate of 79%, an overall tumor progression rate of 1.5%, local residual PTMC detected at 0.4%, new PTMC detection at 0.9%, new lymph node metastasis at 0.2%, and a major complication rate at 0.2% [4].

When compared to surgery, the largest series by Yan et al. found no significant differences in local tumor progression, lymph node metastasis, recurrent PTMC, persistent lesion, and 4-year recurrence-free survival rates between thyroid lobectomy and RFA groups without distant metastasis [5]. RFA offers advantages such as shorter procedure time, lower estimated blood loss, shorter hospitalization, lower cost, and lower complication rates compared to thyroid lobectomy. Furthermore,

RFA has been shown to provide better quality-of-life outcomes, addressing both physical and emotional problems [6].

Several studies have presented favorable outcomes of RFA for PTMC in specific conditions. Song et al. compared the outcomes of RFA and total thyroidectomy in PTMC patients located in the isthmus [7]. The study showed similar outcomes between RFA and total thyroidectomy, challenging the common belief that thyroid cancers in the thyroid isthmus tend to have extrathyroidal extension and advocating for total thyroidectomy.

In older patients with PTMC, there appears to be a lower tumor progression rate but higher mortality compared to younger patients. A study showed that older PTMC patients (≥60 years) had a significantly lower progression rate to clinical disease (1.6% vs. 8.9%, $P < 0.0001$) compared to younger patients (<40 years) [8]. Moreover, among patients who died from PTMCs ≤2 cm, there was a significantly higher proportion of patients aged ≥45 years (92% vs. 52%; $P < 0.01$) [9].

In the study conducted by He et al., it was demonstrated that RFA was safe and effective in PTMC patients aged 55 years or older [10]. Although multifocality is common in PTMC patients and does not exclude them from active surveillance, most RFA studies have reported outcomes in unifocal PTMC cases. A recent study by Yan et al. found that RFA showed similar outcomes between multifocal PTMC and unifocal PTMC [11].

## Primary Thyroid Cancer Other Than Papillary Thyroid Microcarcinoma

Although the majority of studies have focused on PTMC, recent publications have expanded the indication of RFA to other primary thyroid cancers.

### *T1b Papillary Thyroid Cancer (1 cm < Tumor ≤ 2 cm)*

Numerous studies have reported favorable outcomes following RFA or thermal ablation for T1b papillary thyroid cancer (PTC) (Fig. 19.2).

In a retrospective study by Xiao et al., a cohort of 66 patients demonstrated a 100% technical success rate with no major complications [12]. The final follow-up revealed a remarkable 99.11% volume reduction rate, with 57.6% of patients experiencing complete disappearance of the tumor. Malignant cells were detected in 3.0% of the ablation zones, and 1.5% of patients developed cervical lymph node metastasis.

A comparison between T1a and T1b PTC outcomes by Xiao et al. showed no significant difference in the local tumor progression rate [13]. However, the tumor disappearance rate was higher in the T1a group (81.7% vs. 52.7%). Notably, RFA

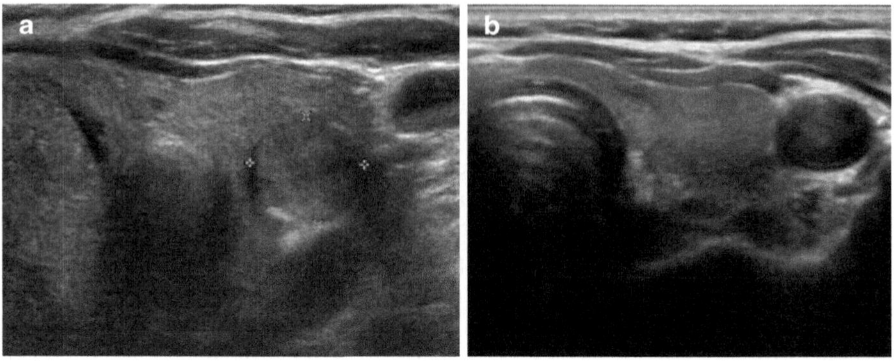


**Fig. 19.2** Outcome of radiofrequency ablation for T1b papillary thyroid carcinoma (PTC) in an 81-year-old woman. Pre-ablation ultrasonography (**a**) reveals a 1.2 × 1.2 × 1.5 cm T1b PTC in the left thyroid gland. Ultrasonography (**b**) obtained 2 years later after radiofrequency ablation (RFA) shows near-complete disappearance of the PTC

for T1b tumors required higher output power and longer duration, and one patient experienced transient recurrent laryngeal nerve injury.

Several studies have also compared the outcomes of RFA and surgery for T1b PTC. Xiao et al. reported comparable tumor progression rates between the two approaches [14]. Notably, permanent hypoparathyroidism was observed only in the surgery group (4.4%), while no major or minor complications occurred in the RFA group. Similarly, He et al. found no significant differences in tumor progression or complication rates between the two treatment modalities [15]. RFA exhibited advantages in terms of lower cost and shorter operation duration compared to surgery.

## *T2 Papillary Thyroid Cancer: (2 cm < Tumor ≤ 4 cm)*

Xiao et al. reported the outcome of RFA in T2 papillary thyroid cancer [16]. All tumors were successfully ablated according to the treatment plan. During a mean follow-up of 24.1 months, there was a significant decrease in tumor volume from 4.4 ± 2.8 to 0.3 ± 0.5 mL. The volume reduction rate at the final follow-up was 93.7 ± 7.6%, and two tumors (16.7%) completely disappeared. There were no instances of new or recurrent tumors, and no local or distant metastasis was detected during the follow-up period. No life-threatening or delayed complications were observed. Xiao et al. reported the outcome of RFA in T2 papillary thyroid cancer [16].

## Follicular Neoplasm

The preoperative diagnosis of follicular neoplasm is challenging, although core-needle biopsy has shown better accuracy compared to fine-needle aspiration. Additionally, distinguishing between follicular adenoma and follicular carcinoma preoperatively is not possible. Therefore, surgery is typically recommended for thyroid nodules with a preoperative Bethesda IV diagnosis of follicular neoplasm/suspicious for follicular neoplasm. However, it is noteworthy that approximately 70–80% of these cases are ultimately diagnosed as follicular adenoma rather than follicular carcinoma.

There have been two studies investigating the use of RFA in patients with follicular neoplasm. Ha et al. reported the outcome of RFA in 10 cases of small follicular thyroid neoplasms [17]. Eight patients underwent a single session of RFA, while two patients required two sessions. During a follow-up period of 66.4 months, the mean volume reduction rate was 99.5%, and 80% of cases (8/10) demonstrated complete disappearance without any instances of recurrence or major complications (Fig. 19.3). Lin et al. performed RFA in 22 patients with follicular thyroid neoplasms and SUVmax <5 on positron emission tomography/computed tomography (PET/CT). The volume reduction ratios at 6–12 months (mean: 10.1 months) after RFA were 73.3 ± 17.7%. One patient experienced transient vocal cord palsy lasting for 3 months, but there were no cases of post-procedural hypothyroidism [18].

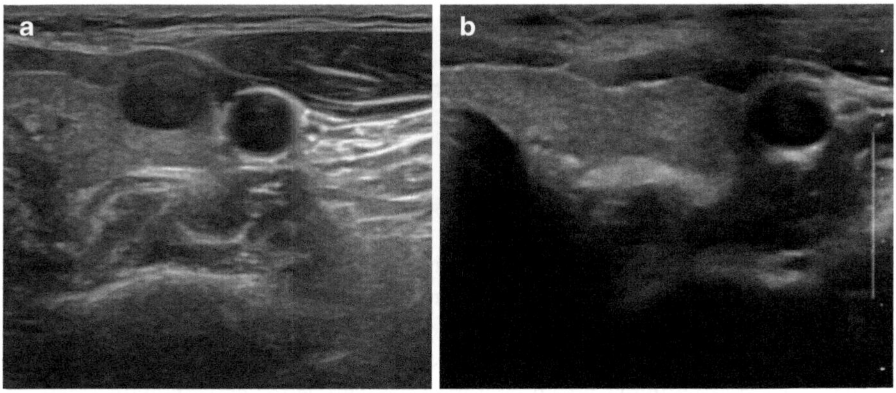


**Fig. 19.3** Outcome of radiofrequency ablation for follicular neoplasm in a 42-year-old woman. Pre-ablation longitudinal ultrasonography (**a**) reveals a 1.0 × 0.9 × 0.6 cm follicular neoplasm in the left thyroid gland. Ultrasonography (**b**) obtained 2 years later after radiofrequency ablation (RFA) shows complete disappearance of the neoplasm

## Medullary Thyroid Carcinoma

Due to its rarity, there have been only two reported cases of RFA for medullary thyroid carcinoma [19, 20]. In a case report by Biamonte et al., a 64-year-old woman with a high serum calcitonin level and a thyroid nodule suspicious for medullary thyroid carcinoma underwent RFA. The treatment resulted in a normalized serum calcitonin level and a marked decrease in the size of the nodule on ultrasonography at 6 months of follow-up [19]. However, RFA was found to be ineffective in a case of advanced medullary thyroid carcinoma (T4N1Amx), even after repeated ablations were performed [20].

### *Inoperable Primary Thyroid Cancer*

The use of RFA for inoperable primary thyroid cancer has been reported extremely rarely. Jeong et al. reported the outcome of RFA in two cases of anaplastic thyroid carcinoma compared to papillary microcarcinomas and macrocarcinomas [21]. Although the anaplastic carcinoma cases underwent multiple RFA treatments, they showed no improvement in clinical symptoms or neck bulging. In contrast, the cases of papillary microcarcinomas and macrocarcinomas showed significant improvement. Based on this limited study, the authors concluded that the effectiveness of RFA on anaplastic thyroid carcinoma remains questionable.

## International Consensus of Thermal Ablation for Primary Thyroid Cancer

Since 2015, several national and international societies have started discussing the potential role of RFA or thermal ablation for PTMC (Table 19.1). In 2015, Italian societies suggested that US-guided techniques might have a role in the future for PTMC when no multifocality or nodal metastasis is present [22]. In 2018, the Korean Society of Radiology also suggested that thermal ablation could be considered as an alternative treatment for patients with primary thyroid cancer, who refuse surgery or are not eligible for an operation, as well as for patients with advanced thyroid cancer for palliative purposes [23]. In 2021, the European Thyroid Association (ETA) and the Cardiovascular and Interventional Radiological Society of Europe (CIRSE) recommended considering thermal ablation for low-risk PTMC in patients who are at surgical risk, have a short life expectancy or comorbidities, refuse surgery, or opt for active surveillance [24]. They also emphasized the importance of informing patients about the advantages and limitations of thermal ablation as an alternative therapeutic option to immediate surgery or active surveillance. Additionally, they suggested considering minimally invasive treatment for palliative

**Table 19.1** National and international consensus of thermal ablation of primary thyroid cancer

| Society | Year | Journal | Indication |
|---|---|---|---|
| A group of physician experts in thyroid pathology and interventional ultrasound, including endocrinologists, surgeons, radiologists, and specialists in nuclear medicine, from the main centers for thyroid disease in Italy and several Italian scientific societies | 2015 | Journal of Ultrasound [20] | Primary unifocal papillary thyroid microcarcinoma without nodal metastasis |
| Korean Society of Thyroid Radiology | 2018 | Korean Journal of Radiology [21] | Patients with primary thyroid cancer, who refuse surgery or who cannot undergo an operation<br>Patients with advanced thyroid cancer for palliative purposes |
| European Thyroid Association (ETA) and the Cardiovascular and Interventional Radiological Society of Europe (CIRSE) | 2021 | European Thyroid Journal [22] | Patients with low-risk papillary thyroid microcarcinoma, mainly if the patient is at surgical risk, is expected to have short life expectancy, has comorbidities that need to be prioritized before thyroid surgery, or is unwilling to undergo surgery or active surveillance<br>For palliative purposes in patients with primary thyroid cancer, other than low-risk papillary thyroid microcarcinoma, preferentially in the context of a multimodality approach |
| An international multidisciplinary consensus statement of the American Head and Neck Society Endocrine Surgery Section with the Asia Pacific Society of Thyroid Surgery, Associazione Medici Endocrinologi, British Association of Endocrine and Thyroid Surgeons, European Thyroid Association, Italian Society of Endocrine Surgery Units, Korean Society of Thyroid Radiology, Latin American Thyroid Society, and Thyroid Nodules Therapies Association | 2021 | Head & Neck [23] | Candidate primary tumors should demonstrate the following characteristics:<br>1. unifocal microcarcinoma confined to the thyroid gland, without evidence of extrathyroidal extension or capsular contact<br>2. cytologic confirmation of papillary thyroid cancer without aggressive subtype<br>3. no evidence of metastatic lymphadenopathy<br>4. high risk, ineligible for, or declines surgery |

purposes. Most recently, in 2021, an international multidisciplinary consensus statement was published for RFA and related ultrasonography-guided ablation technologies for the treatment of benign and malignant thyroid diseases [25]. The consensus statement stated that RFA is currently not considered a first-line treatment for primary thyroid cancer, but it can be considered under certain conditions, including unifocal microcarcinoma without evidence of extrathyroidal extension or capsular contact, cytologic confirmation of papillary thyroid cancer without aggressive subtype, no evidence of metastatic lymphadenopathy, and high-risk patients, who are ineligible for or decline surgery.

## Issues

Despite the promising results of RFA and thermal ablation for primary thyroid cancer, there are several unresolved issues that need to be addressed.

One important issue is the long-term follow-up results for low-risk PTMC. While RFA may have short-term benefits over surgery, the long-term outcomes and comparison with active surveillance are not yet clear [26, 27]. There are concerns of overdiagnosis and overtreatment that need to be carefully considered.

The limitation of pre-procedural diagnosis of lymph node metastasis is another challenge. Hidden nodal micrometastasis has been detected during surgery after laser ablation for PTMC, highlighting the difficulty in accurately diagnosing lymph node involvement preoperatively [28]. Missed macroscopic lymph node metastasis cases are also encountered, emphasizing the need for improved diagnostic techniques.

In real clinical practice, incomplete ablation for primary thyroid cancer can occur, leading to potential problems. A case series of patients, who underwent surgery after RFA for papillary thyroid carcinoma, reported incomplete ablations and cervical lymph node metastasis in many cases [29]. This highlights the importance of operator experience and careful evaluation of treatment outcomes.

While RFA may be feasible for T2 papillary thyroid carcinoma, the potential for extrathyroidal extension and lymph node metastasis in larger cancers should be carefully considered [16]. Long-term follow-up studies and more research are needed to determine the role of RFA in treating T2 papillary thyroid carcinoma.

Sonographic limitations in evaluating tumor disappearance after RFA in calcified carcinomas is another challenge. Many papillary thyroid carcinomas are accompanied by calcifications, which may disappear after RFA [30]. However, persistent or increasing calcifications make it challenging to assess tumor ablation (Fig. 19.4).

The use of RFA for PTMC with extrathyroidal extension is a topic of controversy. While active surveillance may be indicated for PTMC with extrathyroidal extension into the anterior strap muscle, the use of RFA in these cases requires careful consideration and further debate [31].

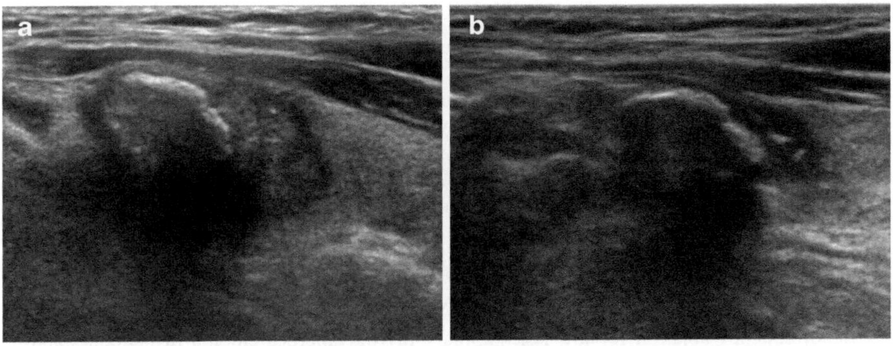


**Fig. 19.4** Outcome of radiofrequency ablation for T2 papillary thyroid carcinoma (PTC) in an 80-year-old woman. Pre-ablation longitudinal ultrasonography (**a**) reveals a 2.7 × 1.6 × 2.8 cm T2 PTC in the left thyroid gland. Ultrasonography (**b**) obtained 1 year later after RFA shows a decrease in the size of the PTC

## Conclusion

For palliative purposes, other than curative purposes, RFA may be beneficial for patients with advanced cancer [32]. However, further, many studies are needed with regard to when, how, with which combination.

Lastly, the location of the publications that reported the efficacy and safety of RFA for primary thyroid cancer showed the great regional bias, mostly China and partly Korea.

To set RFA or thermal ablation as the global standard for treatment of primary thyroid carcinoma, careful approaches and further studies for these many issues are mandatory.

## References

1. Zhang M, Luo Y, Zhang Y, Tang J. Efficacy and safety of ultrasound-guided radiofrequency ablation for treating low-risk papillary thyroid microcarcinoma: a prospective study. Thyroid. 2016;26:1581–7.
2. Cho SJ, Baek SM, Lim HK, Lee KD, Son JM, Baek JH. Long-term follow-up results of ultrasound-guided radiofrequency ablation for low-risk papillary thyroid microcarcinoma: more than 5-year follow-up for 84 tumors. Thyroid. 2020;30:1745–51.
3. Yan L, Lan Y, Xiao J, Lin L, Jiang B, Luo Y. Long-term outcomes of radiofrequency ablation for unifocal low-risk papillary thyroid microcarcinoma: a large cohort study of 414 patients. Eur Radiol. 2021;31:685–94.
4. van Dijk SPJ, Coerts HI, Gunput STG, van Velsen EFS, Medici M, Moelker A, et al. Assessment of radiofrequency ablation for papillary microcarcinoma of the thyroid: a systematic review and meta-analysis. JAMA Otolaryngol Head Neck Surg. 2022;148:317.
5. Yan L, Zhang M, Song Q, Luo Y. Ultrasound-guided radiofrequency ablation versus thyroid lobectomy for low-risk papillary thyroid microcarcinoma: a propensity-matched cohort study of 884 patients. Thyroid. 2021;31:1662–72.

6. Lan Y, Luo Y, Zhang M, Jin Z, Xiao J, Yan L, et al. Quality of life in papillary thyroid microcarcinoma patients undergoing radiofrequency ablation or surgery: a comparative study. Front Endocrinol (Lausanne). 2020;11:249.
7. Song Q, Gao H, Ren L, Tian X, Lan Y, Yan L, et al. Radiofrequency ablation versus total thyroidectomy in patients with papillary thyroid microcarcinoma located in the isthmus: a retrospective cohort study. Int J Hyperthermia. 2021;38:708–14.
8. Ito Y, Miyauchi A, Kihara M, Higashiyama T, Kobayashi K, Miya A. Patient age is significantly related to the progression of papillary microcarcinoma of the thyroid under observation. Thyroid. 2014;24:27–34.
9. Nilubol N, Kebebew E. Should small papillary thyroid cancer be observed? A population-based study. Cancer. 2015;121:1017–24.
10. He H, Song Q, Lan Y, Yan L, Xiao J, Zhang Y, et al. Efficacy and safety of ultrasound-guided radiofrequency ablation for low-risk papillary thyroid microcarcinoma in patients aged 55 years or older: a retrospective study. Int J Hyperthermia. 2021;38:604–10.
11. Yan L, Zhang M, Song Q, Xie F, Luo Y. Clinical outcomes of radiofrequency ablation for multifocal papillary thyroid microcarcinoma versus unifocal papillary thyroid microcarcinoma: a propensity-matched cohort study. Eur Radiol. 2022;32:1216–26.
12. Xiao J, Zhang M, Zhang Y, Yan L, Lan Y, Zhu Y, et al. Efficacy and safety of ultrasonography-guided radiofrequency ablation for the treatment of t1bn0m0 papillary thyroid carcinoma: a retrospective study. Int J Hyperthermia. 2020;37:392–8.
13. Xiao J, Zhang Y, Yan L, Zhang M, Li X, Tang J, et al. Ultrasonography-guided radiofrequency ablation for solitary t1an0m0 and t1bn0m0 papillary thyroid carcinoma: a retrospective comparative study. Eur J Endocrinol. 2021;186:105–13.
14. Xiao J, Zhang Y, Zhang M, Lan Y, Yan L, Luo Y, et al. Ultrasonography-guided radiofrequency ablation vs. surgery for the treatment of solitary t1bn0m0 papillary thyroid carcinoma: a comparative study. Clin Endocrinol (Oxf). 2021;94:684–91.
15. He H, Wu R, Zhao J, Song Q, Zhang Y, Luo Y. Ultrasound-guided radiofrequency ablation versus surgical resection for the treatment of t1bn0m0 papillary thyroid carcinoma in different age groups. Front Endocrinol (Lausanne). 2021;12:734432.
16. Xiao J, Zhang Y, Zhang M, Xie F, Yan L, Luo Y, et al. Ultrasonography-guided radiofrequency ablation for the treatment of t2n0m0 papillary thyroid carcinoma: a preliminary study. Int J Hyperthermia. 2021;38:402–8.
17. Ha SM, Sung JY, Baek JH, Na DG, Kim JH, Yoo H, et al. Radiofrequency ablation of small follicular neoplasms: initial clinical outcomes. Int J Hyperthermia. 2017;33:931–7.
18. Lin WC, Tung YC, Chang YH, Luo SD, Chiang PL, Huang SC, et al. Radiofrequency ablation for treatment of thyroid follicular neoplasm with low SUV in PET/CT study. Int J Hyperthermia. 2021;38:963–9.
19. Biamonte E, Solbiati L, Ierace T, Colombo P, Lavezzi E, Mazziotti G, et al. Medullary thyroid carcinoma treated with percutaneous ultrasound-guided radiofrequency ablation. Endocrine. 2019;65:515–9.
20. Owen RP, Silver CE, Ravikumar TS, Brook A, Bello J, Breining D. Techniques for radiofrequency ablation of head and neck tumors. Arch Otolaryngol Head Neck Surg. 2004;130:52–6.
21. Jeong SY, Baek JH, Choi YJ, Chung SR, Sung TY, Kim WG, et al. Radiofrequency ablation of primary thyroid carcinoma: efficacy according to the types of thyroid carcinoma. Int J Hyperthermia. 2018;34:611–6.
22. Garberoglio R, Aliberti C, Appetecchia M, Attard M, Boccuzzi G, Boraso F, et al. Radiofrequency ablation for thyroid nodules: which indications? The first Italian opinion statement. J Ultrasound. 2015;18:423–30.
23. Kim JH, Baek JH, Lim HK, Ahn HS, Baek SM, Choi YJ, et al. 2017 thyroid radiofrequency ablation guideline: Korean Society of Thyroid Radiology. Korean J Radiol. 2018;19:632–55.
24. Mauri G, Hegedüs L, Bandula S, Cazzato RL, Czarniecka A, Dudeck O, et al. European Thyroid Association and Cardiovascular and Interventional Radiological Society of Europe

2021 clinical practice guideline for the use of minimally invasive treatments in malignant thyroid lesions. Eur Thyroid J. 2021;10(3):185–97.
25. Orloff LA, Noel JE, Stack BC Jr, Russell MD, Angelos P, Baek JH, et al. Radiofrequency ablation and related ultrasound-guided ablation technologies for treatment of benign and malignant thyroid disease: an international multidisciplinary consensus statement of the American Head and Neck Society Endocrine Surgery Section with the Asia Pacific Society of Thyroid Surgery, Associazione Medici Endocrinologi, British Association of Endocrine and Thyroid Surgeons, European Thyroid Association, Italian Society of Endocrine Surgery Units, Korean Society of Thyroid Radiology, Latin American Thyroid Society, and Thyroid Nodules Therapies Association. Head Neck. 2022;44(3):633–60.
26. Kim EK. Re: papillary thyroid carcinoma treated with radiofrequency ablation in a patient with hypertrophic cardiomyopathy: a case report. Korean J Radiol. 2016;17:965.
27. Mauri G, Sconfienza LM. Image-guided thermal ablation might be a way to compensate for image deriving cancer overdiagnosis. Int J Hyperthermia. 2017;33:489–90.
28. Valcavi R, Piana S, Bortolan GS, Lai R, Barbieri V, Negro R. Ultrasound-guided percutaneous laser ablation of papillary thyroid microcarcinoma: a feasibility study on three cases with pathological and immunohistochemical evaluation. Thyroid. 2013;23:1578–82.
29. Sun W, Zhang H, He L, Zhang T, Wang Z, Dong W, et al. Surgery after ultrasound-guided radiofrequency ablation for papillary thyroid carcinoma in 21 patients: a retrospective study from a single center in China. Med Sci Monit. 2020;26:e928391.
30. Yoo RE, Kim JH, Paeng JC, Park YJ. Radiofrequency ablation for treatment of locally recurrent thyroid cancer presenting as a metastatic lymph node with dense macrocalcification: a case report and literature review. Medicine. 2018;97:e0003.
31. Sugitani I, Ito Y, Takeuchi D, Nakayama H, Masaki C, Shindo H, et al. Indications and strategy for active surveillance of adult low-risk papillary thyroid microcarcinoma: consensus statements from the Japan Association of Endocrine Surgery task force on management for papillary thyroid microcarcinoma. Thyroid. 2021;31:183–92.
32. Mauri G, Hegedüs L, Cazzato RL, Papini E. Minimally invasive treatment procedures have come of age for thyroid malignancy: the 2021 clinical practice guideline for the use of minimally invasive treatments in malignant thyroid lesions. Cardiovasc Intervent Radiol. 2021;44:1481–4.

# Chapter 20
# RFA for the Treatment of Recurrent Thyroid Cancer

**Auh Whan Park**

## Introduction

Papillary thyroid cancer (PTC) represents the majority of thyroid cancer cases, comprising approximately 85% of all diagnoses [1–3] Despite successful initial treatment, a considerable proportion of patients experience loco-regional recurrence, with recurrence rates ranging from 20 to 30% [4, 5]. The first-line management of recurrent thyroid cancer is surgery with subsequent radioactive iodine and thyroid hormone suppression therapy. However, performing open surgery in these cases can be technically challenging due to factors such as tissue scarring, fibrosis, and disruption of normal tissue planes, thereby increasing the risk of complications such as injury to the recurrent laryngeal nerve (RLN) and parathyroid glands [6, 7].

In an effort to decrease surgery-related morbidity, ultrasound (US)-guided radiofrequency ablation (RFA) has emerged as a promising minimally invasive alternative for the treatment of PTC (Fig. 20.1) [8–12]. RFA presents several potential advantages, including reduced invasiveness, decreased morbidity, shorter procedural times, and lower complication rates [7, 10].

This chapter is to review RFA as a minimally invasive treatment for recurrent PTC. In particular, the pre-procedural evaluations, clinical efficacy, and safety profile of this modality are reviewed.

A. W. Park (✉)
Department of Radiology, Division of Interventional Radiology, University of Texas Southwestern Medical Center, Dallas, TX, USA



A. W. Park et al. (eds.), *Thyroid Radiofrequency Ablation*,
https://doi.org/10.1007/978-3-031-65288-2_20

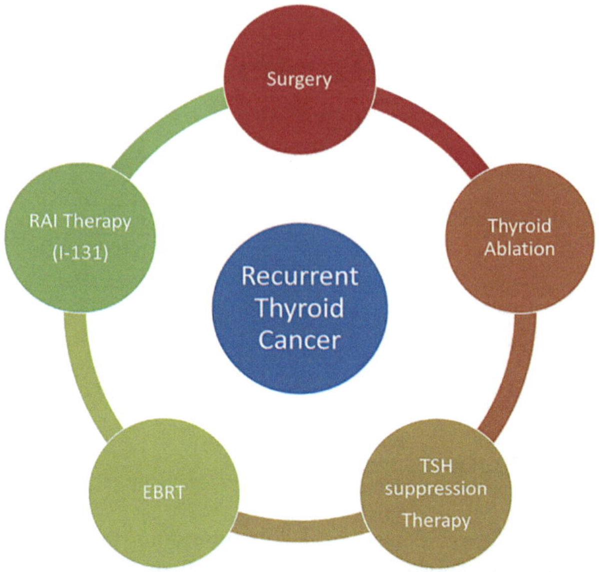


**Fig. 20.1** The Role of Thyroid Ablation in Recurrent Thyroid Cancer. Thyroid ablation can be utilized as a treatment modality in conjunction with other approaches, including surgery, radioactive iodine therapy, hormonal therapy, and external beam radiation therapy (EBRT)

## Indications

The Korean Society of Thyroid Radiology (KSThR) has developed guidelines for the use of US-guided radiofrequency ablation (RFA) in the management of recurrent thyroid cancer [13–15]. According to the KSThR guidelines, RFA is recommended for both curative and palliative purposes in specific patient populations. Patients with a high surgical risk or those who refuse repeated surgery are suitable candidates for RFA [14]. " *Curative ablation*" is defined as the complete ablation of any recurrent cancers observed on imaging. Typically, this is indicated when three or fewer recurrent lesions are visible and there is no evidence of metastatic tumors beyond the neck. On the other hand, "Palliative ablation" is undertaken when recurrent thyroid cancer presents significant symptoms from encroaching on neighboring structures like the trachea, skin, esophagus, nerves, or blood vessels, especially when complete tumor removal is not feasible. In the context of palliative ablation, the significance of a combination therapy becomes evident. Hence, the importance of a multidisciplinary approach cannot be overstated.

## Pre-procedural Evaluations

The presence of a recurrent tumor is typically confirmed through various methods, including fine-needle aspiration (FNA) or core needle biopsy (CNB), as well as increased washout thyroglobulin (Tg) levels. The 2017 KSThR guidelines for the RFA pre-procedural checklist are shown in Table 20.1 [14]. Specific parts of the checklist are further discussed in the sections that follow.

**Table 20.1** Pre-procedural checklist according to the KSThR 2017 guidelines

| Pathologic thyroid nodule | Recurrent thyroid cancer |
|---|---|
| **Pathologic diagnosis** | **Pathologic and/or serologic diagnosis** |
| • Benign diagnosis at least two US-guided FNA or CNB<br>• Benign diagnosis at least one US-guided FNA or CNB in AFTN<br>• Benign diagnosis at least 1 US-guided FNA or CNB in thyroid nodules with highly specific benign US features | • Cancer recurrence at US-guided FNA or CNB<br>• Increased washout Tg level in aspirate or Tg immunostain of CNB specimen<br>• Increased washout calcitonin level in aspirate or calcitonin immunostaining of CNB specimens in patients with medullary cancer |
| **US** | **US** |
| • Features of the nodule and surrounding critical structures<br>• Nodule volume | • Features of the nodule and surrounding critical structures<br>• Tumor volume |
| **Symptom score** | |
| **Cosmetic score** | |
| **Laboratory tests** | **Laboratory tests** |
| • Complete blood count<br>• Blood coagulation battery<br>• Thyroid function test<br>– Serum TSH<br>– Serum T3<br>– Serum fT4 | • Complete blood count<br>• Blood coagulation battery<br>• Thyroid function test<br>– Serum TSH<br>– Serum T3<br>– Serum fT4 |
| **Additional imaging study** | **Additional imaging study** |
| CT or MRI[a]<br>$^{99m}$Tc pertechnetate or $^{123}$I thyroid scan[b] | CT or MRI[a] |

*AFTN* autonomously functioning thyroid nodule, *CNB* core needle biopsy, *CT* computed tomography, *FNA* fine needle aspiration, *fT4* free thyroxine, *MRI* magnetic resonance imaging, *RFA* radiofrequency ablation, *T3* tri-iodothyronine, *Tg* thyroglobulin, *TSH* thyroid stimulating hormone (thyrotropin), *US* ultrasound

[a] Selectively indicated

[b] Indicated for AFTN

## *Imaging*

### Neck US

US imaging is effective in detecting and characterizing recurrent tumors in the neck, encompassing both the thyroidectomy bed and cervical lymph nodes [16–19]. The European Thyroid Association (ETA) has established a US-based classification system for thyroid bed lesions based on their US features (Table 20.2) [20]. For cervical lymph nodes, the imaging features are consistent with the preoperative classification system, categorizing them as suspicious (indicative of malignancy), indeterminate, or probably benign (normal) (Table 20.3) [20, 21].

In 2012, KSThR introduced guidelines which, while having similarities, presented distinct differences from the ETA guidelines. One notable discrepancy pertains to the classification of indeterminate lymph node (LN) metastasis. Specifically, according to ETA guidelines, an LN with an indeterminate feature of 4 mm can be

**Table 20.2** US criteria for diagnosis of tumor recurrence in the thyroid bed after thyroidectomy for thyroid cancer by ETA

| Category | Description |
|---|---|
| Suspicious | Taller than wide orientation<br>Irregular margins<br>Microcalcifications<br>Cystic changes<br>Increased vascularization |
| Indeterminate | Lesions displaying hypoechogenicity alone |
| Normal | Triangular or flattened area, uniformly hyperechoic or isoechoic vs surrounding muscle/tissue |

*ETA* European Thyroid Association

**Table 20.3** US criteria for diagnosis of lymph node metastasis for thyroid cancer by ETA

| Category | US |
|---|---|
| Suspicious | At least one of the following:<br>1. Microcalcifications<br>2. Partially cystic appearance<br>3. Peripheral/diffusely increased vascularization<br>4. Hyperechoic tissue looking like thyroid |
| Indeterminate | Absence of hilum and at least one of the following:<br>1. Round shape<br>2. Increased SD ≥8 mm in level II and ≥5 mm in levels III and IV<br>3. Increased central vascularization |
| Normal | 1. Normal hilum<br>2. Ovoid shape and normal size<br>3. Absent or hilar vascularization<br>4. No suspicious feature |

*ETA* European Thyroid Association

classified as benign, irrespective of its malignant morphological characteristics. However, research indicates that the malignancy rate of indeterminate LNs does not vary based on their size. Given this data, it is rational to argue that LN classification should hinge solely on its morphological characteristics, without size considerations (Table 20.4).

The tumor volume (V) can be measured and calculated using the following formula:

$$V = \pi abc / 6$$

where $a$ is the largest tumor diameter, and $b$ and $c$ are the two perpendicular. diameters.

During US examination, structures near the tumor, like arteries, veins, nerves, and other anatomical landmarks such as esophagus and trachea, are evaluated . This

**Table 20.4** US-based risk stratification for cervical lymph node metastasis in patients with potential or confirmed thyroid carcinomas by KSThR

| Category | Description |
|---|---|
| Suspicious | Any of four suspicious features<br>• Cystic change<br>• Echogenic foci (calcifications)<br>• Cortical hyperechogenicity (focal/diffuse)<br>• Abnormal vascularity (peripheral/diffuse) |
| Indeterminate | Loss of echogenic hilum and hilar vascularity |
| Probably benign | Echogenic hilum<br>Hilar vascularity |

*KSThR* Korean Society of Thyroid Radiology

assessment helps determine the tumor's closeness to vital areas, aiding in treatment planning and risk assessment for ablation.

Color Doppler US can evaluate a tumor's vascularity, giving insights into blood flow changes before and after treatment.

## Neck CT & MRI

Computed tomography (CT) or magnetic resonance imaging (MRI) can be a valuable imaging modality in cases where suspected recurrent disease is not clearly visible on US or when the aerodigestive tract is involved. This is especially relevant for patients who exhibit high levels of serum Tg or Tg antibodies (TgAb) but have negative findings on US [22–24].

Utilizing a dedicated CT protocol for thyroid cancer is essential in both pre- and post-RFA surveillance [21]. The recommended CT protocol is summarized in Table 20.5.

Recent research underscores the complementary nature of CT when used alongside US in detecting recurrent thyroid cancer [25]. Utilizing both imaging modalities enhances the precision in identifying recurrent lesions, especially prior to revision surgery or image-guided interventions [21, 22].

## Nuclear Scan/SPECT

Although it was not addressed by the 2017 KSThR guidelines [14], diagnostic radioactive iodine (RAI) imaging, which includes a whole-body scan combined with the single-photon emission computed tomography (SPECT) technique is a crucial component of nuclear imaging for patients with differentiated thyroid cancer (DTC). This imaging approach allows for the identification of the thyroid remnant, loco-regional nodal disease, and distant metastasis [26].

**Table 20.5** Recommended CT protocol for patients with thyroid cancer[a]

| Items | Parameters |
|---|---|
| Kvp, mAs | Manufacturer's recommended settings |
| Collimation, mm | 64 × 0.5–0.625 |
| Section thickness/increment, mm | 0.5–1/0.5–1 (no overlap) |
| Scan range | Skull base to AP window |
| Scan direction | Craniocaudal direction |
| IV route | Right arm preferred[b] |
| Scan delay, s | 25–40 (using fixed scan delay) |
| Injection rate of contrast media, mL/s | 3.0–3.5 |
| Concentration of contrast media, mg/mL | 300 |
| Amount of contrast media, mL | 75–90 |
| Volume of saline used for flushing, mL | Approximately 30 |
| *Reconstruction parameters* | |
| – Slice thickness, mm | 2–3 |
| – dFOV, mm | 220–230 |
| – Matrix | 512 × 512 |
| – Kernel (filter/algorithm) | Manufacturer's recommended settings (usually standard or smooth kernel) |

Permission from KSThR.
*AP* aortopulmonary, *dFOV* display field of view, *IV* intravenous
[a] This protocol is for multidetector CT scanners with 64 or more channels
[b] Right arm is preferred for IV access to avoid venous reflux of contrast media due to possible physiological compression of the left innominate vein

## *Pathologic and/or Serologic Diagnosis*

When determining the need for US-guided biopsy for potential recurrent lesions in postoperative thyroid cancer patients, several factors must be evaluated. This includes the anatomical positioning of the lymph node (LN) or the questionable lesion, as well as the intended treatment strategy, be it surgical reintervention, non-surgical ablation procedures, or continued monitoring. Given the heightened complication risks associated with successive surgeries, performing an FNA might be deemed unnecessary for small, ambiguous, or dubious LNs that present a short diameter between 8 and 10 mm on both US and CT scans at the postsurgical site. Opting for this strategy might be suitable if using US for continuous monitoring is the selected alternative to surgical or ablation interventions for recurrent suspicious lesions [21, 24].

To bolster the assessment of recurrent malignancies within the cervical region, integrating FNA-Tg washout with cytology has proven to amplify diagnostic sensitivity. Deacu et al. posited that FNA-Tg demonstrates efficacy in evaluating suspicious lymph nodes, supplementing cytological analysis in specific scenarios [27]. The delineated threshold for FNA-Tg stood at 10 ng/mL, achieving a diagnostic sensitivity of 86.6%. Notably, false negative outcomes were observed in two histopathological variants of PTC: the tall cell and the diffuse sclerosing types.

## *Laboratory Tests*

### Serum Tg

Serum (Tg) is a glycoprotein, having a molecular weight of roughly 660 kDa, which is produced by thyrocytes and secreted into thyroid follicles' lumen [28]. Recognized as the paramount biomarker for pinpointing and assessing potential recurrences or metastasis in DTC patients, the American Thyroid Association (ATA) suggests patients with serum Tg levels exceeding 2 ng/mL undergo comprehensive body scans and supplementary tests to trace the Tg source [29–32]. Postoperative serum Tg concentrations beyond 10 ng/mL indicate a heightened likelihood of ongoing or recurrent disease, unsuccessful radioactive iodine (I-131) ablation, distant metastases, and elevated mortality risks. Notably, ATA guidelines abstain from defining an ideal postoperative serum Tg cut-off to the need for I-131 ablation [23], implying that elevated levels necessitate further scrutiny and potential intervention [33].

### Serum Anti-Tg Antibody (TgAb)

Tg antibodies (TgAb) have a molecular weight of 330 kDa. Historically, due to their structure, they were often elusive to older diagnostic techniques. These antibodies, part of the IgG class and primarily of the IgG2 subclass in DTC [34], can misleadingly suppress serum Tg levels in immunometric assays. Notably, TgAb is found in approximately 25% of thyroid cancer patients and approximately 10% of the broader population [35, 36]. This prevalence hampers the clinical utility of Tg measurements, as the presence of TgAb can distort results. To enhance diagnostic accuracy, it is recommended to concurrently measure TgAb and serum Tg using an identical assay method.

Postoperatively, after a total thyroidectomy followed by I-131 remnant ablation, TgAb usually dissipates within a 3-year span in individuals without any persisting disease. A gradual decrease in TgAb concentrations is a promising prognostic marker, suggesting a diminished likelihood of continuous or recurring disease. In contrast, surging TgAb levels or the sudden emergence of new TgAb can signal an elevated risk of the disease persisting or returning [37–40]. Hence, consistent tracking of TgAb levels furnishes crucial insights into disease progression and status in thyroid cancer patients.

### Serum Thyroid Stimulating Hormone (TSH)

Monitoring TSH levels is a valuable diagnostic and prognostic tool in the management of thyroid cancer. Elevated TSH levels may suggest residual or recurrent thyroid cancer. In numerous research studies, a TSH level of 30 mIU/L has been established as the prevailing threshold for achieving adequate Tg stimulation [23, 41]. This threshold holds significant diagnostic value, notably affecting the elevation of Tg levels. Furthermore, it carries therapeutic implications, as evidenced by the increased uptake of I-131 in tumors [42].

## Standard Technique

A comparable method is employed for the ablation of both benign and malignant thyroid nodules. The primary distinction lies in the location of the target lesions outside the thyroid. In particular, recurrent thyroid cancer in the central compartment exhibits a relatively higher likelihood of dense adherence to and/or invasion of adjacent structures, such as the larynx, trachea, esophagus, and RLN. As such, recurrent lesions in the central compartment may present as a challenge with regard to achieving complete ablation with adequate margins. Heterogeneity in thyroid tissue (e.g., from scar tissue and fibrosis due to previous surgery) may also affect the conduction of electricity and heat, thereby reducing RFA efficacy.

Three standard techniques for recurrent cancers are recommended by KSThR RFA guidelines [14]: perilesional lidocaine injection, hydrodissection, and the moving-shot technique. To minimize nerve damage during ablation of a recurrent lesion, the use of a small active tip (i.e., 0.38 or 0.5 cm) and the maintenance of a liquid barrier through the use of hydrodissection with lidocaine, or complementary 5% dextrose in water is recommended [43–46]. Additionally, nerve injury can also be prevented using the moving-shot technique whereby the recurrent tumor can be divided into multiple, small, ablation units, which are individually treated. For the treatment of recurrent thyroid cancer in particular, the moving-shot technique should include the soft tissue surrounding the recurrent tumors [12, 43]. In the event of suspected thermal injury to the RLN during RFA due to voice changes, injection of cold irrigate directly into the region of ablation has been proposed as a management strategy to achieving symptomatic improvement. It should be noted, however, that prior studies have reported hypothermic nerve damage with exposure to cold solutions [47, 48].

## *Advanced Technique*

### Separation Technique: Tilting or Angling of the Electrode

Despite using hydrodissection around the target lesion, there remains an inherent risk of thermal injury. This risk is especially pronounced when the lesion is situated in the central neck compartment, for example, at cervical level 6, near the RLN. One technique to mitigate this risk involves moving the target lesion away from crucial structures by angling the electrode (Fig. 20.2).

### Stenting with Tracheal Involvement

When recurrent thyroid cancer involves the trachea, it can lead to airway obstruction, which in turn can significantly increase mortality and mortality rates [49]. Using RFA early may be more effective for patients with recurrent neck tumors before significant airway invasion [50]. It is crucial to closely assess the depth of the

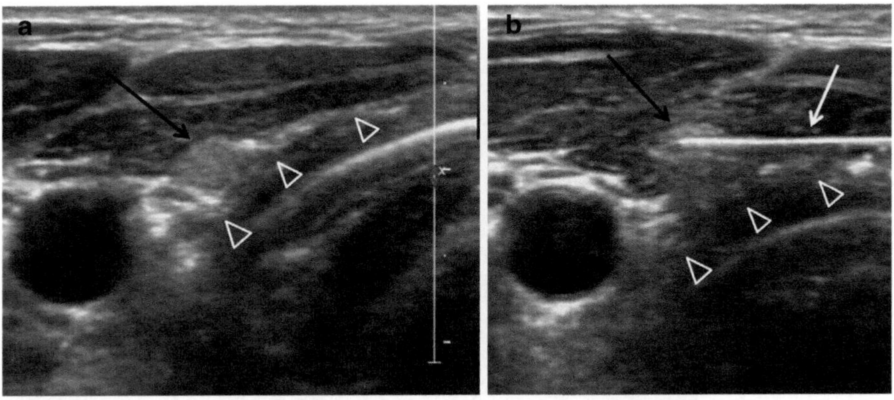


**Fig. 20.2** (**a**) The target lesion (black arrow) is in close pxoximity to the trachea (white arrow heads). (**b**) Following the insersion of an electrode (white arrow) into the target nodule, maintaining a safe distance from the trachea can be achieved by tilting the electrode upward during the thyroid RFA procedure. (Courtesy of Dr. Ji-hoon Kim)

tumor's invasion into the anatomical layers of the trachea. It was noted that the success rate of the hydrodissection technique, designed to create a gap between the tumor and the trachea, significantly decreased with an increase in the angle between the tumor and the trachea [51]. In cases where the tumor invades the tracheal lumen, a tracheal stent may be necessary both to push the tumor aside for a more comprehensive ablation and to support the airway until its anatomical integrity is restored [51].

## Post-procedural Evaluations

Treatment efficacy is usually evaluated by volume reduction rate (VRR), complete disappearance of the recurrent cancer on US and/or CT, reduction of the serum Tg level, and relief of tumor-related symptoms [14, 43, 50].

### *US Follow-Up*

US remains pivotal in post-procedural evaluation, similar to its pretreatment role. The parameters assessed include: tumor size, VRR, calculated as [(initial volume − final volume) × 100/initial volume]), vascularity, and any emergence of new, recurrent thyroid cancers or metastatic lymph nodes [14].

Following RFA, the treated tumor often exhibits hyperechogenicity with diminished vascularity on color Doppler US. An initial increase in tumor volume might be observed due to edema and the larger ablation area, inclusive of the safety margin. This volume subsequently starts to decrease, showing significant reduction over

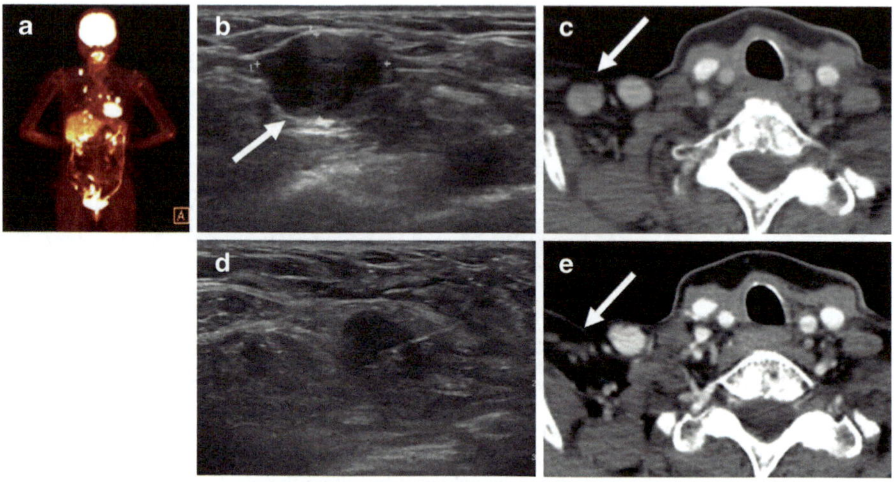


**Fig. 20.3** A 71-year-old female presented with pain due to recurrent thyroid cancer in the right neck (level V) following four surgical operations. (**a**) PET-CT scan displaying positive uptake in the right lower neck. (**b**) US scan revealing a hypoechogenic nodule. (**c**) CT scan illustrating a contrast-enhanced nodule (white arrow). (**d**) Radiofrequency ablation conducted with hydrodissection. (**e**) Follow-up CT scan performed after 6 years, demonstrating nearly complete tumor disappearance (white arrow) along with pain relief. (Courtesy of Dr. Ji-hoon Kim)

a span of 1–3 months [52]. Notably, size diminution and lack of vascularity on US underscore successful treatment. While the precise duration for follow-up US and clinical assessment remains undefined, it should be determined by the patient's treatment status and prospective treatment strategies [43, 50, 52].

## *CT Follow-Up*

An effectively treated tumor on CT is characterized by size reduction and the absence of enhancement, underscoring the importance of CT in treatment efficacy evaluation (Fig. 20.3).

In cases where vascularity is detected on the follow-up color Doppler US or an enhanced section of the treated recurrent cancer is identified on the follow-up CT, it is advisable to contemplate additional treatments.

## Clinical Outcomes

Research into the application of RFA for recurrent thyroid cancer, particularly within thyroid remnants or lymph nodes, remains somewhat limited. Most insights are grounded in small, retrospective studies, often leaving the sample size somewhat constrained, as indicated in Table 20.6.

**Table 20.6** Results of RFA in recurrent thyroid cancer patients

| Authors | Publication year | Number of tumors (patients) | F/U (months) | Volume reduction (%) | Complete disappearance (%) | Recurrence |
|---|---|---|---|---|---|---|
| Dupuy et al. [53] | 2001 | 11 (8) | 10.3 | | 58.2 | 2/8 patients |
| Monchik et al. [54] | 2006 | 24 (16) | 40.7 | | 42 | 2/16 patients |
| Baek et al. [55] | 2011 | 12 (10) | 23.6 | 93 | 50 | 1/12 tumors |
| Park et al. [56] | 2011 | 16 (11) | 6 | 50.9 | | |
| Lee et al. [57] | 2014 | 35 (32) | 30 | 96.4 | 93.3 | 1/35 tumors |
| Wang et al. [58] | 2014 | 20 (8) | 9.4 | 77 | | |
| Lim et al. [43] | 2015 | 61 (39) | 26.4 | 95.1 | 82 | 4/61 tumors |
| Kim et al. [59] | 2015 | 36 (27) | 36 | 98.4 | 86 | 3/26 patients |
| Guang et al. [60] | 2017 | 54 (33) | 21 | 94.9 | 61.1 | 1/33 patients |
| Chung et al. [50] | 2019 | 46 (29) | 80 | 99.5 | 91.3 | 10/29 patients |

In the realm of short-term outcomes, various investigations have reported the efficacy of RFA for recurrent thyroid cancer. A literature review conducted by Jeong et al. showed varied results [61]. Tumor volume displayed a notable decrease, ranging from a substantial 50.9 to 98.4%. The complete disappearance of tumors was reported in a broad spectrum, from 25 to 94% [43, 50, 53–60]. Importantly, about 64% of patients experienced symptom relief. One consistent trend across these studies was the decrease in serum Tg levels following the RFA procedure.

Chung et al., in their research spanning an average of 80 months with 29 patients, documented that the mean tumor volume underwent a drastic reduction of 99.5% [50]. Concurrently, serum Tg levels showed noteworthy drops from 2.55 to 0.75 ng/dL. By the study's end, 91.3% of tumors had disappeared completely, and there were no immediate or delayed complications.

However, several important limitations should be highlighted. The published studies displayed significant heterogeneity, with variations in RFA protocols (e.g., ablation time, power, electrode tip diameters) and imaging follow-up regimens. Consequently, drawing definitive conclusions about local tumor control becomes challenging. It is important to note that RFA cannot eliminate occult, recurrent tumors that are not visible on US images, and it may be difficult to ablate tumors located in inaccessible areas for US imaging, such as the retropharyngeal and superior mediastinal regions. Additionally, large or multiple tumors may require multiple RFA sessions. Therefore, the decision to choose RFA over repeat surgery for controlling recurrent tumors should be made judiciously.

**Table 20.7** Complications of radiofrequency ablation for recurrent thyroid cancer

| Authors | Publication year | Number of patients | Voice change (tumor location) | Other complications |
|---|---|---|---|---|
| Dupuy et al. [53] | 2001 | 8 | 1 (Central) | Skin burn [1] |
| Monchik et al. [54] | 2006 | 16 | 1 (Central) | Skin burn [1] |
| Baek et al. [55] | 2011 | 10 | 1 (Central) | |
| Park et al. [56] | 2011 | 11 | | Skin burn [1] |
| Lee et al. [57] | 2014 | 32 | 6 (Central) | |
| Wang et al. [58] | 2014 | 8 | | |
| Lim et al. [43] | 2015 | 39 | 3 (N/A) | |
| Kim et al. [59] | 2015 | 27 | 1 (N/A) | |
| Guang et al. [60] | 2017 | 33 | 0 | |
| Chung et al. [50] | 2019 | 29 | 3 (N/A) | |

## Complications

The incidence of procedure-related major complications in recurrent thyroid cancer was observed to be significantly greater than in benign thyroid nodules (Table 20.7) [62]. However, when it comes to minor complications and side effects, both recurrent thyroid cancer and benign thyroid nodules demonstrated no significant disparities. One plausible explanation for the heightened major complication rate in recurrent thyroid cancer could be the tumor's inherent location or its desmoplastic transformation, impacting the neighboring vital nerve structures.

Notably, the likelihood of experiencing voice changes is markedly higher for individuals with recurrent thyroid cancers, at a rate of 7.95%, compared to those with benign thyroid nodules, where it stands at a mere 0.94% [62]. This discrepancy can largely be attributed to the restricted buffer of the tissue that usually surrounds the tumor in cases of recurrent thyroid cancer. Hence, for practitioners, understanding the exact positioning of the recurrent tumor becomes critical, especially in the context of its proximity to pivotal neck structures.

## Conclusion

US-guided RFA can serve as a safe and effective alternative treatment for patients with small, recurrent PTC, who are at high risk or ineligible for surgery, or those who refuse surgical intervention. The high rates of complete disappearance and volume reduction suggest successful tumor eradication and reduction of disease burden. Moreover, the observed sustained local tumor control indicates the ability of RFA to effectively treat recurrent PTC over the long term.

Importantly, the safety profile of US-guided RFA was favorable, with minimal major complications and minor complications that were transient and manageable. This supports the notion that RFA is a well-tolerated procedure with low associated risks.

## References


1. Prete A, Borges de Souza P, Censi S, Muzza M, Nucci N, Sponziello M. Update on fundamental mechanisms of thyroid cancer. Front Endocrinol (Lausanne). 2020;11:102.
2. Seib CD, Sosa JA. Evolving understanding of the epidemiology of thyroid cancer. Endocrinol Metab Clin North Am. 2019;48(1):23–35.
3. Tufano RP, Mohamed AK. The year in surgical thyroidology: recent technological developments and future challenges. Thyroid. 2022;32(1):14–8.
4. Guenette JP, Monchik JM, Dupuy DE. Image-guided ablation of postsurgical locoregional recurrence of biopsy-proven well-differentiated thyroid carcinoma. J Vasc Interv Radiol. 2013;24(5):672–9.
5. Ruggiero FP, Fedok FG. Outcomes in reoperative thyroid cancer. Otolaryngol Clin North Am. 2008;41(6):1261–8, xii.
6. Choi Y, Jung SL, Bae JS, Lee SH, Jung CK, Jang J, et al. Comparison of efficacy and complications between radiofrequency ablation and repeat surgery in the treatment of locally recurrent thyroid cancers: a single-center propensity score matching study. Int J Hyperthermia. 2019;36(1):359–67.
7. Kim C, Lee JH, Choi YJ, Kim WB, Sung TY, Baek JH. Complications encountered in ultrasonography-guided radiofrequency ablation of benign thyroid nodules and recurrent thyroid cancers. Eur Radiol. 2017;27(8):3128–37.
8. Bernardi S, Palermo A, Grasso RF, Fabris B, Stacul F, Cesareo R. Current status and challenges of US-guided radiofrequency ablation of thyroid nodules in the long term: a systematic review. Cancers (Basel). 2021;13(11):2746.
9. Min Y, Wang X, Chen H, Chen J, Xiang K, Yin G. Thermal ablation for papillary thyroid microcarcinoma: how far we have come? Cancer Manag Res. 2020;12:13369–79.
10. Muhammad H, Tehreem A, Russell JO. Radiofrequency ablation and thyroid cancer: review of the current literature. Am J Otolaryngol. 2022;43(1):103204.
11. Tufano RP, Pace-Asciak P, Russell JO, Suárez C, Randolph GW, López F, et al. Update of radiofrequency ablation for treating benign and malignant thyroid nodules. The future is now. Front Endocrinol (Lausanne). 2021;12:698689.
12. Orloff LA, Noel JE, Stack BC, Russell MD, Angelos P, Baek JH, et al. Radiofrequency ablation and related ultrasound-guided ablation technologies for treatment of benign and malignant thyroid disease: an international multidisciplinary consensus statement of the American Head and Neck Society Endocrine Surgery Section with the Asia Pacific Society of Thyroid Surgery, Associazione Medici Endocrinologi, British Association of Endocrine and Thyroid Surgeons, European Thyroid Association, Italian Society of Endocrine Surgery Units, Korean Society of Thyroid Radiology, Latin American Thyroid Society, and Thyroid Nodules Therapies Association. Head Neck. 2022;44(3):633–60.
13. Na DG, Lee JH, Jung SL, Kim JH, Sung JY, Shin JH, et al. Radiofrequency ablation of benign thyroid nodules and recurrent thyroid cancers: consensus statement and recommendations. Korean J Radiol. 2012;13(2):117–25.
14. Kim JH, Baek JH, Lim HK, Ahn HS, Baek SM, Choi YJ, et al. 2017 thyroid radiofrequency ablation guideline: Korean Society of Thyroid Radiology. Korean J Radiol. 2018;19(4):632–55.

15. Hahn SY, Shin JH, Na DG, Ha EJ, Ahn HS, Lim HK, et al. Ethanol ablation of the thyroid nodules: 2018 consensus statement by the Korean Society of Thyroid Radiology. Korean J Radiol. 2019;20(4):609.
16. Leboulleux S, Girard E, Rose M, Travagli JP, Sabbah N, Caillou B, et al. Ultrasound criteria of malignancy for cervical lymph nodes in patients followed up for differentiated thyroid cancer. J Clin Endocrinol Metab. 2007;92(9):3590–4.
17. Pacini F, Molinaro E, Castagna MG, Agate L, Elisei R, Ceccarelli C, et al. Recombinant human thyrotropin-stimulated serum thyroglobulin combined with neck ultrasonography has the highest sensitivity in monitoring differentiated thyroid carcinoma. J Clin Endocrinol Metab. 2003;88(8):3668–73.
18. Torlontano M, Crocetti U, Augello G, D'Aloiso L, Bonfitto N, Varraso A, et al. Comparative evaluation of recombinant human thyrotropin-stimulated thyroglobulin levels, 131I whole-body scintigraphy, and neck ultrasonography in the follow-up of patients with papillary thyroid microcarcinoma who have not undergone radioiodine therapy. J Clin Endocrinol Metab. 2006;91(1):60–3.
19. Post-operative neck ultrasound and risk stratification in differentiated thyroid cancer patients with initial lymph node involvement—PubMed [Internet]. [cited 2023 Jul 31]. https://pubmed.ncbi.nlm.nih.gov/24659355/.
20. Leenhardt L, Erdogan MF, Hegedus L, Mandel SJ, Paschke R, Rago T, et al. 2013 European Thyroid Association guidelines for cervical ultrasound scan and ultrasound-guided techniques in the postoperative management of patients with thyroid cancer. Eur Thyroid J. 2013;2(3):147–59.
21. Ha EJ, Chung SR, Na DG, Ahn HS, Chung J, Lee JY, et al. 2021 Korean thyroid imaging reporting and data system and imaging-based management of thyroid nodules: Korean Society of Thyroid Radiology consensus statement and recommendations. Korean J Radiol. 2021;22(12):2094–123.
22. Lee JY, Baek JH, Ha EJ, Sung JY, Shin JH, Kim JH, et al. 2020 imaging guidelines for thyroid nodules and differentiated thyroid cancer: Korean Society of Thyroid Radiology. Korean J Radiol. 2021;22(5):840–60.
23. Haugen BR, Alexander EK, Bible KC, Doherty GM, Mandel SJ, Nikiforov YE, et al. 2015 American Thyroid Association management guidelines for adult patients with thyroid nodules and differentiated thyroid cancer: the American Thyroid Association guidelines task force on thyroid nodules and differentiated thyroid cancer. Thyroid. 2016;26(1):1–133.
24. Expert Panel on Neurologic Imaging, Juliano AF, Policeni B, Agarwal V, Burns J, Bykowski J, et al. ACR appropriateness criteria® ataxia. J Am Coll Radiol. 2019;16(5S):S44–56.
25. Hong EK, Kim JH, Lee J, Yoo RE, Kim SC, Kim MJ, et al. Diagnostic value of computed tomography combined with ultrasonography in detecting cervical recurrence in patients with thyroid cancer. Head Neck. 2019;41(5):1206–12.
26. Avram AM, Giovanella L, Greenspan B, Lawson SA, Luster M, Van Nostrand D, et al. SNMMI procedure standard/EANM practice guideline for nuclear medicine evaluation and therapy of differentiated thyroid cancer: abbreviated version. J Nucl Med. 2022;63(6):15N–35N.
27. Deacu L, Niculescu DA, Caragheorgheopol A, Terzea D, Poiană C. Thyroglobulin in lymph node fine-needle aspiration biopsy washout fluid. A tertiary center experience. Arch Clin Cases. 2021;8(4):106–10.
28. Malthiéry Y, Lissitzky S. Primary structure of human thyroglobulin deduced from the sequence of its 8448-base complementary DNA. Eur J Biochem. 1987;165(3):491–8.
29. Pacini F, Schlumberger M, Dralle H, Elisei R, Smit JWA, Wiersinga W, et al. European consensus for the management of patients with differentiated thyroid carcinoma of the follicular epithelium. Eur J Endocrinol. 2006;154(6):787–803.
30. Kwon H, Jeon MJ, Kim WG, Park S, Kim M, Song DE, et al. A comparison of lobectomy and total thyroidectomy in patients with papillary thyroid microcarcinoma: a retrospective individual risk factor-matched cohort study. Eur J Endocrinol. 2017;176(4):371–8.
31. Castagna MG, Cevenini G, Theodoropoulou A, Maino F, Memmo S, Claudia C, et al. Post-surgical thyroid ablation with low or high radioiodine activities results in similar outcomes in intermediate risk differentiated thyroid cancer patients. Eur J Endocrinol. 2013;169(1):23–9.

32. Reiners C, Hänscheid H, Luster M, Lassmann M, Verburg FA. Radioiodine for remnant ablation and therapy of metastatic disease. Nat Rev Endocrinol. 2011;7(10):589–95.
33. Pelttari H, Välimäki MJ, Löyttyniemi E, Schalin-Jäntti C. Post-ablative serum thyroglobulin is an independent predictor of recurrence in low-risk differentiated thyroid carcinoma: a 16-year follow-up study. Eur J Endocrinol. 2010;163(5):757–63.
34. Caturegli P, Kuppers RC, Mariotti S, Burek CL, Pinchera A, Ladenson PW, et al. IgG subclass distribution of thyroglobulin antibodies in patients with thyroid disease. Clin Exp Immunol. 1994;98(3):464–9.
35. Spencer CA, LoPresti JS, Fatemi S, Nicoloff JT. Detection of residual and recurrent differentiated thyroid carcinoma by serum thyroglobulin measurement. Thyroid. 1999;9(5):435–41.
36. Spencer CA. Challenges of serum thyroglobulin (Tg) measurement in the presence of Tg autoantibodies. J Clin Endocrinol Metab. 2004;89(8):3702–4.
37. Spencer C, Fatemi S. Thyroglobulin antibody (TgAb) methods - Strengths, pitfalls and clinical utility for monitoring TgAb-positive patients with differentiated thyroid cancer. Best Pract Res Clin Endocrinol Metab. 2013 Oct;27(5):701–12.
38. Görges R, Maniecki M, Jentzen W, Sheu SNY, Mann K, Bockisch A, et al. Development and clinical impact of thyroglobulin antibodies in patients with differentiated thyroid carcinoma during the first 3 years after thyroidectomy. Eur J Endocrinol. 2005;153(1):49–55.
39. Seo JH, Lee SW, Ahn BC, Lee J. Recurrence detection in differentiated thyroid cancer patients with elevated serum level of antithyroglobulin antibody: special emphasis on using (18)F-FDG PET/CT. Clin Endocrinol (Oxf). 2010;72(4):558–63.
40. Kim WG, Yoon JH, Kim WB, Kim TY, Kim EY, Kim JM, et al. Change of serum antithyroglobulin antibody levels is useful for prediction of clinical recurrence in thyroglobulin-negative patients with differentiated thyroid carcinoma. J Clin Endocrinol Metab. 2008;93(12):4683–9.
41. Edmonds CJ, Hayes S, Kermode JC, Thompson BD. Measurement of serum TSH and thyroid hormones in the management of treatment of thyroid carcinoma with radioiodine. Br J Radiol. 1977;50(599):799–807.
42. Torres MS, Ramirez L, Simkin PH, Braverman LE, Emerson CH. Effect of various doses of recombinant human thyrotropin on the thyroid radioactive iodine uptake and serum levels of thyroid hormones and thyroglobulin in normal subjects. J Clin Endocrinol Metab. 2001;86(4):1660–4.
43. Lim HK, Baek JH, Lee JH, Kim WB, Kim TY, Shong YK, et al. Efficacy and safety of radiofrequency ablation for treating locoregional recurrence from papillary thyroid cancer. Eur Radiol. 2015;25(1):163–70.
44. Laeseke PF, Sampson LA, Brace CL, Winter TC 3rd, Fine JP, Lee FTJ. Unintended thermal injuries from radiofrequency ablation: protection with 5% dextrose in water. J Roentgenol. 2006;1(5 Suppl):S249–54.
45. Park HS, Baek JH, Park AW, Chung SR, Choi YJ, Lee JH. Thyroid radiofrequency ablation: updates on innovative devices and techniques. Korean J Radiol. 2017;18(4):615.
46. Xiaoyin T, Ping L, Dan C, Min D, Jiachang C, Tao W, et al. Risk assessment and hydrodissection technique for radiofrequency ablation of thyroid benign nodules. J Cancer. 2018;9(17):3058–66.
47. Esposito RA, Spencer FC. The effect of pericardial insulation on hypothermic phrenic nerve injury during open-heart surgery. Ann Thorac Surg. 1987;43(3):303–8.
48. Wu Y, Jia JP, Xu M, Geng ZW, Liu FY, Song JX, et al. [Role of nitric oxide in pathogenesis of cold nerve injury]. Zhonghua Yi Xue Za Zhi. 2009;89(31):2214–2220.
49. Djalilian M, Beahrs OH, Devine KD, Weiland LH, DeSanto LW. Intraluminal involvement of the larynx and trachea by thyroid cancer. Am J Surg. 1974;128(4):500–4.
50. Chung SR, Baek JH, Choi YJ, Lee JH. Longer-term outcomes of radiofrequency ablation for locally recurrent papillary thyroid cancer. Eur Radiol. 2019;29(9):4897–903.
51. Chung SR, Baek JH, Choi YJ, Sung TY, Song DE, Kim TY, et al. Efficacy of radiofrequency ablation for recurrent thyroid cancer invading the airways. Eur Radiol. 2021;31(4):2153–60.
52. Xiao J, Zhang Y, Zhang M, Lan Y, Yan L, Luo Y, et al. Ultrasonography-guided radiofrequency ablation vs. surgery for the treatment of solitary T1bN0M0 papillary thyroid carcinoma: a comparative study. Clin Endocrinol (Oxf). 2021;94(4):684–91.

53. Dupuy DE, Monchik JM, Decrea C, Pisharodi L. Radiofrequency ablation of regional recurrence from well-differentiated thyroid malignancy. Surgery. 2001;130(6):971–7.
54. Monchik JM, Donatini G, Iannuccilli J, Dupuy DE. Radiofrequency ablation and percutaneous ethanol injection treatment for recurrent local and distant well-differentiated thyroid carcinoma. Ann Surg. 2006;244(2):296–304.
55. Baek JH, Kim YS, Sung JY, Choi H, Lee JH. Locoregional control of metastatic well-differentiated thyroid cancer by ultrasound-guided radiofrequency ablation. Am J Roentgenol. 2011;197(2):W331–6.
56. Park KW, Shin JH, Han BK, Ko EY, Chung JH. Inoperable symptomatic recurrent thyroid cancers: preliminary result of radiofrequency ablation. Ann Surg Oncol. 2011;18(9):2564–8.
57. Lee SJ, Jung SL, Kim BS, Ahn KJ, Choi HS, Lim DJ, et al. Radiofrequency ablation to treat loco-regional recurrence of well-differentiated thyroid carcinoma. Korean J Radiol. 2014;15(6):817.
58. Wang L, Ge M, Xu D, Chen L, Qian C, Shi K, et al. Ultrasonography-guided percutaneous radiofrequency ablation for cervical lymph node metastasis from thyroid carcinoma. J Cancer Res Ther. 2014;10(Suppl):C144–9.
59. Kim JH, Yoo WS, Park YJ, Park DJ, Yun TJ, Choi SH, et al. Efficacy and safety of radiofrequency ablation for treatment of locally recurrent thyroid cancers smaller than 2 cm. Radiology. 2015;276(3):909–18.
60. Guang Y, Luo Y, Zhang Y, Zhang M, Li N, Zhang Y, et al. Efficacy and safety of percutaneous ultrasound guided radiofrequency ablation for treating cervical metastatic lymph nodes from papillary thyroid carcinoma. J Cancer Res Clin Oncol. 2017;143(8):1555–62.
61. Jeong SY, Baek JH, Choi YJ, Lee JH. Ethanol and thermal ablation for malignant thyroid tumours. Int J Hyperthermia. 2017;33(8):938–45.
62. Chung SR, Suh CH, Baek JH, Park HS, Choi YJ, Lee JH. Safety of radiofrequency ablation of benign thyroid nodules and recurrent thyroid cancers: a systematic review and meta-analysis. Int J Hyperthermia. 2017;33:1–35.

# Chapter 21
# A Surgeon's Perspective on Thyroid RFA

**Kepal Patel**

## Introduction

The current management of thyroid nodules and well-differentiated thyroid cancers is generally directed toward surgical resection or surveillance. Increasingly, the international literature describes minimally invasive interventional procedures, specifically, radiofrequency ablation (RFA) as a valid treatment option for individuals, who do not want active surveillance and do not wish or are not able to tolerate surgery. Nonsurgical options are attractive for both patients and health-care systems for a multitude of reasons. From a patient perspective, these procedures do not require general anesthesia and rarely necessitate overnight stay in the hospital. Furthermore, patient quality of life can be significantly affected by the need for life-long thyroid hormone supplementation and the presence of a neck scar. Although thyroid surgery is readily available and safe in many institutions, there remains a risk of major complications including recurrent laryngeal nerve damage, hypoparathyroidism, and potentially life-threatening hematoma in 2–10% of patients [1]. Surgery is also associated with increased cost and may not be an option for high-risk patients or those who would prefer nonoperative management.

K. Patel (✉)
Department of Surgery, NYU Langone Health, New York, NY, USA
e-mail: Kepal.Patel@nyulangone.org



A. W. Park et al. (eds.), *Thyroid Radiofrequency Ablation*,
https://doi.org/10.1007/978-3-031-65288-2_21

## Surgery Versus RFA in the Treatment of Benign Thyroid Nodules

The safety of RFA in the treatment of thyroid disease has been well documented. Major complications inherent in both surgery and minimally invasive treatments of the thyroid gland include permanent or transient vocal cord paralysis and neck hematoma, resulting in airway compromise. In the surgical treatment of thyroid disease, transient recurrent laryngeal nerve palsy occurs in up to 9.8% of patients with permanent nerve palsy seen in up to 2.3% of patients [2]. Neck hematoma requiring emergent intervention occurred in 0.6% of patients undergoing thyroid or parathyroid surgery in a Collaborative Endocrine Surgery Quality Improvement Program (CESQIP) study [3]. A recent meta-analysis reviewed a sample of 2421 patients, who underwent RFA for benign nodules and reported an overall complication rate of 2.11%. In this cohort, 21 patients (0.94%) developed transient nerve palsy and one patient (0.04%) sustained permanent nerve damage [4]. Of all RFA studies reviewed, no patient developed a neck hematoma that required operative intervention. Transient and permanent hypoparathyroidism are known complications of thyroid surgery; however they have rarely been reported as complications of minimally invasive techniques used to treat thyroid nodules. Bernardi et al. [5] compared RFA to hemithyroidectomy for the alleviation of nodule-related symptoms and found that though symptomatic and cosmetic outcomes were not statistically different following RFA, patients experienced significantly less procedure-related pain and hypothyroidism. The study demonstrated that RFA and surgery were equivalent in safety; however, RFA was significantly cheaper [5]. In patients treated with RFA, there was a negligible risk of hypothyroidism with 2 of 1468 (0.13%) cases, all of which occurred in patients with a high titer of thyroid peroxidase antibody (TPO) or thyroglobulin (TG) antibodies prior to RFA [6, 7], while 71.5% of surgical patients required thyroid hormone replacement [8].

### *Autonomously Functioning Thyroid Nodules (AFTNs)*

Radioactive iodine (RAI) and surgery are still the first-line treatments for AFTN, though RFA is now commonly recognized as a reasonable second-line option. When comparing RFA and surgery for the definitive treatment of AFTNs, it is necessary to consider resolution of hyperthyroidism in addition to cost and patient satisfaction. In a non-randomized comparative retrospective study, Che et al. demonstrated the efficacy and safety of RFA ($n$ = 200) compared to patients managed surgically ($n$ = 200) for cytological benign symptomatic or functional thyroid nodules [8]. The study demonstrated no cost difference between RFA and surgery; however, it showed a longer hospital stay for those who underwent thyroidectomy. The chance of complications was significantly higher for those who underwent surgery and 71% of the surgical patients required levothyroxine postoperatively. The authors, however, fail to specify what percentage underwent total thyroidectomy versus thyroid lobectomy. Another study revealed that patients who underwent RFA for AFTNs had a significantly higher health-related quality of life at 6 months post-procedure than those who underwent surgery for therapy [9]. Conversely, they noted that surgery was significantly less expensive than RFA. The costs of RFA and surgery vary considerably. For example, in China hemithyroidectomy was reported to cost $2556.95 + $171.88 compared to an average US Medicare cost of $5784 (https://www.medicare.gov/procedure-price-lookup/cost/60210 accessed 8/7/2021) suggesting that cost-benefit comparison is location dependent. Recently, cost comparison between open thyroid lobectomy and RFA for management of thyroid nodules was published [10]. Cost-effectiveness hinged on the simulated price of the RFA probe. In contrast to open lobectomy, the direct cost variation for conducting RFA was $597 (representing a 19% cost reduction) when the simulated probe cost was set at $1500; but, it increased by $403 (equivalent to a 13% cost increase) when the probe cost was $2500. Should the cost per RFA probe fall below $2100—the critical threshold separating open lobectomy and RFA—it would yield significant cost savings in the treatment of thyroid nodules.

Data regarding patient preference suggests that those who underwent surgery were more satisfied with symptom improvement, but less satisfied with cosmesis when compared to RFA for the treatment of AFTNs [11]. Given these findings, we consider RFA to be a viable treatment option for the treatment of autonomous nodules in the appropriate patient. Although RAI is likely more cost-efficient than surgery or RFA, it carries a relatively high risk of permanent hypothyroidism and exposes the patient to radiation. Furthermore, RAI is contraindicated in pregnant women, those who plan to attempt conception, and those who are breastfeeding. Thyroidectomy would be favored in a patient who requires more urgent resolution of hyperthyroidism, has a coexisting thyroid or parathyroid nodule that requires surgery, or a large AFTNs that is less likely to respond to minimally invasive techniques. For health-care systems, RFA may initially be less attractive for AFTNs due to increased costs when compared to surgery and less definitive symptomatic control.

## Surgery Versus RFA in the Treatment of Malignant Thyroid Disease

RFA is also emerging as a useful tool for the management of small, primary, papillary thyroid cancers and loco-regionally recurrent papillary thyroid cancer. Limited data does not support the use of RFA for the treatment of more aggressive thyroid carcinomas such as anaplastic carcinoma and medullary thyroid cancer.

## *Papillary Thyroid Cancer*

The safety and efficacy of RFA for the treatment of papillary thyroid microcarcinoma (PTMC) has been well-demonstrated [12, 13] suggesting that, in addition to observational management, RFA may be another useful nonsurgical alternative. Ding et al. retrospectively examined 38 patients with PTMC, who underwent RFA, and found that 100% of patients demonstrated complete disappearance of lesions without complications, with all patients remaining euthyroid [14]. Complete or near-complete resolution of PTMC has been repeatedly demonstrated [13, 15, 16]. Additionally, RFA has been shown to be effective for the treatment of bilateral PTMC [17]. Emerging data also show efficacy of RFA in the treatment of larger primary tumors up to T1bN0 [18–20]. Studies generally include cytologically confirmed solitary papillary thyroid carcinomas (PTCs) in patients not otherwise suitable for surgical intervention [12]. However, as seen with all modalities for the management of PTC, the risk of recurrence (0–4.16%) [13, 16, 17], new primaries (0–4.1%) [13, 15], and local lymph node metastasis (0–2.13%) [16, 17] have been reported after RFA. Though the literature is limited and additional studies are necessary, it still appears that RFA offers a very useful alternative to surgery for small, low-risk, papillary thyroid cancers.

## *Recurrent Papillary Thyroid Cancer*

A retrospective study by Choi et al. compared RFA and repeat surgical management for the treatment of patients with fewer than three foci of recurrent PTC [21]. There was no statistically significant difference in recurrence-free survival between two groups; however, there was a significantly higher risk of both hypocalcemia and overall complication rate among the patients managed with surgery. The authors conclude that RFA may be a reasonable alternative to standard surgical management for patients with recurrent disease where the surgical risk is high. Chung et al. published a retrospective, single, institution study examining long-term outcomes among 29 patients with a total of 46 recurrent foci of PTC treated with RFA, all of whom had a minimum of 5 years of post-treatment follow-up [22]. They documented complete resolution of the treated lesion in 91% of cases. New loco-regional recurrence developed in 8 of 29 (28%), and distant metastasis developed in 2 of 29 (7%); however, 19 patients (66%) remained disease-free at last follow-up and no patients had long-term complications due to RFA at a mean of 80 months follow-up.

Chung et al. also performed a meta-analysis to determine the safety of RFA for the treatment of benign and recurrent thyroid cancers [4]. In total, 24 studies, 2421 patients and 2786 thyroid nodules were included of which 141 patients had recurrent cancer with 191 discrete lesions. Perhaps not surprisingly, complications occurred more frequently following treatment of recurrent cancer compared to benign nodules: major complications 6.71% vs 1.27%, respectively, and overall complications: 10.98% and 2.11%, respectively. The authors suggest that the absence of normal thyroid tissue that surrounds benign thyroid nodules and perhaps operator experience, which could not be determined in the meta-analysis, may have been factors explaining the difference in complication rates. In total, only 5 of 2421 (0.21%) treated patients had long-term sequelae following the initial treatment complication. This included one patient treated for a benign nodule that required lobectomy for nodule rupture and abscess, and four cases of permanent vocal hoarseness occurred: three cases in patients treated for recurrent thyroid cancer and one patient treated for a benign thyroid nodule. The authors conclude that though the risk of complications for the treatment of recurrent cancer is higher, RFA is nonetheless a safe and effective means of treatment for recurrent disease.

## Other Considerations

A major disadvantage to RFA is that it does not allow for final pathologic analysis of the nodule. Despite having pre-procedural Bethesda II cytology twice, it was noted that 8% of patients, who underwent surgery, had foci of micropapillary thyroid cancer noted on final pathology. Thus, authors have suggested that ablated nodules should be followed up annually for at least 5 years, which lends concerns to both cost and quality of life [5].

Indications for image-guided RFA in benign and malignant thyroid lesions should be evaluated by a multidisciplinary team including experts in both traditional and image-guided interventional treatment modalities. The choice of the appropriate procedure and lesions depends on many factors such as tumor type, size, and location. It can also depend on team experience, resources, and characteristics of the person undergoing the procedure such as age and comorbidities.

Compared to surgical management, it is important to educate patients that the benefit of RFA is not immediate, and instead accrues over the course of months. The volume reduction rate (VRR) within the first 3–6 months occurs at the most rapid rate with continued but more gradual volume reduction over the following 6–18 months. Despite this delay in therapeutic benefit, thyroid nodules treated with RFA demonstrated 84.8% volume reduction at 1 year and had a lower risk of complications compared to those managed surgically, 1% vs 6%, $p = 0.002$ [8].

Though there is no certification process to perform RFA, physicians seeking to responsibly incorporate this technique into their practice should consider attending one or more RFA workshops, wherein there is opportunity to practice the technique on phantoms, as well as the ability to observe an experienced practitioner performing the procedure on a patient. This may be accomplished through courses often associated with professional society meetings or continued education offerings. Identifying a suitable proctor before undertaking procedures independently is also advisable. Literature sources show a lower complication rate among practitioners with 50 or more cases [6].

RFA itself can be performed in a procedural room or as an in-office procedure at the discretion of the provider. The procedure room provides a sterile environment and the ability to deliver moderate sedation, if desired. The office typically offers greater flexibility and efficiency with scheduling as well as comfort for the patient. In either case, a high-quality ultrasound (US) machine is required, and training of support staff should be undertaken to provide peri-procedural assistance [23].

Given the multidisciplinary backgrounds of physicians performing RFA, it is recognized that paths to procedural competence will vary according to training experiences and clinical practice. Overall, the ideal setting in which to incorporate RFA into practice is within one that is equipped to care for the patient through the diagnostic, interventional, and surveillance process, providing an opportunity for follow-up and audit of patients treated. The performing physician may be a member of an integrated team capable of managing post-procedural clinical, radiographic, and biochemical expectations via regular communication [23].

## Conclusion

RFA has emerged as a minimally invasive treatment option for thyroid nodules and cancer with a low risk of major complications. The cost-effectiveness of RFA compared to traditional treatment options has been questioned; however, patients have reported increased health-care associated quality of life following RFA when compared to surgery. In the treatment of AFTNs, RFA can achieve durable symptom control; however, it can take several months for patients to achieve a euthyroid state. The risk of lifelong hypothyroidism is much lower than both RAI and surgery, which is beneficial to patients and to health-care systems. Patients with benign nodules have shown significant volume reduction associated with improved symptoms and cosmesis after a single RFA procedure. A limitation for RFA is the inability to get definitive histologic evaluation of the lesion, which is of concern for the potential risk, albeit low, to miss the diagnosis of thyroid cancer. Overall, RFA provides several advantages over surgery in the properly selected patient.

## References

1. Bergenfelz A, et al. Complications to thyroid surgery: results as reported in a database from a multicenter audit comprising 3660 patients. Langenbecks Arch Surg. 2008;393(5):667–73.
2. Jeannon JP, et al. Diagnosis of recurrent laryngeal nerve palsy after thyroidectomy: a systematic review. Int J Clin Pract. 2009;63(4):624–9.
3. Talutis SD, et al. Evacuation of postoperative hematomas after thyroid and parathyroid surgery: an analysis of the CESQIP database. Surgery. 2019;165(1):250–6.
4. Chung SR, et al. Safety of radiofrequency ablation of benign thyroid nodules and recurrent thyroid cancers: a systematic review and meta-analysis. Int J Hyperthermia. 2017;33(8):920–30.

5. Bernardi S, et al. Radiofrequency ablation compared to surgery for the treatment of benign thyroid nodules. Int J Endocrinol. 2014;2014:934595.
6. Baek JH, et al. Complications encountered in the treatment of benign thyroid nodules with US-guided radiofrequency ablation: a multicenter study. Radiology. 2012;262(1):335–42.
7. Baek JH, et al. Radiofrequency ablation for the treatment of autonomously functioning thyroid nodules. World J Surg. 2009;33(9):1971–7.
8. Che Y, et al. Treatment of benign thyroid nodules: comparison of surgery with radiofrequency ablation. AJNR Am J Neuroradiol. 2015;36(7):1321–5.
9. Yue WW, et al. Quality of life and cost-effectiveness of radiofrequency ablation versus open surgery for benign thyroid nodules: a retrospective cohort study. Sci Rep. 2016;6:37838.
10. Miller JR, et al. Cost comparison between open thyroid lobectomy and radiofrequency ablation for management of thyroid nodules. Head Neck. 2023;45(1):59–63.
11. Bernardi S, et al. Patient satisfaction after thyroid RFA versus surgery for benign thyroid nodules: a telephone survey. Int J Hyperthermia. 2018;35(1):150–8.
12. Tufano RP, et al. Update of radiofrequency ablation for treating benign and malignant thyroid nodules. The future is now. Front Endocrinol (Lausanne). 2021;12:698689.
13. Lim HK, et al. US-guided radiofrequency ablation for low-risk papillary thyroid microcarcinoma: efficacy and safety in a large population. Korean J Radiol. 2019;20(12):1653–61.
14. Ding M, et al. Clinical outcomes of ultrasound-guided radiofrequency ablation for the treatment of primary papillary thyroid microcarcinoma. Clin Radiol. 2019;74(9):712–7.
15. Cho SJ, et al. Long-term follow-up results of ultrasound-guided radiofrequency ablation for low-risk papillary thyroid microcarcinoma: more than 5-year follow-up for 84 tumors. Thyroid. 2020;30(12):1745–51.
16. Zhang C, et al. Comparison of ultrasound guided percutaneous radiofrequency ablation and open thyroidectomy in the treatment of low-risk papillary thyroid microcarcinoma: a propensity score matching study. Clin Hemorheol Microcirc. 2021;80:73.
17. Yan L, et al. The efficacy and safety of radiofrequency ablation for bilateral papillary thyroid microcarcinoma. Front Endocrinol (Lausanne). 2021;12:663636.
18. Xiao J, et al. [Short-term outcome of T1bN0M0 papillary thyroid cancer after ultrasonography-guided radiofrequency ablation]. Zhongguo Yi Xue Ke Xue Yuan Xue Bao. 2020;42(6):771–775.
19. Xiao J, et al. Ultrasonography-guided radiofrequency ablation for solitary T1aN0M0 and T1bN0M0 papillary thyroid carcinoma: a retrospective comparative study. Eur J Endocrinol. 2021;186(1):105–13.
20. Xiao J, et al. Ultrasonography-guided radiofrequency ablation vs. surgery for the treatment of solitary T1bN0M0 papillary thyroid carcinoma: a comparative study. Clin Endocrinol (Oxf). 2021;94(4):684–91.
21. Choi Y, et al. Comparison of efficacy and complications between radiofrequency ablation and repeat surgery in the treatment of locally recurrent thyroid cancers: a single-center propensity score matching study. Int J Hyperthermia. 2019;36(1):359–67.
22. Chung SR, et al. Longer-term outcomes of radiofrequency ablation for locally recurrent papillary thyroid cancer. Eur Radiol. 2019;29(9):4897–903.
23. Orloff LA, et al. Radiofrequency ablation and related ultrasound-guided ablation technologies for treatment of benign and malignant thyroid disease: an international multidisciplinary consensus statement of the American Head and Neck Society Endocrine Surgery Section with the Asia Pacific Society of Thyroid Surgery, Associazione Medici Endocrinologi, British Association of Endocrine and Thyroid Surgeons, European Thyroid Association, Italian Society of Endocrine Surgery Units, Korean Society of Thyroid Radiology, Latin American Thyroid Society, and Thyroid Nodules Therapies Association. Head Neck. 2022;44(3):633–60.

# Chapter 22
# A Multidisciplinary Approach to Developing Thyroid RFA Practice

**Timothy C. Huber**

## Introduction

Radiofrequency ablation (RFA) for thyroid nodules has grown rapidly in the United States in recent years. It is now offered at centers across the country. However, the market of potential patients is much larger than can be accommodated by the present number of practitioners. This creates an opportunity for anyone interested in starting and growing a thyroid nodule RFA practice. While this service line can be championed by a single provider, we propose that developing a thyroid nodule RFA program via a multidisciplinary approach is more effective. This chapter describes how interested interventionalists can build an RFA program in a multidisciplinary fashion.

## Rationale for a Multidisciplinary Approach

We prefer a multidisciplinary approach, including members from radiology, surgery, and endocrinology, for several reasons. Each specialty brings a unique compliment of skills and knowledge. The procedural aspects will be familiar to most interventional radiologists and some surgeons. Patient evaluation and management will be more familiar to surgeons and endocrinologists. Multidisciplinary tumor boards have been shown to improve care, especially for complex patients [1]. As the practice matures, and patients with functional nodules or malignancy are being considered, a breadth of expertise becomes even more valuable.

T. C. Huber (✉)
Department of Vascular and Interventional Radiology, Jefferson Radiology, Hartford, CT, USA



A. W. Park et al. (eds.), *Thyroid Radiofrequency Ablation*,
https://doi.org/10.1007/978-3-031-65288-2_22

Building referrals is critical to the growth and stability of the practice. By having members from multiple specialties organized into a referral program, the practice will gain even more visibility to interested patients and providers. This will help bolster volume and can allow multiple providers to offer RFA. We have found that as referral volume has grown, having more than one provider offering RFA has been essential.

As a newer procedure without a dedicated Current Procedural Terminology (CPT) code, preapproval and reimbursement can be challenging. While efforts are currently underway for a dedicated billable CPT code, most practices currently use unlisted codes, supported by comparator codes. Multidisciplinary review of patients, indications, and treatment options can help in the reimbursement process. By having the decision for RFA be the recommendation of multiple physicians, not just one specialty, the justification for RFA can be strengthened.

## Whom to Involve?

A broad swath of specialty representation is recommended. Interventional radiology, endocrinology, surgical oncology, and otolaryngology all have a stake in caring for patients with nodular thyroid disease and should all be involved, if possible. Local factors will determine the feasibility of this model.

Whom to include in the thyroid nodule RFA program:

- Interventional radiology
- Endocrinology
- Otolaryngology
- Surgical oncology

## What Is the Structure of a Multidisciplinary Program?

The program can be structured in one of two ways. Providers can see patients in a multispecialty clinic. This model has been used in a variety of scenarios including uterine fibroid embolization, venous occlusive disease, and liver tumors. This model is beneficial for patients as it reduces the number of visits and can reduce the length of time to a treatment decision. However, due to scheduling constraints, this model is not practical for most providers.

An alternative is to organize a multidisciplinary tumor board. Such tumor boards can be beneficial but the structure and organization are key to their success [2]. Most institutions have a tumor board for thyroid malignancy, and a benign thyroid nodule board can be established in a similar fashion. Figure 22.1 compares the membership of our thyroid cancer tumor board to that of our thyroid nodule RFA tumor board. By discussing patients as a group, local practice patterns can be developed, and

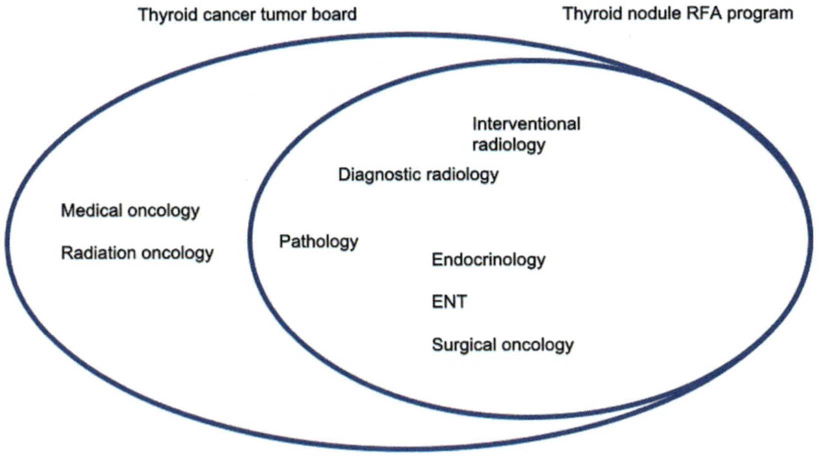


**Fig. 22.1** Comparison of thyroid nodule RFA program versus thyroid cancer tumor board. *ENT* otolaryngology

potential pitfalls can be avoided. Thyroid tumor boards have been shown to change management in 15% of patients presented, with 43% of those changes related to additional imaging [3]. Not all patients, who are referred for RFA, are appropriate candidates, and some may be better served by having surgery.

## How to Start a Thyroid Nodule RFA Program?

First, establish a physician champion to lead efforts to build the program. This will involve negotiating a contract to secure the generator and electrodes, establishing a procedural workflow with nursing staff, and training technologists or other support staff on the operation and setup of the equipment.

As this groundwork is underway, the champion can begin to canvas other specialties for support. Like with any new procedure, expect to be met with resistance. This is where being a clinical expert meets understanding the local political landscape. Perseverance is key.

Once a core group has been identified, it is important to understand everyone's motivation for involvement. Do they want to learn and offer the procedure? Do they want to publish research on the topic? Do they want to be involved in a new and disruptive growth area? Make sure you understand why your colleagues are in the group and make sure you can accommodate them.

Once referrals come in, patients can be discussed in a regular multidisciplinary conference. Not all countries have robust clinical practice guidelines for thyroid nodule RFA. Because of this, multidisciplinary discussion can help to create local practice guidelines based on international guidelines and available evidence in the literature. Table 22.1 outlines topics for review during patient presentations at the

**Table 22.1** Topics for review at thyroid nodule tumor board

| **Imaging** | **Pathology** |
|---|---|
| • Ultrasound<br>• Computed tomography (CT)<br>• Nuclear scan (I-123) | • Number and location of fine-needle aspirations (FNAs)<br>• Review results<br>• Discuss cytologic atypia |
| **Underlying thyroid disease** | **Discussion** |
| • Review thyroid-stimulating hormone (TSH)/T3/T4<br>• Review thyroid medications | • Review patient symptoms and severity<br>• Review cosmetic impact<br>• Discuss treatment options |

**Table 22.2** Template for thyroid nodule tumor board notes

| Patient name/medical record number | Nodule side | Nodule size | FNA/TSH results | Recommendations |
|---|---|---|---|---|
| — | — | — | — | — |
| — | — | — | — | — |

multidisciplinary conference. Assigning roles can be helpful. Identify someone to show imaging, someone to present cases, and someone to record. It is important to document the group's recommendations in the medical record. Table 22.2 outlines a template for recording notes from the conference. It is also important to credit everyone in attendance, and to make sure the final recommendations reflect the discussion and group consensus.

## References

1. Specchia ML, Frisicale EM, Carini E, Di Pilla A, Cappa D, Barbara A, et al. The impact of tumor board on cancer care: evidence from an umbrella review. BMC Health Serv Res. 2020;20(1):73.
2. El Saghir NS, Keating NL, Carlson RW, Khoury KE, Fallowfield L. Tumor boards: optimizing the structure and improving efficiency of multidisciplinary management of patients with cancer worldwide. Am Soc Clin Oncol Educ Book. 2014;(34):e461–e466.
3. Kelley S, Beck AC, Weigel RJ, Howe JR, Sugg SL, Lal G. Influence of endocrine multidisciplinary tumor board on patient management and treatment decision making. Am J Surg. 2022;223(1):76–80.

# Chapter 23
# Financial Considerations in Developing Thyroid RFA Services

**Seung Kwon Kim**

## Introduction

The current standard treatment for benign thyroid nodules is thyroidectomy, which is a surgical procedure. However, thyroidectomy carries certain risks and complications, such as nerve damage, scarring, and the potential need for lifelong hormone medication. Radiofrequency ablation (RFA) is an alternative treatment option that has been extensively studied and utilized for reducing and eliminating benign thyroid nodules without the need for surgery.

RFA for thyroid nodules has been performed in countries like Korea and Europe for over a decade, with clinical studies showing significant and lasting reduction in nodule size ranging from 50 to 80% over years of follow-up. These studies have demonstrated the efficacy and durability of RFA as a treatment option for benign thyroid nodules.

In 2018, RFA for thyroid nodules received clearance from the Food and Drug Administration (FDA) 510(k) process, and it is now being performed at various academic institutions across the United States. The implementation of a thyroid nodule RFA service line can provide patients with a noninvasive alternative to surgery, allowing them to avoid potential complications associated with thyroidectomy. Additionally, offering RFA as a treatment option can generate revenue for the hospital while providing a valuable service to patients.

S. K. Kim (✉)
Department of Radiology, Division of Interventional Radiology, University of Texas Southwestern Medical Center, Dallas, TX, USA
e-mail: seung.kim@utsouthwestern.edu



A. W. Park et al. (eds.), *Thyroid Radiofrequency Ablation*,
https://doi.org/10.1007/978-3-031-65288-2_23

## Strategic Plan

### *Vision*

The vision of the thyroid nodule RFA service line is to promote thyroid health and provide exceptional care to patients by offering an effective treatment option for thyroid disease.

### *Mission*

Our mission is to establish thyroid nodule RFA as a recognized and valuable treatment option for patients with thyroid nodules. We aim to provide comprehensive care and improve patient outcomes through the use of this alternative treatment approach.

### *Objective*

The primary objective of our service line is to develop and implement a successful thyroid nodule RFA practice. This includes ensuring proper infrastructure, training, and resources to deliver high-quality care to patients.

## Value Analysis

### *Thyroid Nodule RFA Procedure*

The thyroid nodule RFA procedure involves the use of ultrasound (US) guidance to position an 18G or 19G needle/electrode directly into the nodule. Under local anesthesia, an external generator generates an alternating electrical current to generate heat, leading to cell death within the nodule. The procedure itself typically takes approximately 15–30 min, during which the patient remains awake and able to communicate. Moderate intravenous (IV) sedation may be administered, and patients can typically be discharged following the procedure according to hospital protocol. Complications are rare, with temporary voice changes ("hoarseness") being the most common [1, 2].

## *Indication for Thyroid Nodule RFA [1, 2]*

**Indication for Thyroid Nodule RFA**

(a) Benign thyroid nodules causing symptomatic or cosmetic issues.
(b) Thyroid nodules confirmed as benign through at least two US-guided fine-needle aspirations (FNA) or core-needle biopsies (CNB) before undergoing RF ablation.
(c) Toxic or pre-toxic autonomously functioning thyroid nodules (AFTNs).
(d) Curative or palliative treatment of recurrent thyroid cancers in the thyroidectomy bed and cervical lymph nodes for patients, who are at high surgical risk or who decline surgery.

## *Effectiveness of RFA for Benign Thyroid Nodules*

Thyroid RFA is considered successful when the nodule shrinks by more than 50%. On average, thyroid RFA can achieve an 80% reduction in the size of solid thyroid nodules, with a range of 65–94% [3, 4]. In some cases, complete disappearance of the nodules can be observed. Patients typically experience significant improvement in symptoms, with complete or nearly complete resolution of compressive symptoms and cosmetic concerns. Approximately 90% of patients can achieve favorable outcomes with a single RFA session [3–5]. However, for patients with large nodules, multiple RFA sessions may be necessary to achieve optimal results and prevent future regrowth [6]. The volume reduction achieved with RFA is also similar for hyperfunctioning thyroid nodules, with resolution of hyperthyroidism observed in 50–80% of patients [7].

## *Benefit of RFA Over Surgical Thyroidectomy*

When comparing thermal ablation (RF, microwave, laser) with conventional thyroidectomy in a meta-analysis, thermal ablation was found to be safer, with a significantly lower incidence of hoarseness, hypothyroidism, and postoperative pain ($p < 0.05$) [8]. Patients who underwent thermal ablation also had better postoperative cosmetic outcomes and shorter hospitalization time compared to those who underwent thyroidectomy ($p < 0.05$) [8]. Another recent trial indicated that thermal ablation is superior to thyroidectomy for benign nodules in terms of patient satisfaction, postoperative quality of life, and shorter hospital stay, although it may take longer to achieve volume reduction of thyroid nodules [9]. Additionally, thyroid

RFA offers a cost reduction by eliminating surgical costs, including general anesthesia and early ambulation.

### *Patient Outcome*

The RFA procedure is minimally invasive and does not result in scarring. The procedure itself typically lasts between 15 and 30 min. After the RFA procedure, patients can resume normal activities immediately, and hospital stay is not required. Since the majority of healthy thyroid tissue remains unaffected during the procedure, patients typically do not require thyroid medications afterward.

## Market Analysis

### *The Potential Market for Thyroid Nodule RFA*

The potential market for thyroid nodule RFA is significant, considering that approximately 130,000 thyroidectomies are performed each year, with an estimated 50% of them being for benign thyroid nodules [5]. Although these nodules are benign, they can grow to a size that causes symptoms such as difficulty swallowing or breathing, hoarseness in the voice, or cosmetic concerns. Currently, thyroidectomy is the standard treatment for benign thyroid nodules.

### *Potential Referrals*

Referrals for thyroid nodule RFA can come from various medical professionals, including primary care physicians, surgeons, endocrinologists, and patients who self-refer. Both thyroid specialists and non-thyroid specialists can refer patients for this procedure.

### *Thyroid Nodule Tumor Board*

Establishing a multidisciplinary tumor board focused on thyroid nodules can be beneficial. This board would consist of experts from various specialties involved in the evaluation and treatment of thyroid nodules, including surgeons, interventional radiologists, and endocrinologists. Collaboration among these experts can lead to more comprehensive and personalized treatment plans for patients.

### *Public and Physician Awareness*

One of the barriers to widespread adoption of thyroid nodule RFA in the United States is the lack of public and physician awareness. To address this, marketing efforts should focus on increasing awareness through various channels. This can include developing informative websites dedicated to the procedure, utilizing social media platforms for marketing purposes, organizing webinars, and delivering lectures to groups of referring physicians. These strategies aim to educate both the public and healthcare professionals about the benefits and availability of thyroid nodule RFA as an alternative treatment option.

## Financial Analysis

### *Cost Analysis*

The clinical workflow of the thyroid nodule RFA procedure is outlined in Fig. 23.1. The procedure will take place in a dedicated procedure room equipped with US guidance. The estimated total procedure time for thyroid RFA, including room preparation between cases, is approximately 1 h.

The costs associated with thyroid RFA were calculated using the following workflow, assumptions, and methods, as outlined in Table 23.1. The staffing for each procedure room includes an interventional radiologist (IR), a dedicated IR nurse, an IR attending physician, and an IR fellow in training. The hourly rates for these positions were determined based on data from the salary.com database.

The cost of consumable materials used during the procedure, such as the RFA probe, angiogram tray, pharmaceuticals, and 25G needles, was calculated based on the hospital purchase prices.

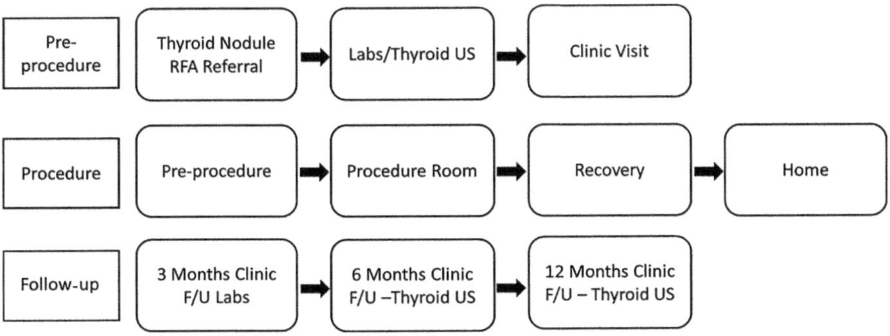


**Fig. 23.1** Clinical workflow of thyroid nodule RFA procedure

**Table 23.1** Cost analysis of thyroid RFA procedure

| Direct costs | | ($) |
|---|---|---|
| *Variable direct costs* | | |
| Supplies | RFA probe | 1490.0 |
| | Other supplies | 49.1 |
| | Pharmaceuticals | 25.5 |
| Salaries (hourly rate) | IR attending physician (1 FTE) | 197.1 |
| | IR fellow | 35.6 |
| | IR technologist (1 FTE) | 28.5 |
| | IR nurse (1 FTE) | 36.9 |
| | IR administrative support (0.7 FTE) | 13.2 |
| | IR coordinator (0.35 FTE) | 12.9 |
| Pre-procedure cost (hourly rate) | | 65.1 |
| Recovery cost (hourly rate) | | 130.1 |
| *Fixed direct costs* | | |
| Equipment depreciation (hourly rate) | US machine | 13.5 |
| | RF generator | 208.0 |
| *Indirect costs* | | |
| Overhead facility costs (hourly rate) | | 25.0 |
| Overhead administrative costs (hourly rate) | | 183.0 |
| *Total costs* | | **2513.4** |

Please note that these costs are estimates based on the provided methodology and assumptions and may vary depending on specific circumstances and healthcare settings
*FTE* Full-Time Equivalent

Direct fixed costs include the expenses for the US machine and RFA generator machine. The US machines were recently purchased at a cost of $225,000, with an 8-year depreciation schedule resulting in a yearly depreciation of $28,125. This cost is divided by the operational hours of the rooms (2080 hours per room, assuming 40 hours per week for 52 weeks), resulting in a cost of $13.50 per hour. The RFA generator machine was purchased at a cost of $40,000, with an 8-year depreciation schedule resulting in a yearly depreciation of $5000. This cost is divided by the total expected number of procedures (24 procedures per year), resulting in a cost of $208 per procedure.

The indirect overhead facility and indirect overhead administration costs were based on a previous study from 2012 regarding operating expenses for conventional transarterial chemoembolization (TACE) in an academic medical center [10]. These costs were adjusted using a Consumer Price Index (CPI) inflation calculator.

The costs associated with the pre-procedure and recovery periods are determined based on the time spent in the IR holding area or the recovery room. The pre-procedure time is estimated at 30 min, and the recovery time after thyroid RFA is less than an hour. The unit costs for pre-procedure and recovery were derived from the same previous study and adjusted using the CPI inflation calculator.

**Table 23.2** Professional fee for thyroid nodule RFA

| CPT code | | Charge |
|---|---|---|
| 60699 | Under other procedures of the endocrine system | $1763 |
| 76940 | Radiology/diagnostic US | $433 |
| 99152 | Moderate sedation services | $95 |
| 99153 | Add-on code for additional time spent administering | $80–320 |
| **Total** | | **$2371–2611** |

## *Reimbursement*

### Professional Fee

Currently, there are no specific CPT codes available for thyroid RFA. As a result, unlisted CPT codes have been utilized to bill for this procedure. The following CPT codes have been used for patients undergoing thyroid RFA, and costs have been calculated accordingly (Table 23.2).

### Technical Fee (Hospital Outpatient)

Although the CPT code 60699 does not have associated relative value units (RVUs), it is cross-referenced with the Ambulatory Payment Classification (APC) code 5361, which carries a dollar value of $5060.44 based on the Medicare National Average reimbursement.

## Future Strategic Plans

In the United States, RFA is currently considered a second-line therapy for metastatic lymph nodes in patients, who are not surgical candidates, as stated in the American Thyroid Association 2015 guidelines [11]. RFA ablation is also recognized as a treatment option for benign symptomatic thyroid nodules in the 2016 American Association of Clinical Endocrinologists guidelines [12]. However, there are significant barriers hindering the widespread adoption of thyroid nodule RFA in the United States.

One major obstacle is the cost of the procedure, as there is currently no specific CPT code for thyroid RFA. As a result, insurance companies often consider this procedure experimental and do not provide reimbursement. Consequently, patients are typically required to pay out-of-pocket for the procedure. Despite this, the total out-of-pocket cost of thyroid RFA, ranging from $3500 to $6000 on average, remains favorable when compared to the estimated national average cost of surgery, which is approximately $19,500 [13, 14]. However, a comparative cost-analysis study between thyroid RFA and thyroidectomy is still needed to provide more comprehensive data.

In addition to the cost barrier, other challenges include the lack of public and physician awareness regarding thyroid nodule RFA and the need for trained physicians to perform the procedure. Increasing public and physician awareness is crucial to improve access to thyroid nodule RFA and reduce patient costs. To address these issues, the Society of Interventional Radiology (SIR) is offering categorical courses, case workshops, and hands-on workshops at their annual meeting to train physicians in performing thyroid nodule RFA. As the procedure becomes more widely accepted and more data becomes available, it is anticipated that obtaining a CPT code will become easier. This, in turn, will facilitate reimbursement by insurance companies, further enhancing accessibility for patients.

## Conclusion

Thyroid nodule RFA is a well-studied and utilized form of treatment that effectively reduces and eliminates benign thyroid nodules without the need for surgery. While RFA has been successfully performed for thyroid nodules in Korea and Europe for over a decade, its adoption in the United States is limited due to reimbursement challenges associated with the absence of a CPT code and the lack of public and physician awareness. Nevertheless, the implementation of a thyroid RFA service line can offer a noninvasive alternative to surgery for patients while generating revenue for the hospital. Continued efforts to raise awareness, train physicians, and address reimbursement issues will contribute to the broader acceptance and utilization of thyroid nodule RFA in the United States.

## References

1. Kim JH, Baek JH, Lim HK, Ahn HS, Baek SM, Choi YJ, Choi YJ, Chung SR, Ha EJ, Hahn SY, Jung SL, Kim DS, Kim SJ, Kim YK, Lee CY, Lee JH, Lee KH, Lee YH, Park JS, Park H, Shin JH, Suh CH, Sung JY, Sim JS, Youn I, Choi M, Na DG, Guideline Committee for the Korean Society of Thyroid Radiology (KSThR) and Korean Society of Radiology. 2017 thyroid radiofrequency ablation guideline: Korean Society of Thyroid Radiology. Korean J Radiol. 2018;19(4):632–55.
2. Papini E, Monpeyssen H, Frasoldati A, Hegedüs L. 2020 European Thyroid Association clinical practice guideline for the use of image-guided ablation in benign thyroid nodules. Eur Thyroid J. 2020;9(4):172–85.
3. Mauri G, Gennaro N, Lee MK, Baek JH. Laser and radiofrequency ablations for benign and malignant thyroid tumors. Int J Hyperthermia. 2019;36(2):13–20.
4. Cho SJ, Baek JH, Chung SR, Choi YJ, Lee JH. Long-term results of thermal ablation of benign thyroid nodules: a systematic review and meta-analysis. Endocrinol Metab (Seoul). 2020;35(2):339–50.

5. Kuo JH, Lee JA. The adoption of ultrasound-guided radiofrequency ablation of thyroid nodules in the United States. Ann Surg. 2021;273(1):e10–2.
6. Sim JS, Baek JH. Long-term outcomes following thermal ablation of benign thyroid nodules as an alternative to surgery: the importance of controlling regrowth. Endocrinol Metab (Seoul). 2019;34(2):117–23.
7. Mauri G, Papini E, Bernardi S, Barbaro D, Cesareo R, De Feo P, Deandrea M, Fugazzola L, Gambelunghe G, Greco G, Messina C, Monti S, Mormile A, Negro R, Offi C, Palermo A, Persani L, Presciuttini F, Solbiati LA, Spiezia S, Stacul F, Viganò M, Sconfienza LM. Image-guided thermal ablation in autonomously functioning thyroid nodules. A retrospective multicenter three-year follow-up study from the Italian Minimally Invasive Treatment of the Thyroid (MITT) Group. Eur Radiol. 2022;32(3):1738–46.
8. Guan SH, Wang H, Teng DK. Comparison of ultrasound-guided thermal ablation and conventional thyroidectomy for benign thyroid nodules: a systematic review and meta-analysis. Int J Hyperthermia. 2020;37(1):442–9.
9. Jin H, Lin W, Lu L, Cui M. Conventional thyroidectomy vs thyroid thermal ablation on postoperative quality of life and satisfaction for patients with benign thyroid nodules. Eur J Endocrinol. 2021;184(1):131–41. https://doi.org/10.1530/EJE-20-0562. PMID: 33112273.
10. Beheshti MV, Meek J. Calculation of operating expenses for conventional transarterial chemoembolization in an academic medical center: a step toward defining the value of transarterial chemoembolization. J Vasc Interv Radiol. 2014;25(4):567–74.
11. Haugen BR, Alexander EK, Bible KC, et al. 2015 American Thyroid Association management guidelines for adult patients with thyroid nodules and differentiated thyroid cancer: the American Thyroid Association guidelines task force on thyroid nodules and differentiated thyroid cancer. Thyroid. 2016;26(1):1–133.
12. Gharib H, Papini E, Garber JR, et al.; AACE/ACE/AME Task Force on Thyroid Nodules. American Association of Clinical Endocrinologists, American College of Endocrinology, and Associazione Medici Endocrinologi medical guidelines for clinical practice for the diagnosis and management of thyroid nodules—2016 update. Endocr Pract. 2016;22(5):622–639.
13. Hussain I, Zulfiqar F, Li X, Ahmad S, Aljammal J. Safety and efficacy of radiofrequency ablation of thyroid nodules-expanding treatment options in the United States. J Endocr Soc. 2021;5(8):10–2.
14. MDsave Incorporated. Thyroidectomy. How much does a thyroidectomy cost? https://www.mdsave.com/procedures/thyroidectomy/d78bfdca. Accessed 2 Feb 2021.

# Part IV
# Miscellaneous

# Chapter 24
# Ethanol Ablation of Thyroid Nodules

**Dong Wook Kim**

Ethanol ablation (EA) is defined as the direct injection of ethanol into the target lesion using a needle or catheter to reduce or remove a lesion within a solid organ. EA is commonly referred to as ethanol injection or ethanol sclerotherapy. Simple needle aspiration of a thyroid cyst was the first interventional approach investigated for a thyroid nodule [1]. Since its introduction, Miller et al. have reported a high recurrence rate of 58% associated with simple aspiration, which is therefore of limited therapeutic utility [2]. EA of benign thyroid nodules was introduced by Rozman et al. for the treatment of thyroid cysts [3]. EA is a relatively safe, simple, and effective procedure and is currently an established therapeutic modality for benign thyroid nodules [4–13]. Although EA is widely accepted for the management of benign thyroid cysts or predominantly cystic thyroid nodules, its usefulness in patients with solid thyroid nodules or hyperfunctioning thyroid nodules remains questionable [10, 14–19].

Currently, ethanol, tetracycline, sodium tetradecyl sulfate, OK-432 (picibanil), and polidocanol are sclerosing agents used to treat thyroid nodules [20–25]. Among these, ethanol is inexpensive, easy to handle, and relatively safe and is therefore the most widely used agent to treat benign thyroid nodules.

## Mechanism of Action

The mechanisms underlying the effects of ethanol include cell dehydration following diffusion and coagulation necrosis of tissue secondary to protein denaturation, hemorrhagic infarction due to small vessel thrombosis, and inhibition of enzyme

D. W. Kim (✉)
Department of Radiology, Busan Paik Hospital, Inje University College of Medicine, Busan, South Korea



A. W. Park et al. (eds.), *Thyroid Radiofrequency Ablation*,
https://doi.org/10.1007/978-3-031-65288-2_24

activity in surrounding tissue, which together result in fibrosis and contraction of the nodule [4, 26, 27]. The primary action mechanism of ethanol in cystic and solid components is known to be coagulation necrosis and hemorrhagic infarction, respectively [12, 19].

The ethanol concentration used for EA is usually 95–100%, and 99% ethanol is the commercial type of ethanol widely used for this purpose [4, 12, 19, 28, 29]. Owing to its toxicity in humans, the maximum recommended dose of ethanol should not be >1 mL/kg or >20 mL/ablation session [11, 30, 31].

## Ethanol Ablation of Benign Thyroid Nodules

### *Introduction*

Usually, asymptomatic benign thyroid nodules do not require treatment. Thyroid hormone suppression therapy was previously recommended for symptomatic benign thyroid nodules but is not currently indicated because the therapeutic effect is unclear, and long-term use is associated with adverse effects such as osteoporosis or atrial fibrillation [15, 16, 32, 33]. However, EA is widely used as nonsurgical treatment in patients with symptoms caused by a mass effect or in those with cosmetic issues secondary to an increase in the size of the benign thyroid nodules.

### *Indications*

The benign nature of the thyroid nodule should be confirmed in at least one specimen evaluated using fine-needle aspiration cytology before performing EA. The following are the indications for EA of benign thyroid nodules in clinical practice: (1) symptoms such as pain, difficulty in swallowing, or airway pressure due to a mass effect, (2) cosmetic issues, and (3) for prevention of complications following an increase in nodule size [13, 15, 16, 19, 29, 33–37]. However, EA is contraindicated if EA cannot be performed owing to nodule position or in cases of paralysis of the contralateral recurrent laryngeal nerve.

Usually, patients with cystic thyroid nodules initially undergo simple needle aspiration for diagnosis and treatment; EA may be performed if the nodule size does not decrease after simple needle aspiration or if follow-up ultrasonography (US) reveals residual cystic components [3–8, 11–13, 35, 38–41]. To date, EA remains the first-line treatment for benign, cystic, thyroid nodules because it is less expensive and its therapeutic efficacy is comparable with thermal ablation [12, 13, 30, 40, 42, 43].

EA may be effective for treatment of symptomatic benign, solid, thyroid nodules and can be considered only after US confirms that nodules are not highly vascular

[39, 44, 45]. EA may be useful in patients with a remnant solid component after radiofrequency ablation (RFA) or if additional RFA is burdensome [39, 45].

The role of EA for treatment of hyperfunctioning thyroid nodules remains controversial, and radioactive iodine therapy is the first-line treatment in such cases [13]. Reports in the literature describe the usefulness of EA in patients with complications such as hypothyroidism after radioisotope therapy or in women of childbearing age [10, 14, 17, 18, 35, 38, 46]. However, recent guidelines do not recommend EA for treatment of hyperfunctioning thyroid nodules, which are best treated using thermal ablation [12, 13].

## *Methods*

Prior to EA, the procedure should be explained in detail and written, informed consent should be obtained from the patient. Instruments used to perform EA are similar to those used for fine-needle aspiration except for the ethanol injection. Instruments used for EA include needles (18–23 gauge), an adequate number of syringes and volume of ethanol, and/or a lidocaine syringe. The patient is placed in a supine position on the bed with mild extension of the neck. The patient's neck is draped after skin sterilization (e.g., using povidone-iodine [10%] solution), and the US probe is covered with a sterilized vinyl cloth. The US probe is adjusted to center the target nodule on the US monitor.

## *Cystic or Predominantly Cystic Thyroid Nodules*

(a) The patient is placed in a supine position on the bed with a towel or other support at the back of the neck for slight neck extension.
(b) The operator sits (or stands) on the patient, facing the US equipment to confirm the site of the nodule using US guidance.
(c) After sterilization of the skin over the neck, the US probe is placed perpendicular to the patient's neck, and the operator holds an empty syringe connected to a needle and punctures the patient's skin and the target nodule and confirms the position of the needle on real-time US.
(d) The operator places the end of the needle at the center of the cystic component, aspirates the fluid content as much as possible, and replaces only the syringe containing ethanol with the needle fixed as it is.
(e) A minimal amount of ethanol is injected to confirm that ethanol jets are visible inside the target nodule, after which the remaining quantity of ethanol is gradually injected. Following ethanol injection, the operator removes the needle without skin compression.

### Solid Thyroid Nodules

(a) The patient is placed in the supine position on the bed with a towel or other support at the back of the neck for slight neck extension.
(b) The operator sits (or stands) on the patient, facing the US equipment to confirm the site of the nodule under US guidance.
(c) After sterilization of the skin over the neck, the US probe in the operator's hand is placed perpendicular to the patient's neck, and the operator holds an empty syringe connected to a needle and punctures the skin and the target nodule and confirms the position of the needle on real-time US.
(d) The operator places the end of the needle at the center of the solid component and replaces the empty syringe with a syringe containing ethanol with the needle fixed as it is.
(e) A minimal amount of ethanol is injected to confirm that ethanol jets are visible inside the target nodule, after which an appropriate quantity of ethanol is gradually injected into the entire portions of a target nodule. The operator places the needle tip at the deepest portion of the target nodule. While ethanol is injected, the needle tip is gradually shifted into a shallow area to facilitate successful ethanol instillation into all zones of the target nodule.
(f) The procedure is immediately terminated if the patient experiences significant pain or if US reveals ethanol leakage into the tissue around the thyroid gland.
(g) After the procedure, the operator promptly removes the needle, and the puncture site is lightly compressed for 5–10 min.

## *Specific Considerations*

### Local Anesthesia

Previous studies that have described EA of thyroid nodules (prior to the use of US-guided procedures) report that local anesthesia was not used because local anesthetics were shown to reduce sensitivity of palpation of the thyroid tissue [3, 6, 11, 16, 32, 47]. Following the introduction of US for such procedures, application of local anesthesia during EA is at the operator's discretion. An advantage of local anesthesia is that patients do not experience much pain even with slight leakage of ethanol along the puncture site during injection [39]. However, administration of local anesthetics is associated with adverse effects such as pain, and fine air bubbles injected along with the anesthetic interfere with accurate visualization of the US window; therefore, local anesthetics are sometimes avoided [48, 49].

## Puncture Technique

Usually, 18–23 gauge needles with a single hole are used; however, various types of needles with several side holes may be used for EA [17]. A needle of an appropriate gauge is selected based on the viscosity of the cystic contents after needle aspiration of cystic thyroid nodules [39, 40]. A long puncture needle is used for deep-seated target nodules [17, 46].

The following puncture methods may be used: (a) the puncture is performed using a needle placed perpendicular to an US image (vertical or perpendicular puncture) or (b) the puncture is performed with the needle placed parallel to the US image (horizontal or oblique puncture). The vertical puncture technique is relatively more accurate and easy to perform; however, the needle position may shift even with minimal movements of the patient's neck, with a high risk of ethanol leakage [8, 39, 46, 50]. In contrast, the horizontal puncture technique requires minimal experience and expertise, and the needle position does not tend to shift even if the patient swallows saliva [8, 39, 46, 50]. Both puncture methods are widely used and either may be selected based on the location or size of the target nodule and the operator's preference.

## Types of Thyroid Nodules

### Cystic Thyroid Nodules

On US, a cystic thyroid nodule appears as a lesion that is completely filled with liquid. EA is the most effective and least expensive method for the treatment of cystic thyroid nodules and serves as the first-line ablation method for these lesions [12, 30, 40, 42, 43, 51]. Before EA, patients should undergo simple aspiration at least once (usually, US-guided fine-needle aspiration) for diagnosis and treatment of symptomatic benign cystic thyroid nodules [12]. Therefore, EA is performed in patients with recurrent, cystic thyroid nodules after simple aspiration. Several studies have reported favorable outcomes following EA for benign cystic thyroid nodules [3–11, 13, 15, 16, 19, 29, 33–35, 37, 39, 42, 52, 53] (Table 24.1).

Complete removal of all cystic contents is preferred before ethanol injection to prevent ethanol dilution in patients, who undergo EA for benign cystic thyroid nodules [5, 10, 11]. However, the needle tip may be invisible on US in patients in whom complete removal of cystic contents is performed; therefore, a minimal amount of cystic contents should be retained in the nodule. Colloid cysts contain a highly viscous gel-like substance, and the cystic contents are not easily aspirated even with the use of an 18-gauge needle. Therefore, a small amount of ethanol (approximately 10% of the total volume) is injected into the colloid cyst before the main procedure [54]. The colloid cyst gradually liquefies over approximately 2–4 weeks, which

**Table 24.1** The published data of EA for benign cystic thyroid nodules

| Name | Year | Number of patients | Follow-up (months) | Number of sessions | Success[a] rate (%) | Major complication |
|---|---|---|---|---|---|---|
| Rozman et al. [3] | 1990 | 13 | 8 | 1 | 77 | No |
| Yasuda et al. [4] | 1992 | 61 | 6 | 1–4 | 72 | No |
| Monzani et al. [6] | 1994 | 20 | 12 | 1–2 | 95 | No |
| Verde et al. [7] | 1994 | 42 | 1–12 | 1 | 80 | No |
| Antonelli et al. [5] | 1994 | 26 | 12 | 1–5 | 77 | No |
| Cho et al. [8] | 2000 | 22 | 1–10 | 1–2 | 68 | No |
| Bennebaek et al. [9] | 2003 | 33 | 6 | 1–4 | 82 | No |
| Guglielmi et al. [10] | 2004 | 58 | 83 | 1–4 | 86.2 | No |
| Kim et al. [11] | 2005 | 60 | 1–24 | 1 | 96.7 | No |
| Sung et al. [42] | 2013 | 21 | 6 | 1 | 100 | No |
| Park et al. [52] | 2019 | 94 | 1–36 | 1 | 93.6 | No |
| Cho et al. [53] | 2021 | 38 | 1–12 | 1 | 100 | No |

[a] Success means complete loss of the cystic components in follow-up ultrasonography

facilitates complete aspiration of the cystic contents. A few authors have reported that connecting a 16-gauge needle to a suction device enables removal of a considerable quantity of colloid substance for successful EA [55].

## Nonfunctioning Thyroid Nodules

Ethanol is gradually instilled into the cystic component after aspiration of the cystic content, followed by ethanol injection into the solid component in patients with nonfunctioning, partially cystic thyroid nodules [37, 39]. The outcomes of EA performed for solid thyroid nodules differ across studies reported in the literature [15, 16, 31, 33, 37, 39, 41, 44, 51] (Table 24.2); therefore, the role of EA in the treatment of nonfunctioning thyroid nodules remains controversial. Combination therapy comprising EA and RFA may be useful for the treatment of nonfunctioning thyroid nodules, particularly to treat predominantly cystic thyroid nodules [12, 44, 56]. Notably, RFA appears to be superior to EA in reducing the volume of benign thyroid nodules during short- and long-term follow-up [41, 51, 57]. In patients with an incomplete response to EA or RFA of a benign solid thyroid nodule, RFA or EA, respectively, is effective [12, 45].

## Hyperfunctioning Thyroid Nodules

EA is proposed as an alternative to surgery and radioiodine therapy for hyperfunctioning nodules. Many authors have reported diverse outcomes following EA of hyperfunctioning thyroid nodules [14, 17, 18, 34, 38, 58–61] (Table 24.3). However,

**Table 24.2** The published data of EA for nonfunctioning solid thyroid nodules

| Name | Published year | Number of nodules | Number of sessions | Success[a] rate (%) | Major complication |
|---|---|---|---|---|---|
| Goletti et al. [15] | 1994 | 20 | 1–3 | 100 | No |
| Bennedbak et al. [16] | 1995 | 13 | 1 | 100 | No |
| Zingrillo et al. [33] | 1998 | 41 | 2–8 | 92.7 | No |
| Lee et al. [31] | 2005 | 198 | 2.2 ± 1.4 | 89 | No |
| Kim et al. [39] | 2012 | 30 | 1–2 | 60 | No |
| Felicio et al. [37] | 2016 | 52 | 2.8 ± 1.9 | 75 | No |
| Karatay et al. [41] | 2020 | 50 | 1 | 100 | No |

[a] Success means 50% or more volume reduction rate

**Table 24.3** The published data of EA for benign, hyperfunctioning thyroid nodules

| Name | Year | Number of nodules | Number of sessions | Success rate (%) | Major complications |
|---|---|---|---|---|---|
| Martino et al. [59] | 1992 | 37 | 1–3 | 100[a] | No |
| Mazzeo et al. [14] | 1993 | 32 | 3–10 | 100[b] | No |
| Papini et al. [60] | 1993 | 20 | 3–8 | 100[b] | No |
| Livraghi et al. [34] | 1994 | 101 | 4–8 | 58.4[b] | No |
| Di Lelio et al. [17] | 1995 | 31 | 3–7 | 77[b] | No |
| Lippi et al. [18] | 1996 | 429 | 2–12 | 74.6[b] | No |
| Monzani et al. [38] | 1997 | 117 | 5–10 | 77.9[b] | No |
| Del Prete et al. [58] | 2001 | 34 | 1–11 | 88.2[b] | No |
| Tarantino et al. [61] | 2008 | 124 | 1–11 | 93[b] | 3.2% |

[a] Success means 50% or more volume reduction rate
[b] Complete cure of toxic nodules means that both free thyroid hormone and thyrotropin serum levels returned to within the normal range

EA plays a limited role in the management of hyperfunctioning nodules owing to the need for multisession therapy and associated complications [12, 13]. Newer ablation techniques including RFA, laser and microwave ablation, and high-intensity focused US are recommended for the treatment of hyperfunctioning nodules [12, 13].

## Volume and Concentration of Ethanol

The volume of ethanol injected is determined by the quantity of cystic contents or the nodule volume. A previous study has reported that injection of a high volume of ethanol was associated with better treatment success rates [8]. In a retrospective single-center study, however, the authors observed that single-session EA using low-dose ethanol (≤5 mL), regardless of the target nodule or aspirate volume, effectively treated symptomatic cystic thyroid nodules [53].

Usually, it is recommended that the total quantity of ethanol injected should not exceed 10 mL to avoid the risk of complications [11, 14, 17, 50]. Therefore, the amount of ethanol injected in cases of cystic thyroid nodules usually corresponds to 50–90% of the aspirated fluid (however, this volume should be <10 mL). The amount of ethanol injected should not exceed 10 mL/session in cases of solid thyroid nodules.

EA is commonly performed using pure 100% ethanol. To our knowledge, no study has investigated the concentration of ethanol required to improve the therapeutic effect of EA in cases of cystic thyroid nodules. An in vitro study performed on endothelial cells showed necrosis of all cells following only 5-second exposure to 30% ethanol [27]. Therefore, in view of the possibility that the concentration of injected ethanol may partially be diluted by the residual cystic fluid, it is reasonable to use an ethanol concentration ≥95%.

## Aspiration Vs. Non-aspiration of Injected Ethanol

Whether the injected ethanol should be aspirated after EA is debatable, and authors' opinions vary in this regard. The method selected depends on the operator's preference or clinical conditions [4, 5, 11, 47, 50, 52]. In a previous study, aspiration of the injected ethanol was shown to prolong the procedure time, although the nodule showed an immediate reduction in size after the procedure [11]. However, no difference was observed in the prevalence of complication or success rates between the aspiration and non-aspiration groups. Another study claimed that aspiration of injected ethanol may be preferred to non-aspiration because of less post-EA pain associated with the aspiration of the injected ethanol [52]. Usually, the indwelling time is approximately 5–10 minutes after ethanol injection [4, 5, 11, 50].

## Follow-Up

The first follow-up US is performed 1–2 months after EA to evaluate the success of the procedure [5, 7, 8, 10, 11, 38, 50]. Switching to an alternative sclerosant or RFA may be considered for lesions that are refractory to one or two trials of EA [11, 35, 39, 62]. Evaluation of serum thyroid hormones and thyroid-stimulating hormone, as well as a thyroid scan and follow-up US, should be performed over at least 6 months of follow-up in patients who undergo EA for functioning thyroid nodules because it is important to evaluate post-EA thyroid function as opposed to merely confirming a reduction in the nodule volume [10, 14, 17, 18, 38, 63].

## *Criteria for Success*

Clinically, patient satisfaction is important for determining a successful outcome of EA; however, no objective criteria are established for this purpose. Many authors recommend that a reduction in the nodule volume by >50% or volume <1 mL on follow-up US be used as a criterion for successful EA [4, 11, 50].

### Cystic Thyroid Nodules

Successful EA is defined as complete disappearance of the cystic component observed on the first follow-up US. Many studies have reported the outcomes of EA, most of which report a relatively high treatment success rate of 68–100% on follow-up US performed over 6 months [3–8, 11, 13, 15, 16, 19, 29, 33–35, 37, 39, 42, 52]. Kim et al. reported EA performed for 60 benign cystic thyroid nodules with a success rate as high as 96.7%, without any recurrence on follow-up US over >12 months, and additional EA yielded favorable results (Fig. 24.1) [11]. Post-EA recurrence is defined as reappearance of the cystic component on follow-up US

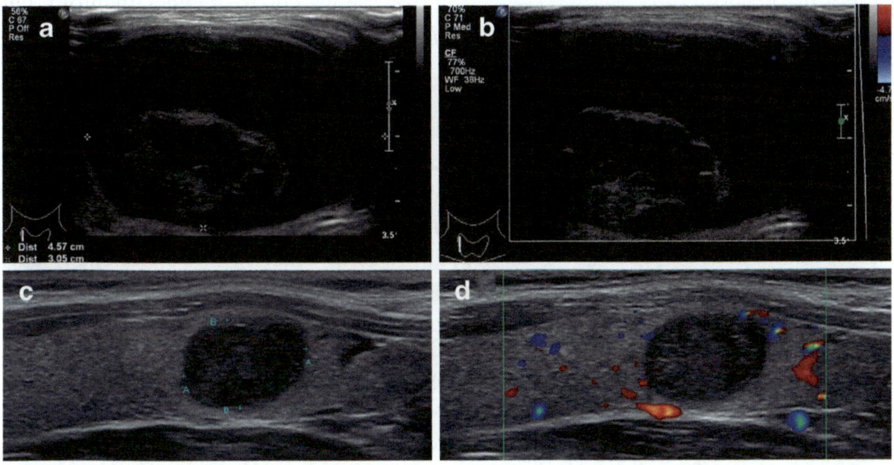


**Fig. 24.1** A case of successful US-guided percutaneous ethanol ablation (EA) of a benign cystic thyroid nodule in a 41-year-old woman. Longitudinal gray-scale (**a**) and color Doppler (**b**) US images of a cystic thyroid nodule in the right lobe show an ovoid shape and scant vascularity (3.1 × 4.6 × 4.7 cm). Follow-up longitudinal gray-scale (**c**) and color Doppler (**d**) US images at 12 months after the one session of EA (injection of 5 mL 100% ethanol after aspiration of 11 mL dark brownish fluid using a 23-gauge needle) show marked shrinkage and no vascularity (1.1 × 1.2 × 1.5 cm)

after complete disappearance of it [9, 64]. EA results in shrinkage of cystic nodules, which are replaced by a solid component of low echogenicity observed on follow-up US; this component histologically consists of scar tissue and old hemorrhage [4]. Clinicians should carefully monitor the nodules after successful EA because post-ablation nodules may mimic findings of thyroid malignancy on follow-up US [64]. Therefore, accurate history taking is important; most lesions can be differentiated following comparison with previous US images.

## Nonfunctioning Thyroid Nodules

Authors vary in their opinion regarding the criterion for successful EA used for the treatment of nonfunctioning thyroid nodules; however, reduction in nodule volume and clinical improvement are important criteria (Fig. 24.2). An US-documented, post-ablation, nodule volume <1 mL during follow-up may be considered successful treatment. A single-center study that compared the therapeutic effects of EA for cystic and solid thyroid nodules observed a volume reduction rate of 64% and 35% for cystic and solid nodules, respectively [50]. The following factors are considered contributors to the lower success rates of EA in solid nodules: (a) the injected ethanol does not spread evenly within solid nodules and (b) most solid nodules measure

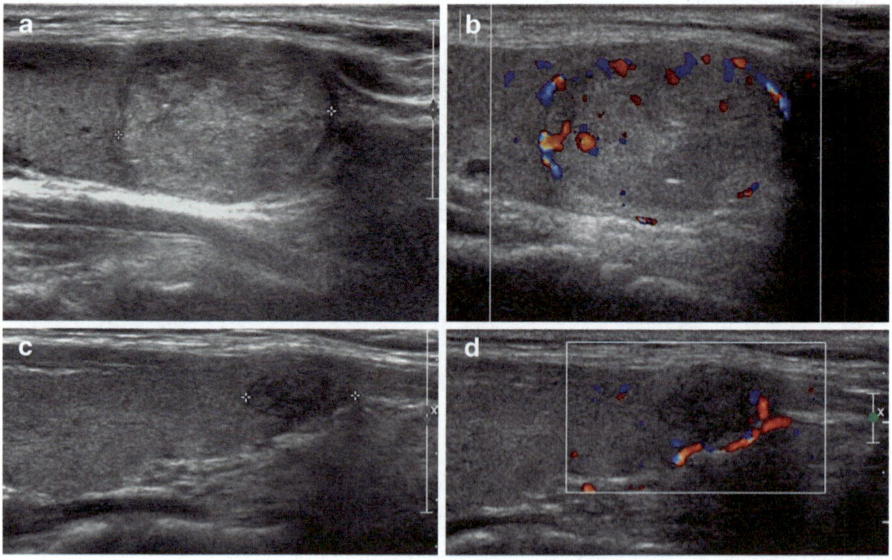


**Fig. 24.2** A case of successful US-guided percutaneous ethanol ablation (EA) of a benign solid thyroid nodule in a 34-year-old woman. Longitudinal gray-scale (**a**) and color Doppler (**b**). US images of a solid thyroid nodule in the right lobe show an ovoid shape, isoechogenicity, and mixed vascularity (1.5 × 2.3 × 2.4 cm). Follow-up longitudinal gray-scale (**c**) and color Doppler (**d**) US images at 6 months after the second session of EA (injection of 2 and 1 mL 100% ethanol in the first and second sessions, respectively) show moderate shrinkage and no vascularity (0.5 × 0.7 × 1.1 cm)

>3 cm in diameter. Therefore, it is important to be aware of the predictors of successful EA used for the treatment of solid thyroid nodules. A previous study observed a high success rate of EA in patients with low vascularity of the solid nodule documented by pre-EA Doppler US and in those in whom microbubbles created by the injected ethanol remained in the nodule over a prolonged period without being flushed down a vein [39].

### Hyperfunctioning Thyroid Nodules

The therapeutic effect of EA performed for hyperfunctioning thyroid nodules differs from that observed in nonfunctioning thyroid nodules; the effect depends on the success of complete remission. Complete remission is defined as post-EA normalization of serum thyroid hormone and thyroid-stimulating hormone levels and normal uptake of tracer by the thyroid parenchyma on a thyroid scan. The complete remission rate varies from 50 to 100% across studies [10, 14, 17, 18, 38, 63]. Studies have shown that the therapeutic effect of EA for the management of hyperfunctioning thyroid nodules is superior in nodules of a smaller volume than in those with nodules of a larger volume; notably, large-sized nodules typically require a greater number of EA sessions [10, 34].

## *Complications*

Most EA-induced complications are mild and temporary [4, 10, 14–18, 39]. The most common complication is pain around the needle puncture site, which lasts for several hours; most patients experience mild pain that does not require analgesic administration, immediately after the procedure. Rarely, pain lasts over 1–2 days after EA; however, it is well controlled with oral analgesics in most cases. Hematoma is a relatively common complication along with pain and occurs secondary to needle injury to veins around the thyroid capsule. Light compression on the puncture site for approximately 10 minutes following the procedure can prevent hematoma formation, and most hematomas completely resolve within 1–2 weeks.

Facial flushing, headache, drunkenness, or dizziness may occur during or after EA. Ethanol leakage from the thyroid gland can injure adjacent organs and cause severe pain; however, this is a rare complication. Post-EA thyroid abscess or thyrotoxicosis may occur in rare cases [65, 66].

## *Conclusion*

EA is considered the first-line therapy for benign, cystic thyroid nodules. Combined therapy using EA and RFA may be useful for the management of nonfunctioning thyroid nodules. However, radioisotope therapy or thermal ablation techniques are preferred over EA for the management of hyperfunctioning thyroid nodules.

## Ethanol Ablation of Malignant Thyroid Nodules

### *Primary Thyroid Cancer*

Since 1993, only three case reports have described EA for the treatment of primary thyroid cancer; notably, this approach was used in patients with inoperable lesions [67–69]. To date, there is lack of evidence to support the use of EA to treat primary thyroid cancer, and this therapeutic approach is not recommended [12].

### *Recurrent Thyroid Cancer*

EA is used as an alternative for locally recurrent thyroid cancer in patients, who are deemed high-risk surgical candidates or in those who refuse repeat surgery [12, 70, 71]. A few studies have reported the efficacy of EA in the treatment of recurrent thyroid cancer [72–76]. EA involves multisession treatment [1–6], and large-sized lesions require a greater number of EA sessions [12, 74, 75]. EA shows limited effectiveness with regard to the complete disappearance of recurrent cancers [12, 77, 78]. EA may be recommended for complete ablation in patients with recurrent thyroid cancer with ≤3 local recurrent nodules without distant metastasis or for palliation in patients with distant metastasis [12]. Further studies are warranted to gain a deeper understanding of this subject to establish the appropriate guidelines for the application of EA in clinical practice.

## References

1. Crile G. Treatment of thyroid cysts by aspiration. Surgery. 1966;59(2):210–2.
2. Miller JM, Zafar S, Karo JJ. The cystic thyroid nodule: recognition and management. Radiology. 1974;110(2):257–61.
3. Rozman B, Bencezigman Z, Tomicbrzac H, Skreb F, Pavlinovic Z, Simonovic I. Sclerosation of thyroid cysts by ethanol. Period Biol. 1990;91(4):453.
4. Yasuda K, Ozaki O, Sugino K, Yamashita T, Toshima K, Ito K, et al. Treatment of cystic lesions of the thyroid by ethanol instillation. World J Surg. 1992;16(5):958–61.
5. Antonelli A, Campatelli A, Di Vito A, Alberti B, Baldi V, Salvioni G, et al. Comparison between ethanol sclerotherapy and emptying with injection of saline in treatment of thyroid cysts. Clin Investig. 1994;72(12):971–4.
6. Monzani F, Lippi F, Goletti O, Del Guerra P, Caraccio N, Lippolis PV, et al. Percutaneous aspiration and ethanol sclerotherapy for thyroid cysts. J Clin Endocrinol Metabol. 1994;78(3):800–2.
7. Verde G, Paplni E, Pacella CM, Gallotti C, Delpiano S, Strada S, et al. Ultrasound guided percutaneous ethanol injection in the treatment of cystic thyroid nodules. Clin Endocrinol. 1994;41(6):719–24.
8. Cho YS, Lee HK, Ahn IM, Lim SM, Kim DH, Choi CG, et al. Sonographically guided ethanol sclerotherapy for benign thyroid cysts: results in 22 patients. Am J Roentgenol. 2000;174(1):213–6.

9. Bennebaek FN, Hegedüs L. Treatment of recurrent thyroid cysts with ethanol: a randomized double-blind controlled trial. J Clin Endocrinol Metabol. 2003;88(12):5773–7.
10. Guglielmi R, Pacella CM, Bianchini A, Bizzarri G, Rinaldi R, Graziano FM, et al. Percutaneous ethanol injection treatment in benign thyroid lesions: role and efficacy. Thyroid. 2004;14(2):125–31.
11. Kim DW, Rho MH, Kim HJ, Kwon JS, Sung YS, Lee SW. Percutaneous ethanol injection for benign cystic thyroid nodules: is aspiration of ethanol-mixed fluid advantageous? Am J Neuroradiol. 2005;26(8):2122–7.
12. Hahn SY, Shin JH, Na DG, Ha EJ, Ahn HS, Lim HK, et al. Ethanol ablation of the thyroid nodules: 2018 consensus statement by the Korean Society of Thyroid Radiology. Korean J Radiol. 2019;20(4):609–20.
13. Papini E, Monpeyssen H, Frasoldati A, Hegedüs L. 2020 European thyroid association clinical practice guideline for the use of image-guided ablation in benign thyroid nodules. Eur Thyroid J. 2020;9(4):172–85.
14. Mazzeo S, Toni M, De Gaudio C, Caramella D, Pinto F, Lencioni R, et al. Percutaneous injection of ethanol to treat autonomous thyroid nodules. AJR Am J Roentgenol. 1993;161(4):871–6.
15. Goletti O, Monzani F, Lenziardi M, Lippolis PV, De Negri F, Caraccio N, et al. Cold thyroid nodules: a new application of percutaneous ethanol injection treatment. J Clin Ultrasound. 1994;22(3):175–8.
16. Bennedbaek F, Hegedüs L. Alcohol sclerotherapy for benign solitary solid cold thyroid nodules. Lancet. 1995;346(8984):1227.
17. Di Lelio A, Rivolta M, Casati M, Capra M. Treatment of autonomous thyroid nodules: value of percutaneous ethanol injection. AJR Am J Roentgenol. 1995;164(1):207–13.
18. Lippi F, Ferrari C, Manetti L, Rago T, Santini F, Monzani F, et al. Treatment of solitary autonomous thyroid nodules by percutaneous ethanol injection: results of an Italian multicenter study. The Multicenter Study Group. J Clin Endocrinol Metabol. 1996;81(9):3261–4.
19. Kim DW. Usefulness of two-stage ethanol ablation in the treatment of benign predominantly cystic thyroid nodules. Endocr Pract. 2014;20(6):548–55.
20. Sykes D. The solitary thyroid nodule. J Br Surg. 1981;68(7):510–2.
21. Ryan WG, Dwarakanathan A. Minor complication of thyroid cyst sclerosis with tetracycline. Arch Intern Med. 1986;146(1):201–2.
22. Hegedüs L, Hansen JM, Karstrup S, Torp-Pedersen S, Juul N. Tetracycline for sclerosis of thyroid cysts: a randomized study. Arch Intern Med. 1988;148(5):1116–8.
23. Chang HS, Yoon JH, Chung WY, Park CS. Sclerotherapy with OK-432 for recurrent cystic thyroid nodule. Yonsei Med J. 1998;39(4):367–71.
24. Kalra N, Ahuja CK, Dutta P, Rajwanshi A, Mittal BR, Bhansali A, et al. Comparison of sonographically guided percutaneous sodium tetradecyl sulfate injection with ethanol injection in the treatment of benign nonfunctioning thyroid nodules. J Vasc Interv Radiol. 2014;25(8):1218–24.
25. Gong X, Wang F, Du H, Chen X, Shi B. Comparison of ultrasound-guided percutaneous Polidocanol injection versus percutaneous ethanol injection for treatment of benign cystic thyroid nodules. J Ultrasound Med. 2018;37(6):1423–9.
26. Crescenzi A, Papini E, Pacella C, Rinaldi R, Panunzi C, Petrucci L, et al. Morphological changes in a hyperfunctioning thyroid adenoma after percutaneous ethanol injection: histological, enzymatic and sub-microscopical alterations. J Endocrinol Investig. 1996;19(6):371–6.
27. Mol W, Furukawa H, Sasaki S, Tomaru U, Hayashi T, Saito A, et al. Evaluation of the sclerotherapeutic efficacy of ethanol, polidocanol, and OK-432 using an in vitro model. Dermatologic Surg. 2007;33(12):1452–9.
28. Papini E, Pacella CM, Verde G. Percutaneous ethanol injection (PEI): what is its role in the treatment of benign thyroid nodules? Thyroid. 1995;5(2):147–50.
29. Kim YJ, Baek JH, Ha EJ, Lim HK, Lee JH, Sung JY, et al. Cystic versus predominantly cystic thyroid nodules: efficacy of ethanol ablation and analysis of related factors. Eur Radiol. 2012;22(7):1573–8.

30. Yang C-C, Hsu Y, Liou J-Y. Efficacy of ethanol ablation for benign thyroid cysts and predominantly cystic nodules: a systematic review and meta-analysis. Endocrinol Metab. 2021;36(1):81.
31. Lee SJ, Ahn I-M. Effectiveness of percutaneous ethanol injection therapy in benign nodular and cystic thyroid diseases: long-term follow-up experience. Endocr J. 2005;52(4):455–62.
32. Livraghi T, Paracchi A, Ferrari C, Bergonzi M, Garavaglia G, Raineri P, et al. Treatment of autonomous thyroid nodules with percutaneous ethanol injection: preliminary results. Work in progress. Radiology. 1990;175(3):827–9.
33. Zingrillo M, Collura D, Ghiggi MR, Nirchio V, Trischitta V. Treatment of large cold benign thyroid nodules not eligible for surgery with percutaneous ethanol injection. J Clin Endocrinol Metabol. 1998;83(11):3905–7.
34. Livraghi T, Paracchi A, Ferrari C, Reschini E, Macchi RM, Bonifacino A. Treatment of autonomous thyroid nodules with percutaneous ethanol injection: 4-year experience. Radiology. 1994;190(2):529–33.
35. Na DG, Lee JH, Jung SL, Kim JH, Sung JY, Shin JH, et al. Radiofrequency ablation of benign thyroid nodules and recurrent thyroid cancers: consensus statement and recommendations. Korean J Radiol. 2012;13(2):117–25.
36. Kim D. Sonography-guided ethanol ablation of a remnant solid component after radiofrequency ablation of benign solid thyroid nodules: a preliminary study. Am J Neuroradiol. 2012;33(6):1139–43.
37. Felício JS, Conceição AMS, Santos FM, Sato MMM, de Arruda Bastos F, de Souza ACCB, et al. Ultrasound-guided percutaneous ethanol injection protocol to treat solid and mixed thyroid nodules. Front Endocrinol (Lausanne). 2016;7:52.
38. Monzani F, Caraccio N, Goletti O, Lippolis PV, Casolaro A, Del Guerra P, et al. Five-year follow-up of percutaneous ethanol injection for the treatment of hyperfunctioning thyroid nodules: a study of 117 patients. Clin Endocrinol. 1997;46(1):9–15.
39. Kim D, Rho M, Park H, Kwag H. Ultrasonography-guided ethanol ablation of predominantly solid thyroid nodules: a preliminary study for factors that predict the outcome. Br J Radiol. 2012;85(1015):930–6.
40. In HS, Kim DW, Choo HJ, Jung SJ, Kang T, Ryu JH. Ethanol ablation of benign thyroid cysts and predominantly cystic thyroid nodules: factors that predict outcome. Endocrine. 2014;46(1):107–13.
41. Karatay E, Javadov M. Comparison of the effectiveness of ethanol and radiofrequency ablation in the treatment of thyroid nodules and their effects on cosmetic scoring. J Invest Surg. 2022;35(3):685–90.
42. Sung JY, Baek JH, Kim KS, Lee D, Yoo H, Kim JK, et al. Single-session treatment of benign cystic thyroid nodules with ethanol versus radiofrequency ablation: a prospective randomized study. Radiology. 2013;269(1):293–300.
43. Deandrea M, Trimboli P, Creanza A, Garino F, Mormile A, Bertolino S, et al. Long-term follow-up of cystic thyroid nodules treated with percutaneous ethanol injection (PEI) using two different approaches. Eur J Endocrinol. 2020;183(5):489–95.
44. Yoon H, Baek J, Lee J, Ha E, Kim J, Yoon J, et al. Combination therapy consisting of ethanol and radiofrequency ablation for predominantly cystic thyroid nodules. Am J Neuroradiol. 2014;35(3):582–6.
45. Park HS, Baek JH, Choi YJ, Lee JH. Innovative techniques for image-guided ablation of benign thyroid nodules: combined ethanol and radiofrequency ablation. Korean J Radiol. 2017;18(3):461–9.
46. Tarantino L, Giorgio A, Mariniello N, de Stefano G, Perrotta A, Aloisio V, et al. Percutaneous ethanol injection of large autonomous hyperfunctioning thyroid nodules. Radiology. 2000;214(1):143–8.
47. Basu N, Dutta D, Maisnam I, Basu S, Ghosh S, Chowdhury S, et al. Percutaneous ethanol ablation in managing predominantly cystic thyroid nodules: an eastern India perspective. Indian J Endocrinol Metab. 2014;18(5):662.

48. Kim DW, Rho MH, Kim KN. Ultrasound-guided fine-needle aspiration biopsy of thyroid nodules: is it necessary to use local anesthesia for the application of one needle puncture? Korean J Radiol. 2009;10(5):441–6.
49. Lee YJ, Kim DW, Jung SJ. Comparison of sample adequacy, pain-scale ratings, and complications associated with ultrasound-guided fine-needle aspiration of thyroid nodules between two radiologists with different levels of experience. Endocrine. 2013;44(3):696–701.
50. Kim JH, Lee HK, Lee JH, Ahn IM, Choi CG. Efficacy of sonographically guided percutaneous ethanol injection for treatment of thyroid cysts versus solid thyroid nodules. Am J Roentgenol. 2003;180(6):1723–6.
51. Baek JH, Ha EJ, Choi YJ, Sung JY, Kim JK, Shong YK. Radiofrequency versus ethanol ablation for treating predominantly cystic thyroid nodules: a randomized clinical trial. Korean J Radiol. 2015;16(6):1332–40.
52. Park HS, Yim Y, Baek JH, Choi YJ, Shong YK, Lee JH. Ethanol ablation as a treatment strategy for benign cystic thyroid nodules: a comparison of the ethanol retention and aspiration techniques. Ultrasonography. 2019;38(2):166.
53. Cho W, Sim JS, Jung SL. Ultrasound-guided ethanol ablation for cystic thyroid nodules: effectiveness of small amounts of ethanol in a single session. Ultrasonography. 2021;40(3):417.
54. Zieleźnik W, Kawczyk-Krupka A, Barlik MP, Cebula W, Sieroń A. Modified percutaneous ethanol injection in the treatment of viscous cystic thyroid nodules. Thyroid. 2005;15(7):683–6.
55. Sung JY, Baek JH, Kim YS, Jeong HJ, Kwak MS, Lee D, et al. One-step ethanol ablation of viscous cystic thyroid nodules. Am J Roentgenol. 2008;191(6):1730–3.
56. Zhu Y, Zhang M, Jin Z, Tian X, Zhang Y, Xie F, et al. Solid benign thyroid nodules (> 10 ml): a retrospective study on the efficacy and safety of sonographically guided ethanol ablation combined with radiofrequency ablation. Int J Hyperthermia. 2020;37(1):157–67.
57. He L, Zhao W, Xia Z, Su A, Li Z, Zhu J. Comparative efficacy of different ultrasound-guided ablation for the treatment of benign thyroid nodules: systematic review and network meta-analysis of randomized controlled trials. PLoS One. 2021;16(1):e0243864.
58. Del Prete S, Russo D, Caraglia M, Giuberti G, Marra M, Vitale G, et al. Percutaneous ethanol injection of autonomous thyroid nodules with a volume larger than 40 ml: three years of follow-up. Clin Radiol. 2001;56(11):895–901.
59. Martino E, Murtas ML, Loviselli A, Piga M, Petrini L, Miccoli P, et al. Percutaneous intranodular ethanol injection for treatment of autonomously functioning thyroid nodules. Surgery. 1992;112(6):1161–5.
60. Papini E, Panunzi C, Pacella C, Bizzarri G, Fabbrini R, Petrucci L, et al. Percutaneous ultrasound-guided ethanol injection: a new treatment of toxic autonomously functioning thyroid nodules? J Clin Endocrinol Metabol. 1993;76(2):411–6.
61. Tarantino L, Francica G, Sordelli I, Sperlongano P, Parmeggiani D, Ripa C, et al. Percutaneous ethanol injection of hyperfunctioning thyroid nodules: long-term follow-up in 125 patients. Am J Roentgenol. 2008;190(3):800–8.
62. Jang SW, Baek JH, Kim JK, Sung JY, Choi H, Lim HK, et al. How to manage the patients with unsatisfactory results after ethanol ablation for thyroid nodules: role of radiofrequency ablation. Eur J Radiol. 2012;81(5):905–10.
63. Monzanl F, Golettl O, Caracclo N, Del Guerra P, Ferdeghinl M, Puccl E, et al. Percutaneous ethanol injection treatment of autonomous thyroid adenoma: hormonal and clinical evaluation. Clin Endocrinol (Oxf). 1992;36(5):491–7.
64. Park JS, Kim DW, Eun CK, Choi SJ, Rho MH. Long-term follow-up sonography of benign cystic thyroid nodules after a percutaneous ethanol injection: the incidence of malignancy-mimicking nodules. J Korean Radiol Soc. 2008;58(1):21–8.
65. Cesareo R, Naciu AM, Pasqualini V, Pelle G, Manfrini S, Tabacco G, et al. A rare complication following thyroid percutaneous ethanol injection: Plummer adenoma. Case Rep Endocrinol. 2017;2017:1026139.
66. Mulita F, Tchabashvili L, Verras G-I, Liolis E, Siouti S, Panagopoulos K, et al. Thyroid abscess as a complication of percutaneous ethanol ablation of cystic thyroid nodules. Endokrynol Pol. 2021;72(3):284–5.

67. Akasu H, Shimizu K, Kitagawa W, Naito Z, Kawanami O, Tanaka S. Histological study of papillary thyroid carcinoma treated with percutaneous ethanol injection therapy. Pathol Int. 2002;52(5–6):406–9.
68. Goletti O, Lenziardi M, De Negri F, Fiorini I, Lippolis P. Inoperable thyroid carcinoma: palliation with percutaneous injection of ethanol. Eur J Surg. 1993;159(11–12):639–41.
69. Isozaki T, Kiba T, Numata K, Saito S, Shimamura T, Kitamura T, et al. Medullary thyroid carcinoma with multiple hepatic metastases: treatment with transcatheter arterial embolization and percutaneous ethanol injection. Intern Med. 1999;38(1):17–21.
70. Fontenot TE, Deniwar A, Bhatia P, Al-Qurayshi Z, Randolph GW, Kandil E. Percutaneous ethanol injection vs reoperation for locally recurrent papillary thyroid cancer: a systematic review and pooled analysis. JAMA Otolaryngol Head Neck Surg. 2015;141(6):512–8.
71. Goyal RM, Jonklaas J, Burman KD. Management of recurrent cervical papillary thyroid cancer. Endocrinol Metab Clin North Am. 2014;43(2):565–72.
72. Hay ID, Charboneau JW. The coming of age of ultrasound-guided percutaneous ethanol ablation of selected neck nodal metastases in well-differentiated thyroid carcinoma, vol. 96. Oxford: Oxford University Press; 2011. p. 2717.
73. Heilo A, Sigstad E, Fagerlid KH, Håskjold OI, Grøholt KK, Berner A, et al. Efficacy of ultrasound-guided percutaneous ethanol injection treatment in patients with a limited number of metastatic cervical lymph nodes from papillary thyroid carcinoma. J Clin Endocrinol Metabol. 2011;96(9):2750–5.
74. Kim BM, Kim MJ, Kim E-K, Park SI, Park CS, Chung WY. Controlling recurrent papillary thyroid carcinoma in the neck by ultrasonography-guided percutaneous ethanol injection. Eur Radiol. 2008;18(4):835–42.
75. Kim SY, Kim S-M, Chang H, Kim B-W, Lim CY, Lee YS, et al. Long-term outcomes of ethanol injection therapy for locally recurrent papillary thyroid cancer. Eur Arch Otorrinolaringol. 2017;274(9):3497–501.
76. Lewis B, Hay I, Charboneau J, McIver B, Reading C, Goellner J. Percutaneous ethanol injection for treatment of cervical lymph node metastases in patients with papillary thyroid carcinoma. Am J Roentgenol. 2002;178(3):699–704.
77. Shin JE, Baek JH, Lee JH. Radiofrequency and ethanol ablation for the treatment of recurrent thyroid cancers: current status and challenges. Curr Opin Oncol. 2013;25(1):14–9.
78. Suh CH, Baek JH, Choi YJ, Lee JH. Efficacy and safety of radiofrequency and ethanol ablation for treating locally recurrent thyroid cancer: a systematic review and meta-analysis. Thyroid. 2016;26(3):420–8.

# Chapter 25
# Embolization of Goiter

**Alan A. Sag and Ravi N. Srinivasa**

The American Thyroid Association (ATA) treatment paradigm for symptomatic benign goiter has maintained that once bulk or hormonal symptoms exhaust nonsurgical management, patients are offered resection. However, some patients are high-risk candidates for surgery, while others are not interested in undergoing the operation. For these patients, goiter embolization is an emerging approach that can palliate goiter symptoms with a minimally invasive, outpatient, titrable, repeatable, thyroid-sparing, parathyroid-sparing, and recurrent laryngeal nerve-sparing procedure. This chapter presents a primer to thyroid artery embolization for goiter reduction (TAEGR) with special emphasis on nuances in pre-, intra-, and post-procedural patient management.

---

No Financial disclosures.

---

A. A. Sag (✉)
Department of Interventional Radiology, University of Miami Miller School of Medicine, Miami, FL, USA
e-mail: alan.sag@med.miami.edu

R. N. Srinivasa
Department of Radiology, Division of Interventional Radiology, University of California, Los Angeles, CA, USA


A. W. Park et al. (eds.), *Thyroid Radiofrequency Ablation*,
https://doi.org/10.1007/978-3-031-65288-2_25

## Background and Role of Radiofrequency Ablation and Embolization

RFA of thyroid nodules is a facile option in patients with one or several nodules [1], but patients with a large, multinodular gland or a difficult to access substernal goiter may benefit from a minimally invasive approach to shrink the entire thyroid gland. Transarterial embolization is a common method to devascularize and subsequently shrink hypervascular tissue. This has been demonstrated by interventional radiologists in the treatment of hypervascular tumors, such as hepatocellular carcinoma and uterine fibroids as well as in patients with enlarged prostate glands (benign prostatic hyperplasia, BPH) [2–4].

Blood supply to the thyroid gland is predictable, offering a simple minimally invasive approach to embolotherapy. Furthermore, in patients with enlarged glands, the blood vessels feeding the hypertrophied gland are generally enlarged themselves, making cannulation relatively easy. Embolization therapy is focused on using calibrated particles to reduce the amount of blood flow to the gland rather than eliminate it. This endpoint increases the odds that the patient will still have functional thyroidal tissue, reducing the risk of metabolic dysfunction requiring future medical therapy. Furthermore, once the gland has been reduced in size, select nodules can still be treated with RFA, if required. Some patients with hyperthyroidism may become euthyroid following thyroid artery embolization. While data for the treatment of benign disease is presently sparse, a recent study by Yilmaz et al. demonstrated 86% success (19/22) in converting hyperthyroid patients to a euthyroid state and a 57% decrease in total thyroid gland volume at 6 months following embolization [5].

TAEGR and RFA are best seen as complementary approaches, and may be used sequentially in the appropriate setting. Some considerations regarding the selection of RFA versus TAEGR are included in Table 25.1.

**Table 25.1** Examples of factors favoring RFA versus TAEGR

| | Favor RFA | Favor TAEGR |
|---|---|---|
| Goiter distribution | Focal nodules<br>AFTN<br>Supraclavicular | Large (>30 mL) clinical target volume<br>Retrosternal |
| Arterial supply | Non-hypertrophic | Hypertrophic vessels |
| Comorbidities | Renal insufficiency | Pacemaker<br>Anticoagulation desiring uninterruption<br>Solitary functional recurrent laryngeal nerve |
| Practice logistics | Office-based practice | Available cone beam CT |

## Pre-embolization Evaluation

Pre-embolization evaluation for patients considering thyroid artery embolization begins with a clinic consultation as well as laboratory workup to determine any baseline thyroid dysfunction. Uncorrectable coagulopathy and active infectious thyroiditis are absolute contraindications to thyroid artery embolization. Patients who are on thyroid medications prior to embolization should generally remain on these medications during the embolization procedure. A basic metabolic panel and blood calcium and/or parathyroid hormone levels should be checked to ensure no abnormalities to suggest parathyroid gland abnormalities. Patients should be evaluated for baseline symptoms including any airway compromise, positional dyspnea, dysphagia, hoarseness, and any evidence for toxic goiter, including palpitations, irritability, insomnia, anxiety, and weight loss. Patients with hypothyroidism may have fatigue, weight gain, constipation, and joint pain.

Evaluation of the thyroid gland arterial supply prior to performing embolization is paramount for patient safety and procedural success. Pre-procedure imaging may include thyroid ultrasound; however, delineation of the arterial supply to the gland and any anatomic variation is important. Any nodules, which have suspicious features on ultrasound imaging, should be biopsied (using fine-needle aspiration, FNA) prior to intervention. The Duke-University of California, Los Angeles algorithm involves obtaining a pre-procedure computed tomography angiography study of the neck to ascertain any anatomic variation. Imaging should be performed in the arterial and venous phase. Typically, the inferior thyroidal arteries (ITA) arise directly from the thyrocervical trunk, which arise from the subclavian arteries bilaterally (Fig. 25.1). The ITA is the dominant supply to the gland and typically first to be embolized. The superior thyroidal arteries (STA) are branches arising from the external carotid artery and are only embolized if ITA embolization fails. In patients who have had prior vertebral artery or carotid artery occlusion, collaterals may potentially develop which may involve the thyrocervical trunk. Determining whether such collaterals may be present is crucial to ensuring the safety of particle embolization of the gland to avoid embolic transgression into the cerebral circulation. Patients who have such collaterals would either need coil embolization of collaterals or may not be suitable candidates for thyroid artery embolization. Branch patterns can also be identified on pre-procedure imaging including the origin of the suprascapular arteries and the transverse cervical artery to plan optimal catheter positioning during the TAEGR procedure.

Pre-procedure imaging also helps with planning the treatment approach. Patients, who have a predominantly unilateral nodule, may have supply from only one vessel (Fig. 25.2). In these cases, sometimes a radial approach may be preferred as the left or right inferior thyroidal artery can be easily selected from an ipsilateral radial access. If nodules are bilateral and large, it is generally necessary to select and embolize both inferior thyroidal arteries. In these cases, a femoral approach may be

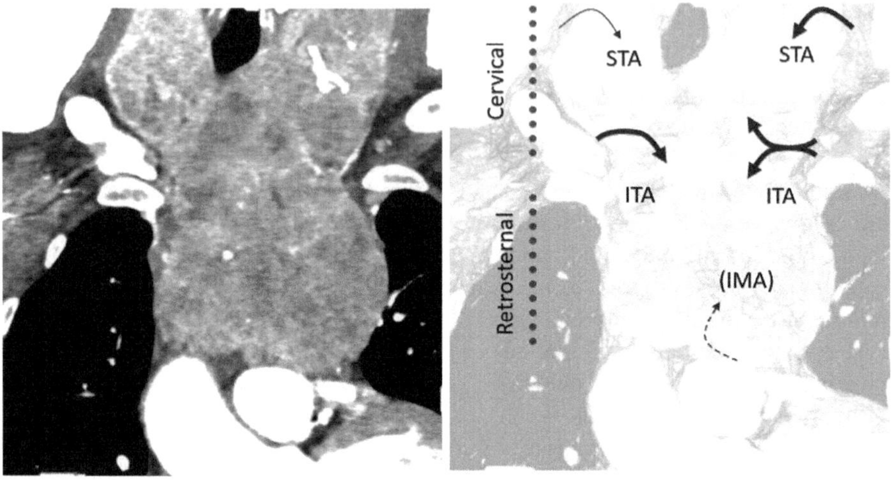


**Fig. 25.1** Standard vascularization of thyroid goiter. The ITA (inferior thyroid artery) typically supplies the posterior–inferior gland accounting for mass effect on aerodigestive structures. The STA (superior thyroid artery) typically supplies the cervical goiter accounting for mass effect as well as cosmesis. Thyroidea ima (IMA) is a variant supply arising rarely directly from the aorta. The above diagram depicts a mixed cervical and retrosternal goiter with dominant supply from the bilateral inferior thyroid arteries and left superior thyroid artery (thick arrows). The diminutive right STA is represented to have a non-hypertrophic arterial supply and would not be targeted with embolization

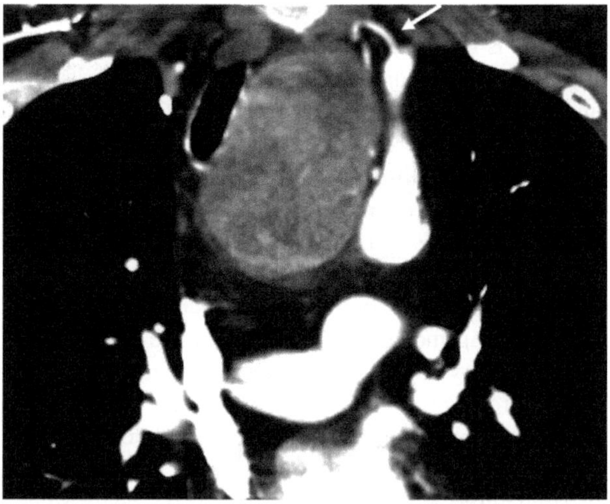

**Fig. 25.2** Pre-procedural CTA demonstrating the vascular anatomy feeding the substernal left thyroid nodule from a dominant left inferior thyroidal artery. This demonstrates that a left radial artery approach would be adequate for the embolization procedure

preferred to avoid crossing multiple arch vessels, which would be necessary from a unilateral radial approach to treat both inferior thyroid arteries. The presence of a substernal glandular component can also be determined with cross-sectional imaging.

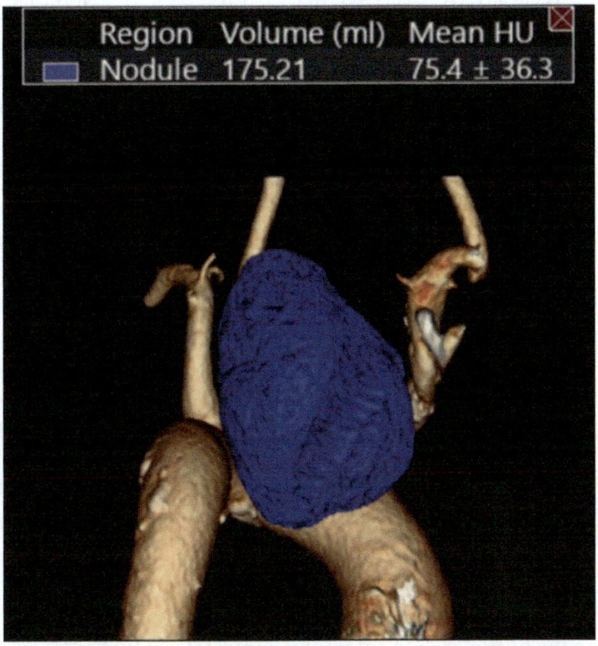


**Fig. 25.3** Three-dimensional reconstruction of the dominant substernal left thyroid nodule on CTA imaging demonstrating a volume of 175 cc

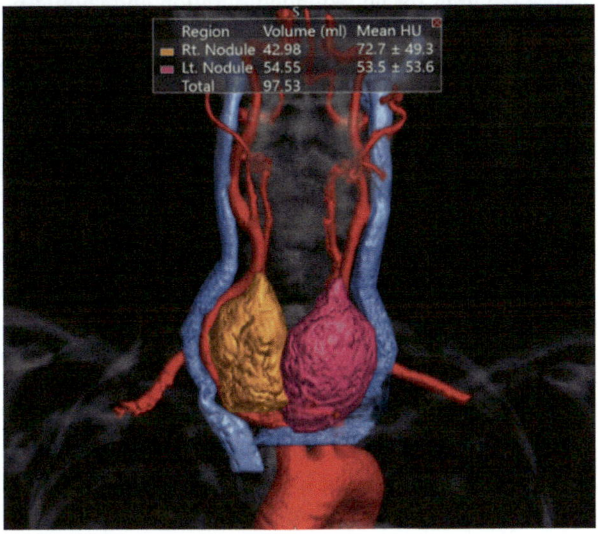


**Fig. 25.4** Three-dimensional reconstructions from CTA imaging demonstrating a bilaterally enlarged gland with a total volume of 97 cc

Additionally, accurate volumetrics of the gland (Figs. 25.3 and 25.4) can be obtained using three-dimensional reconstruction of the pre-procedure CTA imaging allowing for definitive calculation of individual nodular and total glandular volume. This aids in calculating response to therapy following embolization.

Pre-embolization T3, T4, and thyroid stimulation hormone (TSH) levels can be obtained to ensure there is no thyroid dysfunction on the day of the procedure. Just prior to the embolization procedure, patients are treated with dexamethasone 10 mg intravenously to minimize inflammation of the gland during the embolization. They should also be given a pre-procedure intravenous (IV) antibiotic, typically cefazolin 2 g intravenously. As much as 30 mg of ketorolac can be given intravenously before or after embolization.

## Procedural Technique

The arterial approach to the thyroid can take one of three approaches with benefits and risks to both. Optimal planning will start from the pre-procedure imaging, ideally with arterial phase imaging documenting which arteries are hypertrophied. In general, for patients needing treatment of the right and left hemithyroid at the same session (for example, bilateral inferior thyroid artery embolization), a femoral arterial approach will allow access to both arteries from a single site. For isolated unilateral treatments, the respective radial arterial approach can be considered. Finally, a right radial approach can be used with an inverted reverse curve catheter formed in the aortic arch to select the contralateral thyroidal arteries, and while radial access does typically involve heparinization, this approach does leave instrumentation across the arch for an extended duration and should be considered in patients with extremely tortuous aortic arches or arch configurations where selection of the left carotid/subclavian arteries may be challenging (for superior thyroid artery (STA)/ and inferior thyroid artery (ITA) embolizations, respectively). Relative benefits to radial access, in general, are in patients with unfavorable aortofemoral anatomy, habitus, or inability to hold blood thinners (to minimize risk of hematoma).

Operator preference will guide catheter selection. From the groin, a headhunter type catheter is the typical first-line selection for arch navigation. From the radial approach, for an ipsilateral selection of the thyrocervical trunk a Judkins right 2.5 (JR-2.5) base catheter or C2 cobra catheter can be considered. If right arterial access is performed with intent to cross the arch for left hemigoiter embolization, a Simmons 2-shaped catheter can be formed (upside down relative to most visceral IR applications) via the right radial in the aortic arch and brought cranially to select the left carotid and subclavian arteries. Microcatheter selection will depend on the artery size, though, in general, a 2.4-Fr microcatheter (Fig. 25.5) will be small enough to track over the operator's choice of microwire without causing spasm and while leaving sufficient perimicrocatheter flow to carry embolics in a flow-directed fashion, while also being large enough to generate sufficient supraphysiologic intraarterial contrast pressure to visualize aberrant collaterals at the cone beam (described later) and minimize embolic agent clumping (described later). Spasm or occlusive microcatheters may lead to flow redistribution into unsuspected collaterals and, therefore, larger microcatheter systems should be approached with caution but again tailored to the anatomy at hand.

In the Duke-UCLA TAEGR protocol embolization is taken to a five-beat stasis endpoint without additional maneuvers such as PErFecTED [6]. Calibrated embolic

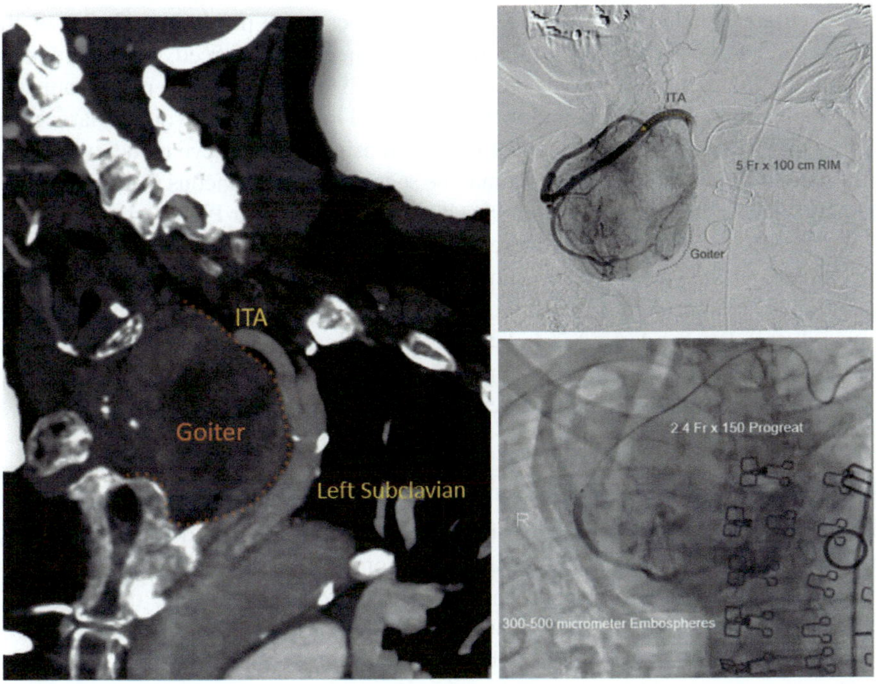


**Fig. 25.5** CT Arteriogram demonstrating dominant inferior thyroid artery (ITA) catheterized with a RIM catheter and superselectively catheterized with 2.4 Fr microcatheter prior to embolization

agents are used to target a tissue bed with capillary size on average 120–250 μm, as described by Xiao et al. [7]. Given the potential for intrathyroidal aberrant collateral networks that may connect to aerodigestive structures, facial tissues, or the spinal cord, two steps are taken in an abundance of caution at the authors' institutions. In the Duke-UCLA TAEGR protocol, every artery that is embolized is first injected with cone beam CT to ensure that there is no collateral flow to dangerous structures. The second safety step is that particles one size larger are used (300–500 μm) to prevent any possible passage of particles across the known intrathyroidal arterio-arterial connections. These connections may be evident at the outset, may be evident at cone beam CT, or may manifest as embolic are delivered in a flow-directed fashion and flow redistribution occurs in the downstream bed. Therefore, the embolization is performed cautiously with dilute particles to minimize embolic clumping and with frequent clearing of the microcatheter and brief angiographic or fluoroscopic contrast injections to ensure the forward flow is intact and rule out interval aberrant flow. A vasodilator can be included in the injectate. As a comparison, in the Yilmaz protocol, a 355–500 μm Contour PVA (Contour; Boston Scientific, Natick, Massachusetts, USA) was diluted 1:1 with contrast into an 80–100 mL volume and mixed with 5 mg papaverine. Of note, in the Duke-UCLA protocol, the preferred embolic is Embospheres (Merit Medical Systems, South Jordan, UT, USA) due to the relative non-compressibility of the embolic agent, which has a few benefits: (1) it further avoids the possibility of clumping sometimes seen with PVA, which could clog the microcatheter, leading to potential loss of microcatheter position to flush out the microcatheter versus risking reflux if further injection is forced, (2) the reduced clumping of particles also avoids premature embolization of the larger upstream arterioles and allows deeper penetration, (3) calibrated microspheres avoid the larger particles that can be seen in PVA (which is created using a serial sieve model with a size minimum cutoff but larger particles may be seen in a heterogeneous fashion), and (4) trisacryl-gelatin beads are less compressible than the Contour PVA particles because Contour SE particles are microporous and release water under compression with incomplete elastic recovery [8] compared to Embospheres. In practical terms, if Contour SE is injected hard enough, it can squeeze into vessels that may be smaller (more distal) than the desired embolic target range. In this territory, that raises the possibility of nontarget embolization. This effect was considered one of the reasons why Embospheres became the preferred embolic agent over Contour SE in the uterus for fibroids, for example, Refs. [8–10].

The choice of which arteries to embolize (assuming there are two superior and two inferior thyroid arteries with no thyroidea ima) has varied in the published protocols. Notably, none of the protocols advocate for whole-thryoid embolization in a single session when the intent of embolization is monotherapy (as compared to preoperative embolization where pan-thyroidal ischemia may be desirable). As such, most operators will treat two or three of the arteries. In general, the STA arises from carotid artery distribution, and for this reason, embolization of the STA may lead to nontarget embolization of the brain. In patients with retrosternal goiter, the dominant artery may be the ITA in most cases. Similarly, patients with cervical goiter may have superior thyroid artery dominant supply. Therefore, the anatomy of the goiter will determine the target vessels for embolization. Finally, the superior parathyroid glands are supplied by the superior thyroid artery only 15% of the time and supplied by the inferior thyroid artery in the remaining 85% of cases [11]. Studies using laser Doppler flowmetry [12] have shown that the parathyroid gland only suffers 40% flow reduction with isolated embolization of the ITA or the STA. However, occlusion of both the ITA and the STA on the same side at the same time creates profound parathyroid ischemia [13]. As a result, in the Duke-UCLA TAEGR protocol treatment usually favors treating the inferior thyroid arteries on one or both sides at the first session to determine whether sufficient shrinkage is achieved. If not, a more aggressive embolization can then be undertaken with superior thyroid artery embolization considered. Since patients undergoing TAEGR are usually not surgical candidates or are refusing surgery, the only comparable available treatment option would include RFA, which would require multiple treatment sessions; therefore, this is generally a tolerated approach by the patient if multiple embolization sessions are required. As previously mentioned, for large retrosternal goiters, thyroid RFA is usually not an option.

In general, TAEGR is not painful, and the entire procedure can be performed with local anesthesia, only if desired. This may be desired if the patient is of sufficient age where a paradoxical reaction to sedation medications is a concern. The procedure usually lasts approximately 60–90 min.

Intraprocedural prophylactic antibiotics are provided (Cefazolin 1 or 2 g IV based on local institutional protocols). Intravenous dexamethasone 10 mg is given before the procedure to prevent the conversion of T4–T3, which helps reduce hyperthyroid symptoms. If a patient was already on a beta blocker, it is continued. But, if they were not using one before the procedure and their heart beats too fast afterward (tachycardia), they might need a short course of metoprolol. For example, they could take 50 mg of metoprolol each day for 1–2 weeks until their thyroid hormone levels stabilize, which usually happens about 30 days after the procedure. Tachycardia and symptomatic hyperthyroidism are rare. Post-procedure pain is also rare; in patients with sufficient renal function, Toradol 15 or 30 mg IV are provided, and the patient is sent home with instructions to take Tylenol and Advil for analgesia at home. This is performed as an outpatient procedure.

## Post-procedure Follow-Up

In the post-procedure recovery room, patients sometimes will already notice an improvement in their compressive symptoms. Patients are counseled regarding the usual post-embolization syndrome symptoms such as low-grade fever, malaise, and pain; however, these are generally very well controlled with non-steroidal anti-inflammatory drugs (NSAIDS) (alternating acetaminophen and ibuprofen). Patients are provided with a steroid taper (Medrol dose pack) to allow continued suppression of T4 activation into T3 while at home. Blood work is obtained on day 7 to assess for peak TSH suppression and the patient is provided clinical follow-up at this time to assess for symptoms of hyperthyroidism, most importantly related to heart rate and rhythm. Blood work in clinical follow-up is then repeated on day 30. Follow-up imaging is based on local protocol and is mainly to document the degree of shrinkage since any decision to re-intervene will mainly be prompted by clinical, persistent or recurrent symptoms and not by imaging findings alone. In particularly aggressive embolizations (STA + ITA) or in patients who have had prior hemithyroidectomy with possibly limited parathyroid reserve, parathyroid blood work can also be obtained. While the patient's symptoms may improve rapidly, the shrinkage of the goiter is expected to occur more gradually with approximately 50% reduction of the clinical target volume at 6 months, based on currently available data [5].

## Conclusion

TAEGR is emerging as a treatment option for inoperable goiter with compressive bulk symptoms. This may be especially helpful in very large (>30 mL) and retrosternal goiters in patients, who are unable or unwilling to undergo surgery, where thyroid RFA is expected to require multiple treatment sessions and/or may not be feasible due to intervening sternum. TAEGR is a thyroid-sparing, parathyroid-sparing, titrable, repeatable, stageable, minimally invasive nonsurgical option that minimizes chance of vocal nerve injury and can improve goiter symptoms including pain, dyspnea, dysphagia, sleep apnea, and cosmetic disfigurement.

**Acknowledgments** The authors acknowledge Dr. Ari Isaacson as the interventional radiologist originally developing the term TAEGR to describe this procedure in 2021.

## References

1. Park HS, Baek JH, Park AW, Chung SR, Choi YJ, Lee JH. Thyroid radiofrequency ablation: updates on innovative devices and techniques. Korean J Radiol. 2017;18(4):615–23.
2. Carnevale FC, de Assis AM, Moreira AM. Prostatic artery embolization: equipment, procedure steps, and overcoming technical challenges. Tech Vasc Interv Radiol. 2020;23(3):100691.
3. Keung JJ, Spies JB, Caridi TM. Uterine artery embolization: a review of current concepts. Best Pract Res Clin Obstet Gynaecol. 2018;46:66–73.
4. Facciorusso A. Drug-eluting beads transarterial chemoembolization for hepatocellular carcinoma: current state of the art. World J Gastroenterol. 2018;24(2):161–9.
5. Yilmaz S, Habibi HA, Yildiz A, Altunbas H. Thyroid embolization for nonsurgical treatment of nodular goiter: a single-center experience in 56 consecutive patients. J Vasc Interv Radiol. 2021;32(10):1449–56.
6. Carnevale FC, Moreira AM, Antunes AA. The "PErFecTED technique": proximal embolization first, then embolize distal for benign prostatic hyperplasia. Cardiovasc Intervent Radiol. 2014;37(6):1602–5.
7. Xiao H, Zhuang W, Wang S, Yu B, Chen G, Zhou M, et al. Arterial embolization: a novel approach to thyroid ablative therapy for Graves' disease. J Clin Endocrinol Metab. 2002;87(8):3583–9.
8. Laurent A. Microspheres and nonspherical particles for embolization. Tech Vasc Interv Radiol. 2007;10(4):248–56.
9. Golzarian J, Lang E, Hovsepian D, Kroncke T, Lampmann L, Lohle P, et al. Higher rate of partial devascularization and clinical failure after uterine artery embolization for fibroids with spherical polyvinyl alcohol. Cardiovasc Intervent Radiol. 2006;29(1):1–3.
10. Spies JB, Allison S, Flick P, Cramp M, Bruno J, Jha RC, et al. Spherical polyvinyl alcohol versus tris-acryl gelatin microspheres for uterine artery embolization for leiomyomas: results of a limited randomized comparative study. J Vasc Interv Radiol. 2005;16(11):1431–7.
11. Lyden ML, Wang TS, Sosa JA. Surgical anatomy of the thyroid gland. In: Carty SE, editor. MA: UpToDate Inc. Accessed 16 Sept 2018.
12. Sanabria A, Kowalski LP, Tartaglia F. Inferior thyroid artery ligation increases hypocalcemia after thyroidectomy: a meta-analysis. Laryngoscope. 2018;128(2):534–41.
13. Johansson K, Ander S, Lennquist S, Smeds S. Human parathyroid blood supply determined by laser-Doppler flowmetry. World J Surg. 1994;18(3):417–20.

# Chapter 26
# Minimal Interventions for Head and Neck Neoplasms Beyond the Thyroid

**Wan Ni Lin and Wei-Che Lin**

## Introduction

Neck masses can develop from various sources, including infectious, inflammatory, congenital, benign, or malignant processes. In pediatric patients, unlike adults, the most common causes of neck masses are infections and congenital abnormalities [1, 2]. A list of common neck mass differential diagnoses is presented in Table 26.1 [1–8].

Management of benign neck neoplasms typically involves surgical excision, sclerotherapy, or trans-arterial embolization (TAE), depending on the nature and location of the lesion. Complete surgical excision is considered the ideal treatment for benign lesions. However, anatomical factors can pose challenges and potential morbidity associated with surgical treatment. The risks of scar formation, morphological deformity, and potential nerve or vascular injury have led to recent exploration of less invasive surgical approaches as well as nonsurgical therapies.

In recent years, minimally invasive interventions, such as ablation therapy, have been proposed to address the challenges of head and neck area lesions, aiming to minimize complications and resolve aesthetic issues associated with bulky lesions.

W. N. Lin (✉)
Department of Otolaryngology Head and Neck Surgery, Chung Gung Memorial Hospital, Linkou Medical Center, Taoyuan, Taiwan
e-mail: y1829@cgmh.org.tw

W.-C. Lin (✉)
Department of Diagnostic Radiology, Kaohsiung Chang Gung Memorial Hospital, Chang Gung University College of Medicine, Kaohsiung, Taiwan

Thyroid Head and Neck Ablation Center, Kaohsiung Chang Gung Memorial Hospital, Kaohsiung, Taiwan

College of Medicine, National Sun Yat-Sen University, Kaohsiung, Taiwan


A. W. Park et al. (eds.), *Thyroid Radiofrequency Ablation*, https://doi.org/10.1007/978-3-031-65288-2_26

**Table 26.1** Differential diagnosis of common neck masses

| Infectious | Congenital anomaly | Benign neoplasm | Malignancy |
|---|---|---|---|
| – Viral infection<br>– *Bartonella henselae* (cat-scratch disease)<br>– Tuberculous cervical lymphadenitis<br>– Ludwig's angina<br>– Sialadenitis | – Thyroglossal duct cyst<br>– Brachial cleft cyst<br>– Lymphatic or venous malformations<br>– Hemangioma<br>– Teratoma | – Lipoma<br>– Neurofibroma<br>– Schwannoma<br>– Plunging ranula | – Metastatic lymph node<br>– Lymphoma<br>– Salivary gland cancer<br>– Thyroid cancer |

Tumor ablation involves the direct application of chemical or thermal energy to induce cellular necrosis within the tumor. Various modalities have been employed for ablation, including ethanol ablation (EA), microwave ablation, and radiofrequency ablation (RFA). The choice of treatment modality depends on clinical characteristics, disease location, tumor size, and the overall condition of the patient.

Pretreatment evaluation for neck masses typically includes ultrasound (US), computed tomography (CT), and magnetic resonance (MR) imaging to assess the relationships between the lesion and the surrounding soft tissues.

This introductory section offers a concise overview of the common application of minimal intervention therapy for head and neck benign neoplasms other than thyroid lesions.

## Ethanol Ablation (EA) in Head and Neck

Ethanol, with its low side-effect profiles, affordability, and widespread availability, is a valuable therapeutic agent. It has found new indications, particularly as an embolization, sclerosing, or ablation agent. Ethanol induces cellular dehydration and protein denaturation, resulting in coagulation necrosis, small vessel thrombosis, hemorrhagic infarction, and reactive fibrosis, ultimately leading to regression of cysts [9].

Ethanol sclerotherapy for benign neck neoplasms had been introduced from treating venous malformation in the 1990s [10]. Treatment options for venous malformations (VM) include surgical excision, sclerotherapy, and a combination of both approaches. Venous malformations located diffusely in superficial areas or with ill-defined margins are less effectively managed through surgery alone. Total excision of large VMs can be a significant challenge and may lead to severe complications, including hemorrhage and undesirable scar formation [11]. Ethanol sclerotherapy has been reported as an effective treatment for head and neck venous malformations, reducing both functional and cosmetic impairments, in both pediatric and adult patients [12–26]. Treatment can be performed percutaneously for aesthetic purposes, or through directed injection to deep lesions to relieve symptoms (such as tongue VM injection [17]). Besides VMs, ethanol sclerotherapy is commonly used in the neck region for the treatment of cystic neoplasms, including conditions such as thyroglossal duct cyst (TGDC), brachial cleft cyst (BCC), ranula, and lymphatic malformations [10, 19, 20, 24, 25, 27–34].

The most common method for neck cyst ablation is percutaneous ethanol injection under an ultrasound (US)-guided procedure. US-guided aspiration of the cystic fluid was followed by injection of absolute ethanol (95–99%). The injected ethanol might be removed completely afterward [28, 29, 31], or little volume of ethanol injected was left inside the cyst after the procedure was completed [28, 30, 32, 34, 35].

Reported volume reductions for thyroglossal duct cyst (TGDC) and brachial cleft cyst (BCC) have approached nearly 100% in some cases [20, 28, 29, 34]. EA for TGDC and BCC has shown successful treatment outcomes in approximately 60–80% of patients [10, 20, 27, 29]. However, repeat EA procedures have demonstrated low efficacy [20, 32]. Patients with BCC typically require more EA sessions than those with thyroid cysts or TGDC [29, 32]. This difference may be attributed to the presence of watery or cheesy secretions with exfoliated cells within the BCC lumen, hindering direct contact of ethanol with the inner epithelial surface. According to a cohort study on ethanol injection for neck cystic neoplasms by Liao et al. [32], the recurrence rate and the number of ethanol injections tend to increase with larger cystic volumes.

EA can be considered as an alternative nonsurgical approach for ranulas, especially in cases with recent onset symptoms, where the complete response rate was significantly higher in patients with symptoms lasting less than or equal to 12 months [31]. However, it exhibits a higher recurrence rate when compared to other cystic lesions. A plunging ranula is a pseudocyst or mucocele caused by the leakage of saliva from the sublingual or minor salivary gland through the mylohyoid muscle into the upper neck region. This continuous secretion of saliva contributes to the observed high recurrence rate [32].

## Radiofrequency Ablation (RFA) in Head and Neck

Radiofrequency ablation RFA remains the most widely used ablative technique [36].

RFA for head and neck neoplasm had been reported preliminary from 1999 [37]. This technique can be performed percutaneously (as shown in Fig. 26.1) or through

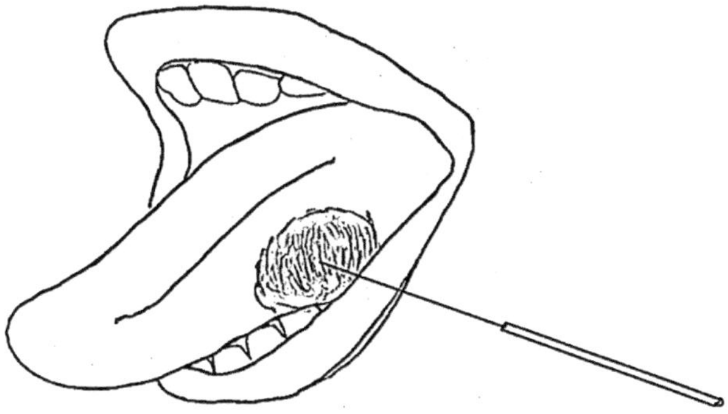

**Fig. 26.1** Ablation tip directly puncturing into a lesion

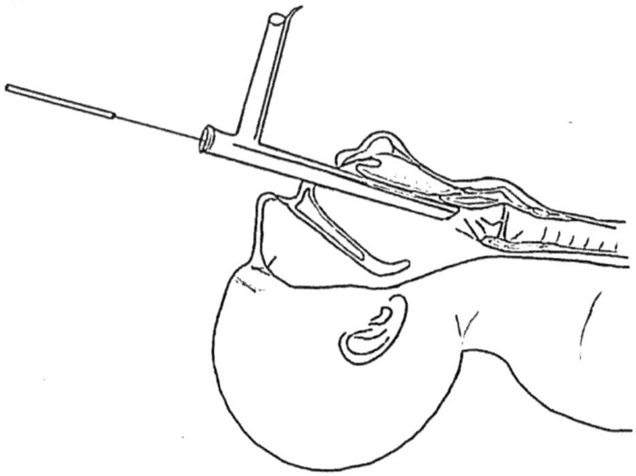

**Fig. 26.2** Ablation therapy under endoscopic guidance

directed puncturing under endoscopic guidance (as illustrated in Fig. 26.2), CT guidance, or ultrasonography (US) guidance, all of which can be done under local anesthesia or general anesthesia [38]. Percutaneous RFA guided by ultrasound (US) is often the preferred first option for head and neck neoplasms due to its ease of availability, absence of radiation exposure, and the ability to provide real-time imaging. It is worth noting that RFA with monopolar generators is contraindicated in patients with cardiac pacemakers or other nerve pacing devices due to the potential for unwanted physiological effects [39].

Vascular anomalies are commonly present from birth or early childhood. These anomalies are categorized into hemangiomas and vascular malformations following the classification by Mulliken and Glowacki [40]. Surgeries for patients with larger or poorly defined margin head and neck VM have often yielded less effective outcomes [11]. Percutaneous sclerotherapy had been replacing surgery in first-line treatment for VM; however, there is potential risk of lesion re-expansion, skin necrosis, nerve damage, and pulmonary embolism [41]. RFA may be offered as an alternative treatment option for symptomatic head and neck VM [42]. Several studies have shown that RFA can achieve good results in terms of VRRs and cosmetic satisfaction, with a minimal rate of complications [42–47].

Cranio-orbital neurofibromatosis is a subtype of neurofibromatosis type 1, which was initially described by von Recklinghausen in 1882 [48]. Head and neck neurofibromatosis often showed craniofacial deformities caused by bone alterations and soft-tissue infiltration. Surgical procedures usually cannot completely eradicate the disease. Neurofibromatosis progresses slowly and irregularly, with occasional accelerations during puberty and pregnancy. RFA has been introduced as a method to relieve symptoms, such as airway compression, and slow the natural progression of plexiform neurofibroma [49, 50]. In the limited clinical reports, RFA has a fair result in tumor shrinkage with symptoms' relief and no neurologic complication [47, 51, 52]. Fig. 26.3 demonstrates RFA treatment for a 5-year-old female patient, who had right temporal fossa plexiform neurofibroma. The lesion nearly completely disappeared 2 months after RFA.

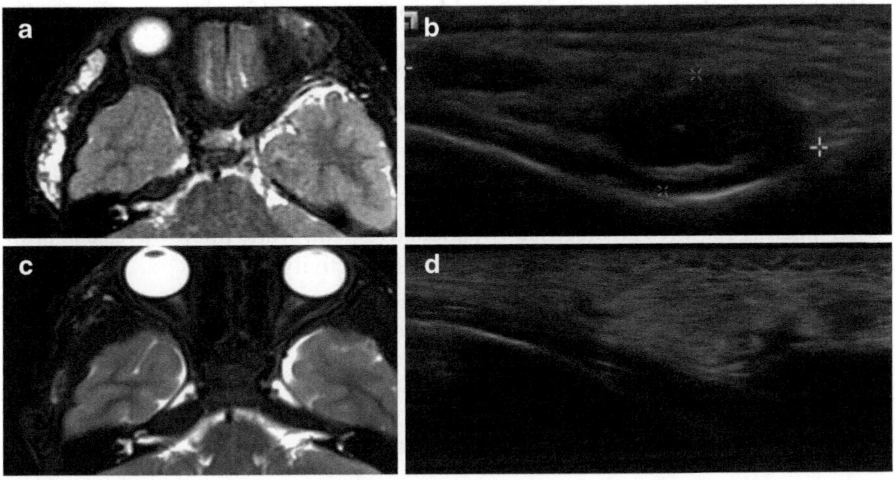


**Fig. 26.3** A 5-year-old female patient presented with a progressively bulging lesion in the right temporal area. Images **a** and **b** show a plexiform neurofibroma in the right temporal fossa before treatment. Images **c** and **d** demonstrate nearly complete lesion disappearance 2 months after RFA

## Microwave Ablation (MWA) in Head and Neck

A microwave generator emits an electromagnetic wave through the exposed, non-insulated portion of the antenna. Electromagnetic microwaves agitate water molecules in the surrounding tissue, producing friction and heat, ultimately inducing cellular death via coagulation necrosis [53] Microwave technology offers several key advantages, including consistently higher intra-tumoral temperatures, the ability to ablate larger tumor volumes, shorter ablation times, and an improved convection profile [54]. This technique has proven to be a valuable tool in managing highly vascularized lesions such as angiolipoma [55], epistaxis, [56] or nasal cavity hemangioma [57]. Ablation of pharyngeal lesions, such as a papilloma or a cyst, under an endoscopic-guide [58] has also been reported. MWA enables both lesion removal and hemostasis with the same instrument under local anesthesia.

In the case of ultrasound-guided percutaneous microwave ablation, it has been shown to be a safe and effective treatment for parotid gland adenolymphoma [59], with tumor VRRs at the 1- and 3-month follow-up being 53% and 82%, respectively, and the remnant finally disappeared at 8 months with no recurrence at 2 years.

**Differences Between RFA and MWA in Treating Head and Neck Lesion**

- RFA is more commercially available worldwide.
- Microwaves (MWA) offer deeper tissue heating, and multiple antenna arrays provide the advantage of constructive interference between antennae. This can

lead to a quicker creation of larger ablation zones, making it more effective for treating tumors located in proximity to blood vessels [60].
- MVA results appear to be similar to RFA for lesions smaller than 3 cm. For tumors larger than 3 cm, MWA can be conducted using multiple probes simultaneously [61].
- MVA seems to be more effective for the ablation of cystic tumors and lesions located close to vessels larger than 3 mm [62].
- RF heating requires an electrically conductive path, while microwaves can propagate through materials with low or zero conductivity [63].
- MWA can benefit patients with electrical implants, such as a pacemaker, or those who cannot be treated with either bipolar or monopolar cautery with suction [64].

## Minimal Intervention for Parotid Tumor

Salivary gland tumors are among the most common tumors in the oral and maxillofacial regions. Warthin tumors (WT) have been identified as the second most-frequent benign tumor of the parotid gland, following pleomorphic adenoma, accounting for 4–25% of all salivary gland tumors [65]. The risk of malignant transformation is extremely low (less than 1%), and the growth rate can be slow. Due to the low risk of malignant transformation, combined with the risks of surgery, minimal intervention treatments have been proposed, such as microwave ablation, RFA, and ultrasound-guided ethanol sclerotherapy for selected cases [66–69]. Ablation, whether through chemical or thermal mechanisms, of the tissue within the tumor capsule can be effective for volume reduction as well as reducing the risk of facial nerve injury by surgical intervention.

The sclerosing effect of ethanol is efficacious in partial and near-total reduction of parotid tumors, especially in cystic-type lesions [32, 35, 69, 70]. Ethanol sclerotherapy (ES) has been previously performed in conjunction with partial parotidectomy for patients, who wish to achieve a definitive diagnosis while also minimizing the risk of complications associated with extensive parotidectomy [35]. ES has been used in human immunodeficiency virus (HIV)-positive patients with benign lymphoepithelial parotid cysts [70]. Good volume reduction efficiency also provides satisfactory cosmetic results [69]. C.-H.C. and S.-D.L et al. report the long-term outcome of RFA for Warthin tumors, indicating that cystic WT had better volume reduction VRRs than solid WT. Figure 26.4 demonstrates RFA treatment for a 58-year-old male patient with a right parotid Warthin tumor. The lesion decreased in size 5 months after radiofrequency ablation (RFA), resulting in cosmetic satisfaction.

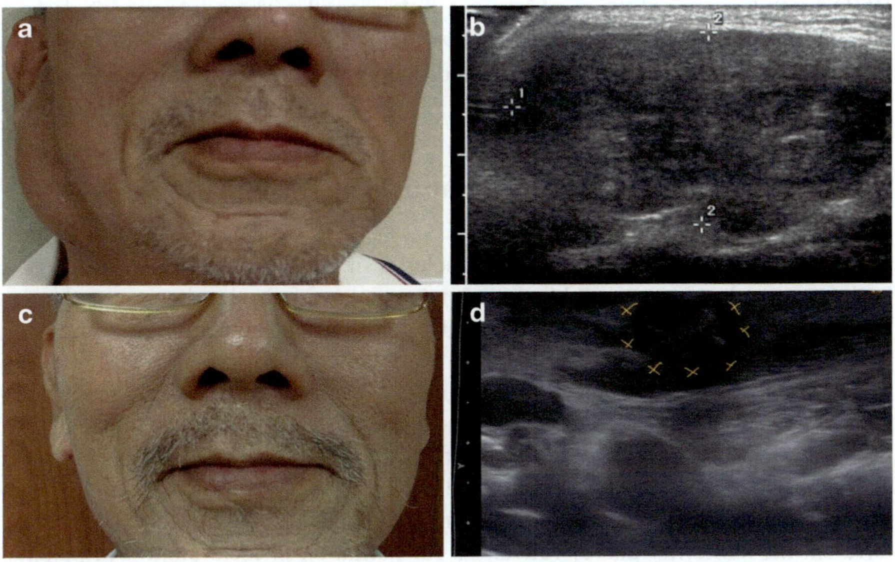

**Fig. 26.4** A 58-year-old male patient presented with a progressively bulging lesion in the right infra-auricular area. Images **a** and **b** depict the pretreatment image of a right parotid Warthin tumor. Images **c** and **d** show the condition 5 months after RFA

## Minimal Intervention for Parathyroid Gland

While surgical parathyroidectomy remains the optimal treatment for symptomatic hyperparathyroidism, it may not be suitable for patients at high surgical risk, such as those with head and neck deformities or a history of neck surgery with soft tissue fibrosis, or for patients who are hesitant about surgery. In such cases, minimally invasive treatment becomes an alternative choice. Ultrasound-guided EA for parathyroid treatment was initially proposed in the 1980s. [71–73] However, the early 2000s saw a rapid development in ultrasound-guided thermal ablation techniques for parathyroid lesions [36], including laser ablation [74, 75], microwave ablation [76, 77], and radiofrequency ablation (RFA) [78]. Due to its availability and low complication rate, RFA has become the most common thermal ablation option for parathyroid lesions. These minimally invasive parathyroid therapies, after long-term follow-up, have demonstrated fair results in terms of volume reduction rates and symptomatic relief, with minor or transient complications. However, the most critical aspect is accurately identifying the target lesion before treatment. C.-Y. L. and

W.-C. L et al. proposed the combination of ultrasound with four-dimensional computed tomography (4D-CT) for optimal preoperative localization before ablation therapy in patients with primary or secondary hyperparathyroidism [79].

## Minimal Intervention for Head and Neck Malignancy

The complete resection of neck malignancies is of utmost importance, considering both functional and anatomical factors. It is crucial to emphasize that minimal intervention is not intended to replace potentially curative management in head and neck malignancies.

Previously reported articles have introduced local invasive ablation techniques designed to provide local control of unresectable tumors and enhance the quality of life for patients, who have not responded to standard curative treatments. The application of RFA to treat malignant head and neck tumors was introduced in 2002 [38, 80]. Thermal ablation methods, including RFA and microwave ablation (MVA), have shown feasibility and effectiveness for palliation or local control in patients with incurable head and neck malignancies [80–86]. Figure 26.5 demonstrates the use of RFA treatment for tumor bulking in a 49-year-old male patient with a history of multiple head and neck cancers, who had previously undergone multiple surgical resections and concurrent chemoradiation therapy (CCRT). One month after the treatment, there is clear evidence of tumor regression, along with relief from symptoms.

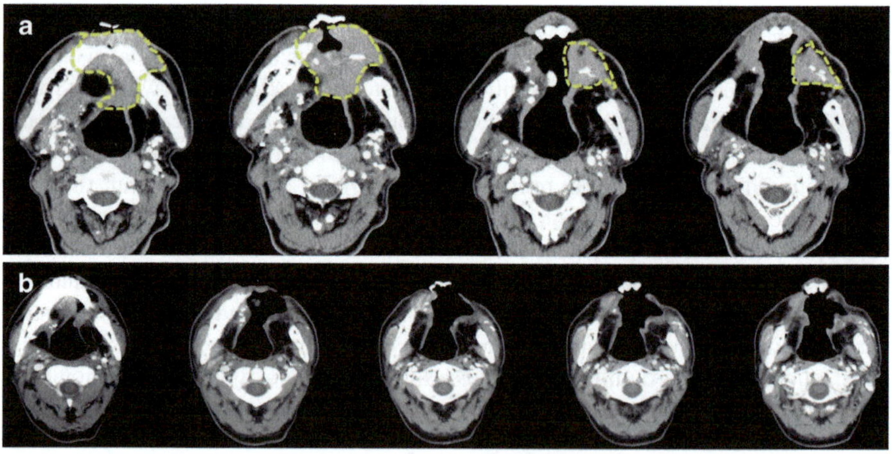


**Fig. 26.5** A 49-year-old male patient had multiple oral and oropharyngeal cancer (tonsil cancer, tongue cancer, buccal cancer, gum cancer, and low lip cancer) status post multiple surgical resections and concurrent chemoradiation therapy (CCRT) . A pretreatment image of tumor recurrent in the oral cavity. The yellow dotted line indicated the tumor area. B showed of local tumor regression 1 month after RFA

## Conclusion

Minimally invasive treatment may serve as an alternative option for managing neck neoplasms with the aim of providing symptomatic relief or improving aesthetics. It can also be used in conjunction with major surgical procedures to minimize the extent of resection. Ablation techniques can be guided using ultrasound (US), CT, or endoscopy, depending on the lesion's characteristics and the operator's preference. Numerous published reports highlight favorable VRRs and minimal complications.

## References


1. Spinelli C, Ricci E, Berti P, Miccoli P. [Neck masses in childhood. Surgical experience in 154 cases]. Minerva Pediatr. 1990;42:169–172.
2. Park YW. Evaluation of neck masses in children. Am Fam Physician. 1995;51:1904–12.
3. McGuirt WF. The neck mass. Med Clin North Am. 1999;83:219–34. https://doi.org/10.1016/s0025-7125(05)70098-5.
4. Schwetschenau E, Kelley DJ. The adult neck mass. Am Fam Physician. 2002;66:831–8.
5. Ramakrishnan K. Identifying and diagnosing the adult neck mass. Am Fam Physician. 2003;67:1190, 1192, 1195.
6. Chorath K, Rajasekaran K. Evaluation and management of a neck mass. Med Clin North Am. 2021;105:827–37. https://doi.org/10.1016/j.mcna.2021.05.005.
7. Ruhl C. Evaluation of the neck mass. Med Health R I. 2004;87:307–10.
8. Pynnonen MA, et al. Clinical practice guideline: evaluation of the neck mass in adults. Otolaryngol Head Neck Surg. 2017;157:S1–S30. https://doi.org/10.1177/0194599817722550.
9. Albanese G, Kondo KL. Seminars in interventional radiology, pp 391–399 (© Thieme Medical Publishers).
10. Fukumoto K, et al. Ethanol injection sclerotherapy for Baker's cyst, thyroglossal duct cyst, and branchial cleft cyst. Ann Plast Surg. 1994;33:615–9. https://doi.org/10.1097/00000637-199412000-00009.
11. Ryu JY, et al. Surgical approach for venous malformation in the head and neck. Arch Craniofac Surg. 2019;20:304–9. https://doi.org/10.7181/acfs.2019.00416.
12. Yakes WF, et al. Symptomatic vascular malformations: ethanol embolotherapy. Radiology. 1989;170:1059–66. https://doi.org/10.1148/radiology.170.3.2916057.
13. Yakes WF, et al. Ethanol embolization of vascular malformations. Radiographics. 1990;10:787–96. https://doi.org/10.1148/radiographics.10.5.2217971.
14. Pappas DC Jr, Persky MS, Berenstein A. Evaluation and treatment of head and neck venous vascular malformations. Ear Nose Throat J. 1998;77:914–6, 918–922.
15. Berenguer B, Burrows PE, Zurakowski D, Mulliken JB. Sclerotherapy of craniofacial venous malformations: complications and results. Plast Reconstr Surg. 1999;104:1–11; discussion 12–15.
16. Gelbert F, et al. Percutaneous sclerotherapy for venous malformation of the lips: a retrospective study of 23 patients. Neuroradiology. 2000;42:692–6. https://doi.org/10.1007/s002340000364.
17. Johnson PL, Eckard DA, Brecheisen MA, Girod DA, Tsue TT. Percutaneous ethanol sclerotherapy of venous malformations of the tongue. AJNR Am J Neuroradiol. 2002;23:779–82.
18. Rimon U, et al. Ethanol sclerotherapy of peripheral venous malformations. Eur J Radiol. 2004;52:283–7. https://doi.org/10.1016/j.ejrad.2003.09.010.
19. Impellizzeri P, et al. Sclerotherapy for cervical cystic lymphatic malformations in children. Our experience with computed tomography-guided 98% sterile ethanol insertion and a review of the literature. J Pediatr Surg. 2010;45:2473–8. https://doi.org/10.1016/j.jpedsurg.2010.07.023.

20. Kim SM, et al. Efficacy and safety of ethanol ablation for thyroglossal duct cysts. AJNR Am J Neuroradiol. 2011;32:306–9. https://doi.org/10.3174/ajnr.A2296.
21. Wiegand S, Eivazi B, Zimmermann AP, Sesterhenn AM, Werner JA. Sclerotherapy of lymphangiomas of the head and neck. Head Neck. 2011;33:1649–55. https://doi.org/10.1002/hed.21552.
22. Pekkola J, et al. Head and neck arteriovenous malformations: results of ethanol sclerotherapy. AJNR Am J Neuroradiol. 2013;34:198–204.
23. Ierardi AM, Colletti G, Biondetti P, Dessy M, Carrafiello G. Percutaneous sclerotherapy with gelified ethanol of low-flow vascular malformations of the head and neck region: preliminary results. Diagn Interv Radiol. 2019;25:459–64. https://doi.org/10.5152/dir.2019.18542.
24. Le Dare B, Gicquel T. Therapeutic applications of ethanol: a review. J Pharm Pharm Sci. 2019;22:525–35. https://doi.org/10.18433/jpps30572.
25. Lee E, et al. Efficacy of ethanol ablation as a treatment of benign head and neck cystic lesions. Am J Otolaryngol. 2021;42:103082. https://doi.org/10.1016/j.amjoto.2021.103082.
26. Lee C-H, Chen S-G. Direct percutaneous ethanol instillation for treatment of venous malformation in the face and neck. Br J Plast Surg. 2005;58:1073–8.
27. Baskin HJ. Percutaneous ethanol injection of thyroglossal duct cysts. Endocr Pract. 2006;12:355–7. https://doi.org/10.4158/EP.12.4.355.
28. Lee DK, et al. Efficacy of ethanol ablation for thyroglossal duct cyst. Ann Otol Rhinol Laryngol. 2015;124:62–7. https://doi.org/10.1177/0003489414542845.
29. Ha EJ, et al. Efficacy and safety of ethanol ablation for branchial cleft cysts. AJNR Am J Neuroradiol. 2017;38:2351–6. https://doi.org/10.3174/ajnr.A5373.
30. Nguyen MT, Orloff LA. Successful ablation of plunging ranula by ultrasound-guided percutaneous ethanol injection. Laryngoscope. 2017;127:2239–41. https://doi.org/10.1002/lary.26505.
31. Ryu KH, et al. Ethanol ablation of ranulas: short-term follow-up results and clinicoradiologic factors for successful outcome. AJNR Am J Neuroradiol. 2017;38:1794–8. https://doi.org/10.3174/ajnr.A5292.
32. Liao L-J, Wang C-T, Huang T-W, Cheng P-W, Lo W-C. Ultrasound-guided-fine-needle aspiration drainage and percutaneous ethanol injection for benign neck cysts. J Med Ultrasound. 2020;28:225.
33. Park SI, et al. Chemical ablation using ethanol or OK-432 for the treatment of thyroglossal duct cysts: a systematic review and meta-analysis. Eur Radiol. 2021;31:9048–56. https://doi.org/10.1007/s00330-021-08033-2.
34. Chow TL, Choi CY, Hui JY. Thyroglossal duct cysts in adults treated by ethanol sclerotherapy: a pilot study of a nonsurgical technique. Laryngoscope. 2012;122:1262–4. https://doi.org/10.1002/lary.23254.
35. Lee E, et al. Ultrasound-guided ethanol sclerotherapy for multifocal unilateral Warthin's tumor after partial parotidectomy. Ultrasound. 2022;30:158–61.
36. Gazelle GS, Goldberg SN, Solbiati L, Livraghi T. Tumor ablation with radio-frequency energy. Radiology. 2000;217:633–46. https://doi.org/10.1148/radiology.217.3.r00dc26633.
37. Dupuy D, Mayo-Smith W, Monchik J, Cronan J. In: Radiology, pp 278–278 (Radiological Soc North Amer 20th and Northampton STS, Easton, PA).
38. Owen RP, et al. Radiofrequency ablation of head and neck tumors: dramatic results from application of a new technology. Head Neck. 2002;24:754–8.
39. Back LJ, et al. When is radiofrequency ablation not indicated in head and neck squamous cell carcinoma management? Eur Arch Otorrinolaringol. 2015;272:1045–6. https://doi.org/10.1007/s00405-014-3102-7.
40. Mulliken JB, Glowacki JJP. Hemangiomas and vascular malformations in infants and children: a classification based on endothelial characteristics. Plast Reconstr Surg. 1982;69:412–20.
41. Castrén E, et al. Complications of sclerotherapy for 75 head and neck venous malformations. Eur Arch Otorhinolaryngol. 2016;273:1027–36.
42. Kim AH, Ko HK, Won JY, Lee DYJ. Percutaneous radiofrequency ablation: a novel treatment of facial venous malformation. J Vasc Surg. 2009;50:424–7.

43. van der Linden E, Overbosch J, Kroft L. Radiofrequency ablation for treatment of symptomatic low-flow vascular malformations after previous unsuccessful therapy. J Vasc Interv Radiol. 2005;16:747–50. https://doi.org/10.1097/01.RVI.0000157245.60426.7B.
44. Ko HK, et al. Experience at 1 year with the moving tip technique of radiofrequency ablation for the treatment of symptomatic venous malformations in the head and neck. J Vasc Surg Venous Lymphat Disord. 2013;1:263–9. https://doi.org/10.1016/j.jvsv.2013.01.001.
45. Koo H, et al. Ethanol and/or radiofrequency ablation to treat venolymphatic malformations that manifest as a bulging mass in the head and neck. Clin Radiol. 2016;71:1070.e1–7. https://doi.org/10.1016/j.crad.2016.03.012.
46. Cho SJ, Lee JH, Chung SR, Choi YJ, Baek JH. Radiofrequency ablation of facial venolymphatic malformations: assessment of efficacy and safety and the role of injectable electrodes. J Vasc Interv Radiol. 2020;31:544–50. https://doi.org/10.1016/j.jvir.2019.04.006.
47. Lin WC, et al. Ultrasound-guided moving shot radiofrequency ablation of benign soft tissue neoplasm. Medicina (Kaunas). 2021;57:830. https://doi.org/10.3390/medicina57080830.
48. von Recklinghausen F. Ueber die multiplen Fibrome der Haut und ihre Beziehung zu den multiplen Neuromen: Festschrift zur Feier des fünfundzwanzigjährigen Bestehens des pathologischen Instituts zu Berlin. Herrn Rudolf Virchow. Hirschwald; 1882.
49. Wise JB, Cryer JE, Belasco JB, Jacobs I, Elden L. Management of head and neck plexiform neurofibromas in pediatric patients with neurofibromatosis type 1. Arch Otolaryngol Head Neck Surg. 2005;131:712–8. https://doi.org/10.1001/archotol.131.8.712.
50. Baujat B, et al. Radiofrequency in the treatment of craniofacial plexiform neurofibromatosis: a pilot study. Plast Reconstr Surg. 2006;117:1261–8. https://doi.org/10.1097/01.prs.0000204863.40195.dd.
51. Zhao M, Li X, Wang J, Li W, Huang Z. Retroperitoneal schwannoma treated with percutaneous computed tomography–guided radiofrequency ablation: report of 2 cases. J Neurosurg Spine. 2012;17:173–6.
52. Mrowczynski O, et al. Percutaneous radiofrequency ablation for the treatment of peripheral nerve sheath tumors: a case report and review of the literature. Cureus. 2018;10(4):e2534.
53. Simon CJ, et al. Intraoperative triple antenna hepatic microwave ablation. AJR Am J Roentgenol. 2006;187:W333–40.
54. Simon CJ, Dupuy DE, Mayo-Smith WW. Microwave ablation: principles and applications. Radiographics. 2005;25(Suppl 1):S69–83. https://doi.org/10.1148/rg.25si055501.
55. Ramirez AS, Gutierrez SVE, Rodriguez PA, Ortiz OAS, Heredia JNS. Juvenile angiolipoma in the subtemporal region, zygomatic, and pterygomaxillary fossa treated by microwave ablation—A case study and literature review. Surg Neurol Int. 2022;13:409. https://doi.org/10.25259/SNI_501_2022.
56. Lou ZC, Dong Y, Lou ZH. Int Forum Allergy Rhinol. pp. 702–706 (Wiley Online Library).
57. Min HJ, Mun S-K, Lee SY, Kim KS. The possible role of endoscopy in diagnosis of benign tumors of the nasal cavity. J Craniofac Surg. 2017;28:973–5.
58. OuYang Z, et al. Microwave ablation for the removal of pharyngeal benign lesions: a prospective pilot case series. Am J Otolaryngol. 2021;42:102916. https://doi.org/10.1016/j.amjoto.2021.102916.
59. Jin M, et al. Ultrasound-guided percutaneous microwave ablation of parotid gland adenolymphoma: a case report. Medicine (Baltimore). 2019;98(35):–e16757.
60. Haemmerich D, Lee F. Multiple applicator approaches for radiofrequency and microwave ablation. Int J Hyperthermia. 2005;21:93–106.
61. Carrafiello G, et al. Microwave tumors ablation: principles, clinical applications and review of preliminary experiences. Int J Surg. 2008;6(Suppl 1):S65–9. https://doi.org/10.1016/j.ijsu.2008.12.028.
62. Brace CL. Microwave tissue ablation: biophysics, technology, and applications. Crit Rev Biomed Eng. 2010;38(1):65–78.
63. Brace CL. Radiofrequency and microwave ablation of the liver, lung, kidney, and bone: what are the differences? Curr Probl Diagn Radiol. 2009;38(3):135–43.
64. Crossley GH, et al. The Heart Rhythm Society (HRS)/American Society of Anesthesiologists (ASA) expert consensus statement on the perioperative management of patients with implant-

able defibrillators, pacemakers and arrhythmia monitors: facilities and patient management: this document was developed as a joint project with the American Society of Anesthesiologists (ASA), and in collaboration with the American Heart Association (AHA), and the Society of Thoracic Surgeons (STS). Heart Rhythm. 2011;8:1114–54.
65. El-Naggar AK, Chan JK, Grandis JR. WHO classification of head and neck tumours. 2017.
66. Quer M, et al. Current trends and controversies in the management of Warthin tumor of the parotid gland. Diagnostics (Basel). 2021;11:1467. https://doi.org/10.3390/diagnostics11081467.
67. Tung YC, et al. Evaluation of outcomes following radiofrequency ablation for treatment of parotid tail Warthin tumors. J Vasc Interv Radiol. 2019;30:1574–80. https://doi.org/10.1016/j.jvir.2019.04.031.
68. Cha CH, et al. Long-term outcomes of radiofrequency ablation for treatment of cystic Warthin tumors versus solid Warthin tumors. Int J Environ Res Public Health. 2021;18:6640. https://doi.org/10.3390/ijerph18126640.
69. Mamidi IS, et al. Ultrasound-guided ethanol sclerotherapy for non-surgical treatment of Warthin's tumor. Am J Otolaryngol. 2021;42:102813.
70. Meyer E, Lubbe D, Fagan JJ. Alcohol sclerotherapy of human immunodeficiency virus related parotid lymphoepithelial cysts. J Laryngol Otol. 2009;123:422–5.
71. Solbiati L, et al. Percutaneous ethanol injection of parathyroid tumors under US guidance: treatment for secondary hyperparathyroidism. Radiology. 1985;155:607–10.
72. Günther R, Beyer J, Hesch H, Reinwein D. Percutaneous transcatheter ablation of parathyroid gland tumors by alcohol injection and contrast media infusion. Rofo. 1984;140:27–30.
73. Charboneau JW, Hay ID, van Heerden JA. Mayo Clinic Proc. pp. 913–917 (Elsevier).
74. Bennedbaek F, Karstrup S, Hegedus L. Ultrasound guided laser ablation of a parathyroid adenoma. 2001;74:905–907.
75. Adda G, et al. Ultrasound-guided laser thermal ablation for parathyroid adenomas: analysis of three cases with a three-year follow-up. Horm Res. 2006;65:231–4.
76. Yu M-A, et al. Safety and efficiency of microwave ablation for recurrent and persistent secondary hyperparathyroidism after parathyroidectomy: a retrospective pilot study. Int J Hyperthermia. 2016;32:180–6.
77. Liu C, et al. US-guided percutaneous microwave ablation for primary hyperparathyroidism with parathyroid nodules: feasibility and safety study. J Vasc Interv Radiol. 2016;27:867–75.
78. Xu S, Wang Y, Xie Q, Wu H. Percutaneous sonography-guided radiofrequency ablation in the management of parathyroid adenoma. Singapore Med J. 2013;54:e137–40.
79. Lee C-Y, et al. Localization strategy prior to radiofrequency ablation for primary and secondary hyperparathyroidism. Biomedicines. 2023;11:672.
80. Bui QT, Dupuy DE. Percutaneous CT-guided radiofrequency ablation of an adenoid cystic carcinoma of the head and neck. AJR Am J Roentgenol. 2002;179:1333–5.
81. Owen RP, et al. Techniques for radiofrequency ablation of head and neck tumors. Arch Otolaryngol Head Neck Surg. 2004;130:52–6.
82. Liukko T, et al. Radiofrequency induced thermotherapy: an alternative palliative treatment modality in head and neck cancer. Eur Arch Otorhinolaryngol. 2006;263:532–6.
83. Brook AL, et al. CT-guided radiofrequency ablation in the palliative treatment of recurrent advanced head and neck malignancies. J Vasc Interv Radiol. 2008;19:725–35. https://doi.org/10.1016/j.jvir.2007.12.439.
84. Owen RP, et al. Radiofrequency ablation in advanced head and neck cancer. Eur Arch Otorrinolaringol. 2014;271:207–10. https://doi.org/10.1007/s00405-013-2681-z.
85. Belfiore MP, et al. Preliminary results in unresectable head and neck cancer treated by radiofrequency and microwave ablation: feasibility, efficacy, and safety. J Vasc Interv Radiol. 2015;26:1189–96. https://doi.org/10.1016/j.jvir.2015.05.021.
86. Liao J, et al. A preliminary study on ultrasound-guided percutaneous microwave ablation for palliative treatment of advanced head and neck malignancies. Int J Hyperthermia. 2021;38:479–87.

# Chapter 27
# Ultrasound Phantoms for Thyroid RFA

**Steven P. Hodak**

Though thyroid radiofrequency ablation (RFA) is minimally invasive, it is nonetheless a complex procedure that requires multiple procedural competencies. These include a thorough understanding of cervical ultrasound anatomy as well as specific technical and dexterity skills, all of which are necessary to ensure safe and successful outcomes. As demonstrated by a growing list of publications, attaining these competencies involves a substantial learning curve that must be negotiated to ensure effective delivery of care [1–3].

Gel-matrix phantoms are frequently employed as training tools for ultrasound-guided soft-tissue interventional procedures. Practice phantoms allow for skill repetition, provide real-time feedback, and improve learning retention, and do so as the learner gains procedure proficiency without exposing actual patients to potential harm [4]. A suitable ultrasound phantom model would therefore be valuable to learners attempting to master thyroid RFA.

The ideal phantom would be easily and inexpensively prepared, allow close approximation of the ultrasonographic appearance of a live target and surrounding tissue, and provide haptic feedback during the mock treatment session. Commercially available phantoms are usually relatively expensive and we know of none suitable for real-time RFA training because of the heat created by the electrode during energy delivery. A variety of more suitable gel-matrix phantoms can be prepared from a variety of ingredients available through online retailers or even some specialty food stores. These include food-grade gelatin, ballistic gel, agarose, bean starch, alginate, as well as numerous organic compounds [5–8]. A variety of objects including vegetables, animal protein, and plastic objects may also be used within these phantoms to simulate treatment targets. Simpler phantoms with relatively few ingredients offer ease of preparation but often have limitations related to quality of

S. P. Hodak (✉)
NYU Langone Health, New York, NY, USA



A. W. Park et al. (eds.), *Thyroid Radiofrequency Ablation*,
https://doi.org/10.1007/978-3-031-65288-2_27

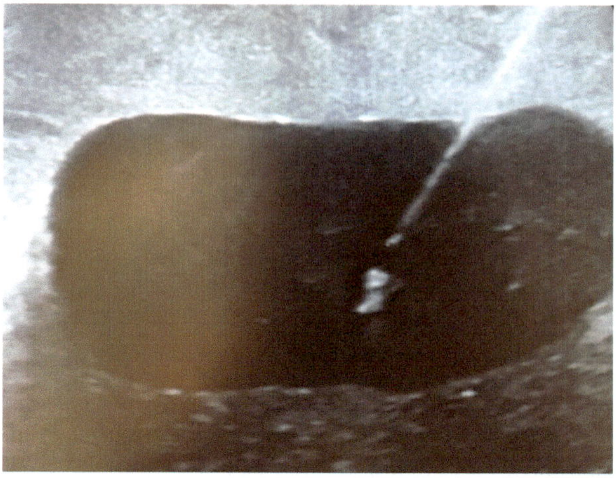

**Fig. 27.1** Ultrasound appearance of nodule in phantom with 19G RFA needle

acoustic transmission, stability at room temperature, and in the specific case of gelatin—a characteristically foul smell that many find distasteful [9]. Additives such as calcium silicate, chalk, cornstarch, milk, oil and other organic agents are employed to modify acoustic properties, phantom stability, and texture.

For the purpose of learning RFA techniques, we wanted to create a phantom that would be relatively simple to produce from readily available nontoxic ingredients with excellent acoustic and tactile qualities. We based our model on a gel-matrix phantom developed by Aoyagi et al. [10] specifically designed to be durable and closely approximate the acoustic and tactile properties of human tissue. This phantom produces excellent ultrasonographic images (Fig. 27.1), has a realistic "feel," and remains stable at room temperature with good tolerance of the considerable heat produced during extended RFA practice sessions. We enhanced this model by incorporating a mock "nodule" made from pork loin, which allows excellent visualization of the target with realistic ultrasonographic changes that nearly duplicate those typically seen during actual RFA. Further, the "nodule" can be excised and examined following the practice treatment session allowing the learner to assess the effectiveness of the mock ablation: specifically, how completely the bulk of the lesion is treated, including the nodule's marginal zones, which are frequently the most challenging portions of a targeted lesion in a live patient (Fig. 27.2).

Though water and four reagents, along with several easily available pieces of equipment, are required to produce this phantom, our experience is that the amount of practice needed to achieve competence with RFA requires multiple practice sessions and multiple phantoms. These materials will therefore be repeatedly used and the effort and relatively small expenses involved will be more than offset by the benefits this phantom will provide. The reagents are available through any laboratory supply company but may also be easily purchased through online retailers. Additional items required for the phantom mold and tools for preparation are available at hardware and cooking stores and from online retailers as well.

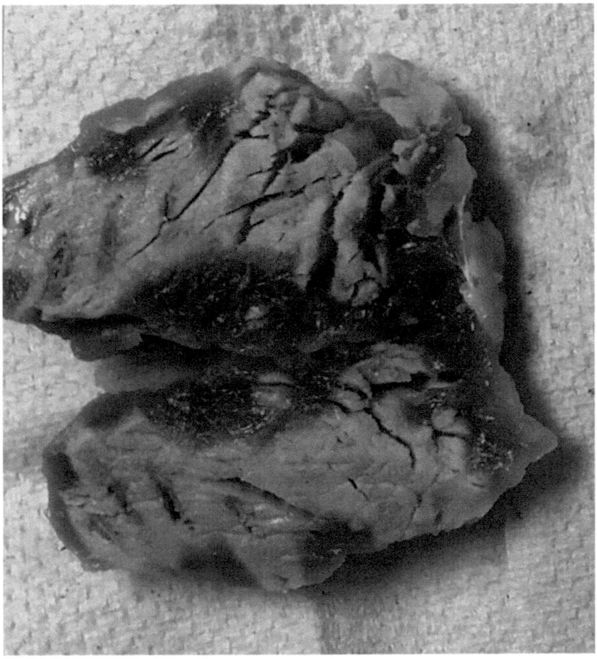

**Fig. 27.2** Practice nodule sliced to allow assessment of completeness of treatment: Note the raw/untreated marginal areas

## Necessary Materials

1. Reagents:
   (a) Sodium alginate
   (b) Food- or reagent grade glycerol (glycerin)
   (c) Calcium sulfate dihydrate
   (d) Trisodium phosphate-12-hydrate
   (e) Tap water heated to 40 °C (100 °F)
2. Lean pork cut into 2–3 cm (20–25 g) cubes to form the "nodule"
3. Plastic wrap
4. 3″–4″ #6 sheet metal screws; 1 screw per nodule
5. An approximately 1.5–2 L flat bottom loaf pan for use as the phantom mold
6. Screwdriver
7. Some 2″ × 8″ wood strips such as a paint stirrer available at hardware store are perfect. Stiff corrugated cardboard can also be substituted
8. 6″ or longer sharp kitchen knife
9. Hot plate
10. Pot large enough to heat the required volume of water per the recipe
11. Containers and tools for mixing
    - Two 3-gallon plastic buckets for mixing
    - Power drill with paint mixer attachment

## Keys to Success

- The original protocol by Aoyagi et al. [10] called for reagent grade glycerin (>99.5% pure glycerol). We have found that food grade glycerin works just as well and is far less expensive.
- Use buckets at least 2–3 times the volume of the gel you will prepare to prevent splashing during vigorous mixing. Three-gallon plastic buckets work well for preparation of up to 6 L of gel.
- It is nearly impossible to quickly and homogeneously mix the phantom gel by hand. An electric drill with paint mixer attachment is strongly recommended.
- The pork "nodules" should be partially rather than completely frozen when you are ready to pour the phantom. The gel requires some warmth to set correctly, and completely frozen nodules may impair correct setting of the gel around the "nodules."

## Prepare the Pork "Nodules"

1. Place each prepared "nodule" into the center of a square of plastic wrap (sometimes doubling the wrap is needed to prevent tearing).
2. Clinch the plastic wrap around the nodule forcing out all the air and twist the nodule so it is tightly compacted into a roughly rounded shape. A 20–25 g piece of lean pork will produce "nodules" that are ~2.5–3.5 cm in diameter.
3. Place the nodule in the freezer and freeze completely.

## Place Nodules on the Screw

The goal is to position the pork nodules so they are approximately 1–2 cm from the bottom surface of the mold when the gel is poured. When the finished mold is eventually inverted, the bottom surface will be your working surface and the nodules will be located at a depth of about 1–2 cm (Fig. 27.3).

1. Drive the screw through a board, or piece of cardboard, or strip of wood.
2. Remove the pork nodules from the freezer and unwrap.
3. Mount the nodule(s) on the screw(s) so that:
   (a) The nodules will be about 1–2 cm from the bottom of the mold.
   (b) The surface of the nodules farthest from the wood or cardboard strip is at roughly the same level (Fig. 27.4).
4. Nodules should remain partially frozen when pouring the phantom. Refreeze if necessary.

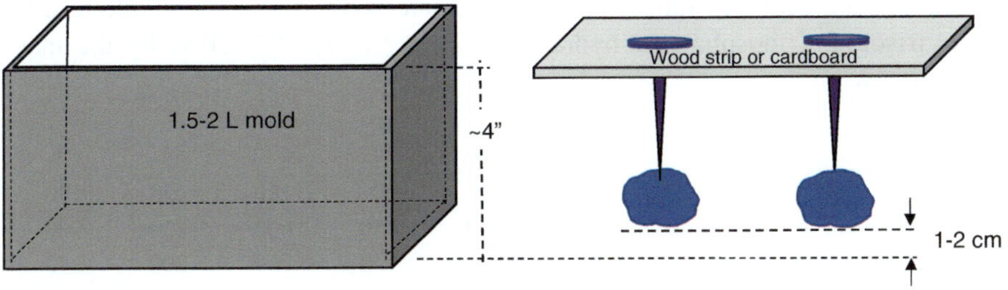


**Fig. 27.3** Schematic representation of how the mock nodules should be mounted and positioned in the phantom mold

**Fig. 27.4** Frozen mock pork "nodules" being unwrapped and mounted on positioning screws

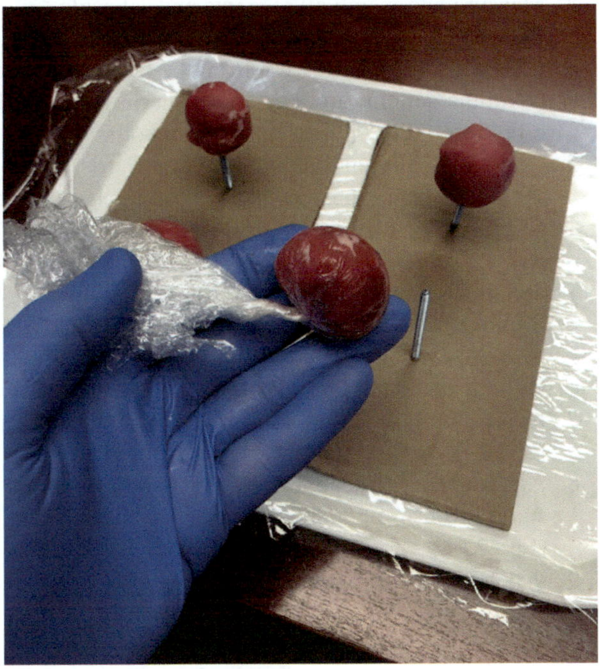

## Prepare the Phantom Gel Material

You will require enough gel to fill each mold about half way. Use the table below to calculate the amount of gel needed based on the number and size of molds you will pour.

The standard mixing ratio of sodium alginate, glycerin, calcium sulfate dihydrate, trisodium phosphate-12-hydrate, and water is 1.5:7.5:2:1:50 by the mass, respectively.

| | 2 L | 3 L | 4 L | 5 L | 6 L |
|---|---|---|---|---|---|
| Sodium alginate | 60 | 90 | 120 | 150 | 180 |
| Food- or reagent-grade glycerol (glycerin) | 300 | 450 | 600 | 750 | 900 |
| Calcium sulfate dihydrate | 80 | 120 | 160 | 200 | 240 |
| Trisodium phosphate-12-hydrate | 40 | 60 | 80 | 100 | 120 |
| Tap water (40 °C/100 °F) | 2000 | 3000 | 4000 | 5000 | 6000 |

1. Heat the required volume of water to 40 °C/100 °F and keep it covered to prevent evaporation during heating.
2. Measure and weigh all reagents and set aside.
3. Place the nodules suspended on the screws into the phantom mold and adjust as needed so they are 1–2 cm from the floor of the mold and set aside (Fig. 27.1).
4. Combine sodium alginate and glycerin in a 3-gallon bucket **labeled "A"** and mix thoroughly until completely smooth.
5. Combine calcium sulfate dihydrate, trisodium phosphate-12-hydrate, and 100 °F water in the second 3-gallon bucket **labeled "B"** and mix thoroughly. Use a power drill with a paint mixer for 15–20 s. *Once mixed move to the next step immediately*. Calcium sulfate dehydrate (gypsum) is poorly water soluble and this mixture will separate if left standing.
6. Rapidly pour contents of container **B** (gypsum and trisodium phosphate-12-hydrate) into container **A** (glycerol and sodium alginate) and use a paint mixer on high speed to combine until completely homogeneous—about 20–30 s.
7. Immediately pour enough gel into the mold to cover the nodules by at least 2–3 cm.
8. Allow the gel to set at room temperature for at least 3–4 hours until the gel has started to firm up, and then place the mold in the refrigerator to cure for 24 h (Fig. 27.5).
9. When mold is completely set, remove "nodule" positioning screws.

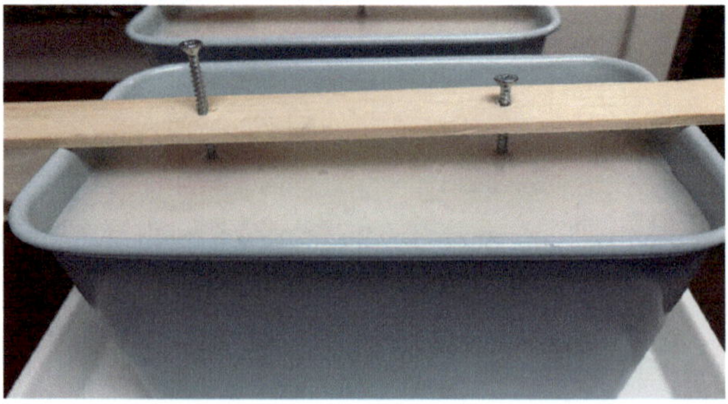

**Fig. 27.5** Poured phantom ready for refrigeration

10. Run a sharp knife around the edge of the mold to separate the phantom from the walls of the mold.
11. Invert mold to release phantom.

## References


1. Bom WJ, Joosten FBM, van Borren M, Bom EP, van Eekeren R, de Boer H. Radiofrequency ablation for symptomatic, non-functioning, thyroid nodules: a single-center learning curve. Endocr Connect. 2022;11(1):e210304.
2. Kuo CY, Liu CL, Tsai CH, Cheng SP. Learning curve analysis of radiofrequency ablation for benign thyroid nodules. Int J Hyperthermia. 2021;38(1):1536–40.
3. Russ G, Ben Hamou A, Poiree S, Ghander C, Menegaux F, Leenhardt L, et al. Learning curve for radiofrequency ablation of benign thyroid nodules. Int J Hyperthermia. 2021;38(1):55–64.
4. Nhan C, Chankowsky J, Torres C, Boucher LM. Creating low-cost phantoms for needle manipulation training in interventional radiology procedures. Radiographics. 2021;41(4):1230–42.
5. Amini R, Kartchner JZ, Stolz LA, Biffar D, Hamilton AJ, Adhikari S. A novel and inexpensive ballistic gel phantom for ultrasound training. World J Emerg Med. 2015;6(3):225–8.
6. Hunt A, Ristolainen A, Ross P, Opik R, Krumme A, Kruusmaa M. Low cost anatomically realistic renal biopsy phantoms for interventional radiology trainees. Eur J Radiol. 2013;82(4):594–600.
7. Qurash MT, Yaacob NY, Azuan N, Khaleel YS, Zakaria R. Special ultrasound phantom for interventional training: construction, advantages, and application. J Med Ultrasound. 2018;26(4):210–4.
8. Selame LA, Risler Z, Zakaria SJ, Hughes LP, Lewiss RE, Kehm K, et al. A comparison of homemade vascular access ultrasound phantom models for peripheral intravenous catheter insertion. J Vasc Access. 2021;22(6):891–7.
9. Abraham D. A method using superconcentrated gelatin and a novel phantom suspension system for ultrasound-guided thyroid biopsy training. Thyroid. 2014;24(11):1662–3.
10. Aoyagi M, Hiraguri T. Ultrasound phantom using sodium alginate as a gelling agent. J Ultrasound Med. 2017;36(11):2345–53.

# Index




A. W. Park et al. (eds.), *Thyroid Radiofrequency Ablation*,
https://doi.org/10.1007/978-3-031-65288-2

**U**



**V**

GPSR Compliance

*The European Union's (EU) General Product Safety Regulation (GPSR) is a set of rules that requires consumer products to be safe and our obligations to ensure this.*

*If you have any concerns about our products, you can contact us on ProductSafety@springernature.com*

In case Publisher is established outside the EU, the EU authorized representative is:

Springer Nature Customer Service Center GmbH
Europaplatz 3
69115 Heidelberg, Germany

**Batch number: 10732090**

Printed by Printforce, the Netherlands